INFLUENZA PANDEMIC - PREPAREDNESS AND RESPONSE TO A HEALTH DISASTER

PUBLIC HEALTH IN THE 21ST CENTURY

Additional books in this series can be found on Nova's website at:

https://www.novapublishers.com/catalog/index.php?cPath=23_29&seriesp=Public+Health+in+the+21st+Century

Additional E-books in this series can be found on Nova's website at:

https://www.novapublishers.com/catalog/index.php?cPath=23_29&seriespe=Public+Health+in+the+21st+Century

INFLUENZA PANDEMIC - PREPAREDNESS AND RESPONSE TO A HEALTH DISASTER

EMMA S. BROUWER
EDITOR

Nova
Nova Science Publishers, Inc.
New York

NOTICE TO THE READER

The Publisher has taken reasonable care in the preparation of this book, but makes no expressed or implied warranty of any kind and assumes no responsibility for any errors or omissions. No liability is assumed for incidental or consequential damages in connection with or arising out of information contained in this book. The Publisher shall not be liable for any special, consequential, or exemplary damages resulting, in whole or in part, from the readers' use of, or reliance upon, this material. Any parts of this book based on government reports are so indicated and copyright is claimed for those parts to the extent applicable to compilations of such works.

Independent verification should be sought for any data, advice or recommendations contained in this book. In addition, no responsibility is assumed by the publisher for any injury and/or damage to persons or property arising from any methods, products, instructions, ideas or otherwise contained in this publication.

This publication is designed to provide accurate and authoritative information with regard to the subject matter covered herein. It is sold with the clear understanding that the Publisher is not engaged in rendering legal or any other professional services. If legal or any other expert assistance is required, the services of a competent person should be sought. FROM A DECLARATION OF PARTICIPANTS JOINTLY ADOPTED BY A COMMITTEE OF THE AMERICAN BAR ASSOCIATION AND A COMMITTEE OF PUBLISHERS.

LIBRARY OF CONGRESS CATALOGING-IN-PUBLICATION DATA
Influenza pandemic : preparedness and response to a health disaster /
editor, Emma S. Brouwer.
p. ; cm.
 Includes bibliographical references and index.
 ISBN 978-1-60692-953-7 (hardcover)
 1. Influenza--Government policy--United States. I. Brouwer, Emma S.
 [DNLM: 1. Influenza, Human--prevention & control--United States. 2.
Disease Outbreaks--prevention & control--United States. 3. Federal
Government--United States. 4. Health Planning--United States. 5.
Influenza, Human--epidemiology--United States. WC 515 I4323 2010]
 RA644.I6I533 2010
 362.196'.203--dc22
2010012202

Published by Nova Science Publishers, Inc. ✛ New York

CONTENTS

PREFACE

Global pandemic preparedness and response efforts are coordinated by the World Health Organization (WHO). Domestic preparedness efforts are led by the White House Homeland Security Council, with the U.S. Department of Health and Human Services (HHS) playing a major role. Domestic response efforts would be carried out under the all-hazards blueprint for a coordinated federal, state and local response laid out in the National Response Plan, overseen by the Department of Homeland Security (DHS). The federal government has released several pandemic flu plans to govern federal, state, local and private preparedness activities. This book discusses pandemic flu in general, WHO and U.S. preparedness and response plans, and a number of relevant policy issues.

Chapter 1 - When there is a catastrophe in the United States, state and local governments lead response activities, invoking state and local legal authorities to support these activities. When state and local response capabilities are overwhelmed, the President, acting through the Secretary of Homeland Security, can provide assistance to stricken communities, individuals, governments, and not-for-profit groups to assist in response and recovery. Aid is provided under the authority of the Robert T. Stafford Disaster Relief and Emergency Assistance Act (the Stafford Act) upon a presidential declaration. The Secretary of Health and Human Services (HHS) also has both standing and emergency authorities in the Public Health Service Act, by which he or she can provide assistance in response to public health and medical emergencies. At this time, however, the Secretary has limited means to finance activities that are ineligible, for whatever reason, for Stafford Act assistance.

The flawed response to Hurricane Katrina, and preparedness efforts for an influenza ("flu") pandemic, have each raised concerns about existing federal response mechanisms for incidents that result in overwhelming public health and medical needs. These concerns include the delegation of responsibilities among different federal departments, and whether critical conflicts or gaps exist in these relationships. In particular, there are some concerns about federal leadership and delegations of responsibility as laid out in the recently published National Response Framework (NRF).

There is no federal assistance program designed purposely to cover the uninsured or uncompensated costs of individual health care that may be needed as a consequence of a disaster, nor is there consensus that this should be a federal responsibility. Following Hurricane Katrina, Congress provided short-term assistance to host states, through the Medicaid program, to cover the uninsured health care needs of eligible Katrina evacuees. Some have proposed establishing a mechanism to cover certain uninsured health care costs of responders and others who are having health problems related to exposures at the World Trade Center site in New York City following the 2001 terrorist attack. Legislation introduced in the 110th Congress (H.R. 6569/S. 3312) would authorize the Secretary of HHS to use a special fund to provide temporary emergency health care coverage for uninsured individuals affected by public health emergencies.

This chapter examines (1) the authorities and coordinating mechanisms of the President and the Secretary of HHS in providing routine assistance, and assistance pursuant to emergency or major disaster declarations and/or public health emergency determinations; (2) mechanisms to assure a coordinated federal response to public health and medical emergencies, and overlaps or gaps in agency responsibilities; and (3) existing mechanisms, potential gaps, and proposals for financing the costs of a response to public health and medical emergencies. A listing of federal public health emergency authorities is provided in the **Appendix**.

Chapter 2 - In 1997, a new avian influenza ("flu") virus emerged in Asia and jumped directly from birds to humans, killing six people. The virus has since spread to more than 50 countries in Asia, Europe and Africa, where it has killed millions of birds and infected more than 270 people, killing more than 160 of them. The virus bears some similarity to the deadly 1918 Spanish flu, which caused a global pandemic estimated to have killed more than 50 million people worldwide. The current spread of avian flu raises concerns about another human flu pandemic.

Global pandemic preparedness and response efforts are coordinated by the World Health Organization (WHO). Domestic preparedness efforts are led by the White House Homeland Security Council, with the U.S. Department of Health and Human Services (HHS) playing a major role. Domestic response efforts would be carried out under the all-hazards blueprint for a coordinated federal, state and local response laid out in the National Response Plan, overseen by the Department of Homeland Security (DHS). HHS officials would have the lead in the public health and medical aspects of a response. The federal government has released several pandemic flu plans to govern federal, state, local and private preparedness activities.

There are concerns about how a domestic public health and medical response would be managed during a flu pandemic. There is precedent, under the Stafford Act, for the President to declare an infectious disease threat an emergency (which provides a lower level of assistance), but no similar precedent for a major disaster declaration (which provides a higher level of assistance). In any case, many of the needs likely to result from a flu pandemic could not be met with the types of assistance provided pursuant to the Stafford Act, even if a major disaster declaration applied.

Vaccination is the best flu prevention measure. But because of continuous changes in the genes of flu viruses, vaccines must be "matched" to specific strains to provide good protection. A pandemic flu strain would, by definition, be novel. Stockpiled vaccine would not match, so stockpiling in anticipation of a pandemic is of limited value. In addition, global and domestic capacity to produce flu vaccine is limited. The U.S. government, primarily through HHS, has launched an aggressive effort to expand domestic vaccine production capacity, and to develop technologies to support more rapid production of a matched vaccine at the onset of a pandemic.

Since matched vaccine would not be available at the outset of a flu pandemic that occurred within the next several years, planning efforts focus on measures to slow the spread of disease, and mitigate its effects. These include stockpiling of antiviral drugs to prevent or treat flu infection, planning for medical surge capacity, and continuity planning for businesses and utilities.

This chapter discusses pandemic flu in general, WHO and U.S. preparedness and response plans, and a number of relevant policy issues. The focus of this chapter is U.S. domestic public health preparedness and response planning, and the projected impacts of an influenza pandemic on Americans.

Chapter 3 - States are the seat of most authority for public health emergency response. Much of the actual work of response falls to local officials. However, the federal government can impose requirements upon states as a condition of federal funding. Since 2002, Congress has provided funding to all U.S. states, territories, and the District of Columbia, to enhance federal, state and local preparedness for public health threats in general, and an influenza ("flu") pandemic in particular. States were required to develop pandemic plans as a condition of this funding.

This chapter describes an approach to the analysis of state pandemic plans, and presents the findings of that analysis. State plans that were available in July 2006 were analyzed in eight topical areas: (1) leadership and coordination; (2) surveillance and laboratory activities; (3) vaccine management; (4) antiviral drug management; (5) other disease control activities; (6) communications; (7) healthcare services; and (8) other essential services. A history of federal funding and requirements for state pandemic planning is provided in an **Appendix**. This analysis is not intended to grade or rank individual state pandemic plans or capabilities. Rather, its findings indicate that a number of challenges remain in assuring pandemic preparedness, and suggest areas that may merit added emphasis in future planning efforts.

Generally, the plans analyzed here reflect their authorship by public health officials. They emphasize core public health functions such as disease detection and control. Other planning challenges, such as assuring surge capacity in the healthcare sector, the continuity of essential services, or the integrity of critical supply chains, may fall outside the authority of public health officials, and may require stronger engagement by emergency management officials and others in planning.

Since different threats — such as hurricanes, earthquakes or terrorism — are expected to affect states differently, many believe that states should have flexibility in emergency planning. This complicates federal oversight of homeland security grants to states, however. Which requirements should be imposed on all states? When is variability among states desirable, and when is it not? A flu pandemic is perhaps unique in that it would be likely to affect all states at nearly the same time, in ways that are fairly predictable. This may argue for a more directive federal role in setting pandemic preparedness requirements. But the matter of what the states should do to be prepared for a pandemic is not always clear. For example, uncertainties about the ways in which flu spreads, the lack of national consensus in matters of equity in rationing, and a long tradition of federal deference to states in matters of public health, all complicate efforts to set uniform planning requirements for states.

In addition to assuring the strength of planning efforts, readiness also depends on assuring that states can execute their plans. This assurance can be provided through analysis of the response during exercises, drills, and relevant real-world incidents. Such an analysis is not within the scope of this chapter.

Chapter 4 - This chapter provides a legal analysis of the eligibility of an influenza pandemic (flu pandemic) to be declared by the President as a major disaster under the Robert T. Stafford Disaster Relief and Emergency Assistance Act. In 1997, the discovery of a virulent H5N1 strain of avian influenza (bird flu) raised the possibility of a flu pandemic occurring in the United States. In such an event, the Stafford Act could provide authority for federal assistance. Although it is widely agreed that emergency assistance under the Stafford Act could be provided by the President in the event of a flu pandemic, questions remain as to whether major disaster assistance would be available. An analysis of the Stafford Act suggests that this issue was not addressed by Congress when it drafted the current definition of a major disaster, and that neither inclusion nor exclusion of flu pandemics from major disaster assistance is explicitly required by the current statutory language.

In the 109th Congress, § 210 of S. 3721 would have made any outbreak of infectious disease explicitly eligible for major disaster assistance, but it was not enacted.

Chapter 5 - The emergence of the H5N1 avian influenza virus (also known as "bird flu") has raised concerns that it or another virus might mutate into a virulent strain that could lead to an influenza pandemic. Experts predict that a severe pandemic could overwhelm the nation's health care system, requiring the rationing of limited resources. GAO was asked to provide information on the progress of the Department of Health and Human Services's (HHS) plans for responding to a pandemic, including analyzing how HHS plans to (1) use pharmaceutical interventions to treat infected individuals and protect the critical workforce and (2) use nonpharmaceutical interventions to slow the spread of disease. To conduct this work, GAO reviewed government documents and scientific literature, and interviewed HHS officials, state and local public health officials, and subject-matter experts on pandemic response.

Chapter 6 - Public health officials are concerned that a particular strain of influenza, known as H5N1, or "avian flu," which has caused widespread infection of poultry flocks in Asia, Europe, the Near East, and Africa, might become easily transmissible among humans, causing illness and death at rates unseen at least since the early 20th century. In the "Spanish flu" pandemic of 1918 and 1919, more than 500,000 people died in the United States and some 50 million perished worldwide. By contrast, in a typical year, seasonal influenza causes about 36,000 deaths in the United States. Public health officials worry that an influenza pandemic today could cause some 2 million deaths in the United States. It also could lead to substantial adverse economic consequences both here and abroad (CBO 2005, 2006a).

Against the prospect of such an event, the Department of Health and Human Services (HHS) has developed a plan to prepare for and combat an influenza pandemic and has budgeted about $7.9 billion since 2004 for influenza preparedness activities (HHS 2005b). Most of that money— about $5.6 billion—was provided through supplemental appropriation bills in 2006 in response to the HHS plan. About $3.2 billion of the supplemental funds, along with some additional funds that are part of HHS's annual appropriation, is being spent for vaccine-related activities, reflecting the strong consensus among public health officials that vaccination is the best tool for reducing the consequences—and the costs—of an influenza pandemic.[1]

HHS planners initially confronted two problems: inadequate capacity for vaccine production and delays in producing vaccine. The emergence of H5N1 as a human health risk found a U.S. production base that had been reduced to a single domestic manufacturer, using an egg- based process developed in the 1940s to produce the vaccine. The current process for delivery of seasonal- influenza vaccine takes about six months from the initial step of isolating the virus strain to the final delivery of the vaccine to the clinic or doctor's office.

Step one in HHS's plan was to promote an increase in capacity as rapidly as possible by encouraging the expansion and refurbishing of existing plants. The second, and current, step is to introduce cell-based manufacturing technology to the domestic production of influenza vaccine. (That method uses cells rather than chicken eggs as the medium in which to grow the active ingredient in the vaccine; it is a standard method for manufacturing most vaccines against childhood diseases, for example.)

Because production requires about six months, and an influenza pandemic could spread much faster than that, HHS's plan includes short- and longer-term approaches to the problem of making vaccines available quickly. In the short run, a small stockpile of vaccines could be used for a limited initial response. Longer-term plans call for the development of "next-generation vaccines," which will draw on advances in biotechnology to speed production. Because developing safe and effective vaccines could take years—perhaps a decade or more—HHS is encouraging pharmaceutical manufacturers to start development now.

In parallel with the efforts to scale up production of egg- and cell-based vaccines, HHS is funding the development of new adjuvants, substances that can be added to influenza vaccines to reduce the amount of active ingredient (also called antigen) needed per dose of vaccine. The use of adjuvants for egg-based and cell-based vaccines could allow domestic manufacturers to produce more doses in existing facilities, and so fewer new facilities would be needed to manufacture cell-based formulations. Moreover, smaller stockpiles could be used to protect larger numbers of people. But adjuvanted vaccines can induce more pronounced side effects than ordinary vaccines can, a definite downside because vaccines, unlike most other pharmaceuticals, are given to healthy people. To date, the Food and Drug Administration has not approved an adjuvanted vaccine for influenza. In contrast, adjuvanted influenza vaccines have been approved for use in Europe.

This paper from the Congressional Budget Office (CBO) focuses on the government's role, under HHS's plan, in the development of new vaccines and the capacity to manufacture them. It provides information on progress and on the potential cost of achieving HHS's vaccine- related goals, the continuing expenditures that are likely to be needed to maintain preparedness, and the experience of other countries in preparing for a possible pandemic. It also presents options for modifying HHS's 2005 plan. The work is based on a review of the academic literature, on industry data, and on interviews with government and industry experts who are working to improve the response of vaccine producers to a potential influenza pandemic.

In: Influenza Pandemic - Preparedness and Response to ...   ISBN: 978-1-60692-953-7
Editor: Emma S. Brouwer pp.1-33   © 2010 Nova Science Publishers, Inc.

Chapter 1

THE PUBLIC HEALTH AND MEDICAL RESPONSE TO DISASTERS: FEDERAL AUTHORITY AND FUNDING

Sarah A. Lister

SUMMARY

When there is a catastrophe in the United States, state and local governments lead response activities, invoking state and local legal authorities to support these activities. When state and local response capabilities are overwhelmed, the President, acting through the Secretary of Homeland Security, can provide assistance to stricken communities, individuals, governments, and not-for-profit groups to assist in response and recovery. Aid is provided under the authority of the Robert T. Stafford Disaster Relief and Emergency Assistance Act (the Stafford Act) upon a presidential declaration. The Secretary of Health and Human Services (HHS) also has both standing and emergency authorities in the Public Health Service Act, by which he or she can provide assistance in response to public health and medical emergencies. At this time, however, the Secretary has limited means to finance activities that are ineligible, for whatever reason, for Stafford Act assistance.

The flawed response to Hurricane Katrina, and preparedness efforts for an influenza ("flu") pandemic, have each raised concerns about existing federal response mechanisms for incidents that result in overwhelming public health and medical needs. These concerns include the delegation of responsibilities among different federal departments, and whether critical conflicts or gaps exist in these relationships. In particular, there are some concerns about federal leadership and delegations of responsibility as laid out in the recently published National Response Framework (NRF).

There is no federal assistance program designed purposely to cover the uninsured or uncompensated costs of individual health care that may be needed as a consequence of a disaster, nor is there consensus that this should be a federal responsibility. Following Hurricane Katrina, Congress provided short-term assistance to host states, through the Medicaid program, to cover the uninsured health care needs of eligible Katrina evacuees.

Some have proposed establishing a mechanism to cover certain uninsured health care costs of responders and others who are having health problems related to exposures at the World Trade Center site in New York City following the 2001 terrorist attack. Legislation introduced in the 110th Congress (H.R. 6569/S. 3312) would authorize the Secretary of HHS to use a special fund to provide temporary emergency health care coverage for uninsured individuals affected by public health emergencies.

This chapter examines (1) the authorities and coordinating mechanisms of the President and the Secretary of HHS in providing routine assistance, and assistance pursuant to emergency or major disaster declarations and/or public health emergency determinations; (2) mechanisms to assure a coordinated federal response to public health and medical emergencies, and overlaps or gaps in agency responsibilities; and (3) existing mechanisms, potential gaps, and proposals for financing the costs of a response to public health and medical emergencies. A listing of federal public health emergency authorities is provided in the **Appendix**.

INTRODUCTION

When there is a catastrophe in the United States, state and local governments take the lead in response activities. State and local legal authorities are the principal means to support these activities. In response to catastrophes, the President can provide certain additional assets and personnel to aid stricken communities, and can provide funding to individuals and to government and not-for-profit entities to assist them in response and recovery.[1] This aid is provided under the authority of the Robert T. Stafford Disaster Relief and Emergency Assistance Act (the Stafford Act), upon a presidential declaration of an emergency (providing a lower level of assistance) or a major disaster (providing a higher level of assistance).[2]

Recent incidents — the September 11 and anthrax attacks of 2001, and several Gulf Coast hurricanes in 2005 — have shown the limitations of existing funding mechanisms in supporting public health and medical incident responses. First, it is not clear that Stafford Act major disaster assistance is available for the response to infectious disease threats, whether intentional (bioterrorism) or natural (e.g., pandemic influenza, or "flu"). Second, the Secretary of Health and Human Services (HHS) has authority to draw upon a special fund to support departmental activities in response to unanticipated public health emergencies, but there is at present no money in the fund. Finally, there is no existing comprehensive mechanism to provide federal assistance for uninsured or uncompensated individual health care costs that may be incurred as a result of a natural disaster or terrorist incident, though there is not general agreement that such assistance should be a federal responsibility.

This chapter examines (1) the statutory authorities and coordinating mechanisms of the President (acting through the Secretary of Homeland Security) and the Secretary of HHS in providing routine assistance, and in providing assistance pursuant to emergency or major disaster declarations and/or public health emergency determinations; (2) mechanisms to assure a coordinated federal response to public health and medical emergencies, and overlaps or gaps in agency responsibilities; and (3) existing mechanisms, potential gaps, and proposals for financing the costs of a response to public health and medical emergencies. A listing of federal public health emergency authorities is provided in the **Appendix**. For more information on aspects of public health and medical preparedness and response in general, and in the context of specific disasters or threats, see the following CRS Reports:

- RS22602, *Public Health and Medical Preparedness and Response: Issues in the 110th Congress;*
- RL33589, *The Pandemic and All-Hazards Preparedness Act (P.L. 109-41 7): Provisions and Changes to Preexisting Law;*
- RL33927, *Selected Federal Compensation Programs for Physical Injury or Death;*
- RL3 1719, *An Overview of the U.S. Public Health System in the Context of Emergency Preparedness;*
- RL33096, 2005 *Gulf Coast Hurricanes: The Public Health and Medical Response;*
- RL3 3083, *Hurricane Katrina: Medicaid Issues;*
- RL33738, *Gulf Coast Hurricanes: Addressing Survivors' Mental Health and Substance Abuse Treatment Needs;*
- RL3 3145, *Pandemic Influenza: Domestic Preparedness Efforts; and*
- RL34190, *Pandemic Influenza: An Analysis of State Preparedness and Response Plans.*

FEDERAL AUTHORITY AND PLANS FOR DISASTER RESPONSE

Federal Statutory Authorities for Disaster Response

Stafford Act: Major Disaster Declaration
A major disaster declaration issued pursuant to the Stafford Act authorizes the President to provide a variety of types of assistance to eligible entities.[3] A major disaster declaration must meet three tests — *definition, need,* and *action.* The statute defines a major disaster as follows:

> ...any natural catastrophe (including any hurricane, tornado, storm, high water, winddriven water, tidal wave, tsunami, earthquake, volcanic eruption, landslide, mudslide, snowstorm, or drought), or, regardless of cause, any fire, flood, or explosion, in any part of the United States, which in the determination of the President causes damage of sufficient severity and magnitude to warrant major disaster assistance under this chapter to supplement the efforts and available resources of States, local governments, and disaster relief organizations in alleviating the damage, loss, hardship, or suffering caused thereby.[4]

Second, the incident must result in damages significant enough to exceed the resources and capabilities not only of the affected local governments, but the state as well. The requirement is set forth as follows:

> All requests for a declaration by the President that a major disaster exists shall be made by the Governor of the affected State. Such a request shall be based on a finding that the disaster is of such severity and magnitude that effective response is beyond the capabilities of the State and the affected local governments and that Federal assistance is necessary.[5]

Third, the state must implement its authorities, dedicate sufficient resources, and commit to meet its share of the costs, as follows:

> As part of such request, and as a prerequisite to major disaster assistance under this chapter, the Governor shall take appropriate response action under State law and direct execution of the State's emergency plan. The Governor shall furnish information on the nature and amount of State and local resources which have been or will be committed to alleviating the results of the disaster, and shall certify that, for the current disaster, State and local government obligations and expenditures (of which State commitments must be a significant proportion) will comply with all applicable cost-sharing requirements of this chapter. Based on the request of a Governor under this section, the President may declare under this chapter that a major disaster or emergency exists.[6]

Stafford Act: Emergency Declaration

By comparison with a major disaster declaration, considerably less assistance is authorized under an emergency declaration.[7] However, the Stafford Act gives the President considerably broader discretion in issuing an emergency declaration. First, the definition of "emergency" does not include the specific causal events listed in the definition of "major disaster." The President instead may determine whether circumstances are sufficiently dire for the affected state to call for an emergency declaration. Also, of importance to a flu pandemic or other public health threat, the protection of public health is to be considered by the President, as seen in the following:

> "Emergency" means any occasion or instance for which, in the determination of the President, Federal assistance is needed to supplement State and local efforts and capabilities to save lives and to protect property and public health and safety, or to lessen or avert the threat of a catastrophe in any part of the United States.[8]

Like those for a major disaster, statutory provisions governing procedures by which an emergency declaration will be considered by the President also contain requirements pertaining to *need* and *action*. However, as with the definition of "emergency," the procedures provide for a wider degree of discretion on the part of the President. While governors requesting assistance must take required actions, they do not have to identify that state and local resources have been committed. Governors must, however, identify the type and extent of federal aid required. The President also has discretion to act in the absence of a gubernatorial request if the emergency creates a condition that primarily or solely constitutes a federal responsibility. The Stafford Act procedure for an emergency declaration follows:

> (a) Request and declaration. All requests for a declaration by the President that an emergency exists shall be made by the Governor of the affected State. Such a request shall be based on a finding that the situation is of such severity and magnitude that effective response is beyond the capabilities of the State and the affected local governments and that Federal assistance is necessary. As a part of such request, and as a prerequisite to emergency assistance under this chapter, the Governor shall take appropriate action under State law and direct execution of the State's emergency plan. The Governor shall furnish information describing the State and local efforts and resources which have been or will be used to

alleviate the emergency, and will define the type and extent of Federal aid required. Based upon such Governor's request, the President may declare that an emergency exists.

(b) Certain emergencies involving Federal primary responsibility. The President may exercise any authority vested in him by Section 5192 of this Title or Section 5193 of this Title with respect to an emergency when he determines that an emergency exists for which the primary responsibility for response rests with the United States because the emergency involves a subject area for which, under the Constitution or laws of the United States, the United States exercises exclusive or preeminent responsibility and authority. In determining whether or not such an emergency exists, the President shall consult the Governor of any affected State, if practicable. The President's determination may be made without regard to subsection (a) of this section.[9]

The emergency declaration authority in the Stafford Act has previously been used by a President to respond specifically to a public health threat. In the fall of 2000, President Clinton issued emergency declarations for New York and New Jersey to help the states contain the threatened spread of the West Nile virus.[10]

Public Health Emergency Authorities

State and local governments, rather than the federal government, are the seats of responsibility and authority for public health activities, both in general, and in response to public health and medical emergencies. As with catastrophes in general, the federal government may provide various forms of assistance to state and local governments, non-profit entities, families, and others, in response to public health threats. Section 319 of the Public Health Service Act (PHS Act) grants the Secretary of HHS broad authority to determine that a public health emergency exists. Pursuant to such a determination, the Secretary may waive certain administrative requirements, provide additional forms of assistance, and take certain other actions to expand federal aid to state and local governments, not-for-profit entities, and others. The Secretary's statutory authority to determine a public health emergency is as follows:

> If the Secretary determines, after consultation with such public health officials as may be necessary, that — (1) a disease or disorder presents a public health emergency; or (2) a public health emergency, including significant outbreaks of infectious diseases or bioterrorist attacks, otherwise exists, the Secretary may take such action as may be appropriate to respond to the public health emergency, including making grants, providing awards for expenses, and entering into contracts and conducting and supporting investigations into the cause, treatment, or prevention of a disease or disorder as described in paragraphs (1) and (2).[11]

The Secretary has a variety of additional authorities to provide assistance. Some of these authorities require a concurrent determination of public health emergency pursuant to the PHS Act authority above, some require a concurrent declaration pursuant to the Stafford Act and/or the National Emergencies Act,[12] and some are independent of any other authority. A listing of various federal public health emergency authorities is provided in the **Appendix**.

The emergency authorities of the Secretary of HHS are not strictly comparable to authorities in the Stafford Act. Stafford Act major disaster assistance is intended to assist states and individuals with needs that exceed the scope of assistance routinely provided by federal agencies, and is often triggered by large-scale infrastructure damage. In contrast, the response to public health emergencies (such as infectious disease outbreaks) often involves extensions of routine program activities, such as technical assistance for epidemiologic and laboratory investigation, workforce assistance, or the provision of special drugs or tests.

In response to public health threats, the Secretary of HHS can provide a considerable degree of assistance to states, upon their request, through the Secretary's standing (i.e., non-emergency) authorities. There is neither a defined threshold, nor a requirement to demonstrate need, as with the Stafford Act. For example, simply upon the request of a State Health Official, and without the involvement of the President, the Centers for Disease Control and Prevention (CDC) can provide financial and technical assistance to states for outbreak investigation and disease control activities. These activities are carried out under the Secretary's general authority to assist states, pursuant to Section 311 of the PHS Act.[13]

Public health emergency determinations are less common than disaster or emergency declarations under the Stafford Act. The Secretary of HHS has determined that a public health emergency exists on only four occasions since 2000: (1) nationwide, in response to the terrorist attacks on September 11, 2001; (2) in several states affected by Hurricane Katrina in August and September 2005 (including states that were directly affected, and a number of states that hosted evacuees); (3) in Texas and Louisiana, affected by Hurricane Rita in September 2005; and (4) in Iowa and Indiana, affected by severe flooding in June 2008.[14]

Two factors may explain the rarity of public health emergency determinations. First, the Secretary of HHS has standing (non-emergency) authority to render many forms of aid to state and local governments and others, without the need to meet a defined threshold of need or impact. Also, although making such a determination authorizes the Secretary to draw from a Public Health Emergency Fund (PHEF), the fund has not had a balance in it for many years.[15] Consequently, none of the determinations issued since 2000 had the effect of mobilizing any additional funds beyond what would otherwise have been available. It is possible that if funds were available to the Secretary in the PHEF, it could influence the decision to make a public health emergency determination, or the pressures put upon the Secretary to do so.[16] Given that, the Congress may consider whether the degree of discretion afforded to the HHS Secretary in making such a determination, and the accompanying reporting requirements, are appropriate.

Although the Secretary of HHS does not, at this time, have access to additional funding if he or she makes a public health emergency determination, the authority appears to have be useful, nonetheless, in addressing the widespread evacuations that resulted from Hurricanes Katrina and Rita in 2005, and the Midwest floods in 2008. When a public health emergency determination is made, the Secretary has authority to waive a number of requirements that typically apply to health care providers as a condition of their receipt of federal reimbursement (through the Medicare program, for example.) Among other things, these waivers allow beneficiaries to receive services despite having lost their documentation of eligibility, and providers to provide services in alternate temporary facilities.[17]

Legislation introduced in the 110th Congress (H.R. 6569/S. 3312) would authorize the Secretary, when he or she has determined there to be a public health emergency pursuant to Section 319 of the PHS Act, to use the PHEF to provide temporary emergency health care coverage for uninsured individuals affected by the emergency. The proposals would require the Secretary to consider, in making such a determination, the extent to which the situation has or is likely to overwhelm health care providers in the affected area, and the potential financial burdens those providers may face as a result.[18]

Intersection of Stafford Act and Public Health Emergency Authority

Disaster and emergency authorities pursuant to the Stafford Act are generally independent of public health emergency authorities. Only one provision in current law — allowing for the waiver of a number of HHS statutory, regulatory and program requirements, discussed above — requires a simultaneous public health emergency determination, *and* a declaration pursuant to either the Stafford Act or the National Emergencies Act. When multiple declarations are in effect as a result of a specific incident, as they were following Hurricane Katrina, it can pose a greater challenge for officials in understanding the scope and interaction of their response authorities.[19]

Federal Coordinating Mechanisms for Disaster Response

National Response Framework

Pursuant to congressional mandate, the Department of Homeland Security (DHS) released the *National Response Plan* (NRP) in December 2004 to establish a comprehensive framework for the coordination of federal resources under specified emergency conditions.[20] In January 200 8, the NRP was replaced by the *National Response Framework* (NRF), following a lengthy stakeholder engagement intended, among other things, to capture lessons learned from the flawed response to Hurricane Katrina.[21] The NRF is under the overall coordination of the Secretary of Homeland Security, and its implementation is delegated to FEMA. It sets forth the responsibilities and roles of federal agencies; identifies tasks to be performed by specified federal officials; and includes annexes with details on support resources and mechanisms that are integral to its implementation. It is not a source of new authority for incident response. While it may be used to guide response activities that flow from Stafford Act declarations, it is not a source of funding for these activities.[22] It is applicable to incidents whether or not they have led to a Stafford Act declaration.[23] Finally, it is intended to be a *national* coordinating blueprint, describing and integrating roles for state, local, territorial and tribal governments and the private sector, as well as federal agencies.

National Response to an Influenza Pandemic

In addition to the NRF, which guides a coordinated national *all-hazards* response (i.e., to a variety of catastrophes), numerous federal and other planning documents that are specific for a flu pandemic have been published. Selected planning documents are listed below. Unless otherwise noted, they can be found on a government-wide pandemic flu website managed by HHS.[24]

- The *National Strategy for Pandemic Influenza,* November 2005: outlines general responsibilities of individuals, industry, state and local governments, and the federal government in preparing for and responding to a pandemic.

- *National Strategy for Pandemic Influenza, Implementation Plan,* May 2006: assigns more than 300 preparedness and response tasks to departments and agencies across the federal government; includes measures of progress and timelines for implementation; provides initial guidance for state, local, and tribal entities, businesses, schools and universities, communities, and non-governmental organizations on the development of institutional plans; provides initial preparedness guidance for individuals and families.

- The *HHS Pandemic Influenza Plan,* November 2005: provides guidance to national, state and local policy makers and health departments, outlining key roles and responsibilities during a pandemic and specifying preparedness needs and opportunities. This plan emphasizes specific preparedness efforts in the public health and health care sectors.

- *Department of Defense Implementation Plan for Pandemic Influenza,* August 2006: provides policy and guidance for the following priorities: (1) force health protection and readiness; (2) the continuity of essential functions and services; (3) Defense support to civil authorities (i.e., federal, state, and local governments); (4) effective communications; and (5) support to international partners.

- *VA Pandemic Influenza Plan,* March 2006: provides policy and instructions for Department of Veterans Affairs (VA) in protecting its staff and the veterans it serves, maintaining operations, cooperating with other organizations, and communicating with stakeholders.

- *Pandemic Influenza Preparedness, Response, and Recovery Guide for Critical Infrastructure and Key Resources,* September 2006: provides business planners with guidance to assure continuity during a pandemic for facilities comprising critical infrastructure sectors (e.g., energy and telecommunications) and key resources (e.g., dams and nuclear power plants).

- *State pandemic plans:* All states were required to develop and submit specific plans for pandemic flu preparedness, as a requirement of grants provided by HHS.[25]

Would the Stafford Act Apply in a Flu Pandemic?

Each of the pandemic influenza plans listed above was written with the premise that the NRP would have been applicable to guide a coordinated federal response to a flu pandemic. The NRF, which was published subsequently, similarly notes that it could serve as the blueprint for a coordinated national response to this incident.[26]

As noted earlier, the NRF serves as a coordinating mechanism, but it does not confer any additional executive authorities, or serve as a source of funding for response activities. When a Stafford Act emergency or major disaster is declared, the Disaster Relief Fund may be used to pay for authorized response activities and assistance.[27] There is precedent for a Stafford emergency declaration in response to an infectious disease threat: as noted earlier, emergency declarations pursuant to the Stafford Act were made in response to West Nile virus in 2000. However, there is no relevant precedent regarding whether Stafford Act major disaster assistance could be provided in response to a flu pandemic. FEMA has in the past, in the context of the national TOPOFF exercises, interpreted biological disasters as ineligible for major disaster assistance pursuant to the Stafford Act.[28] However, the Administration's view is that the President's authority to declare a major disaster pursuant to the Stafford Act could be applied to a flu pandemic,[29] and FEMA has issued a Disaster Assistance Policy regarding major disaster assistance that may be provided in response to this threat.[30]

The matter of the applicability of a Stafford Act declaration to a flu pandemic is important for two reasons. First, the level of funding that may be available to support federal activities, and provide assistance to state and local governments and individuals, is substantially greater following a major disaster declaration than it is for an emergency declaration.[31] Second, the federal leadership structure for incident response may be different depending on whether the incident results in a Stafford Act declaration, or is a "non-Stafford" incident. The Stafford Act requires the President, upon making an emergency or major disaster declaration, to appoint a Federal Coordinating Officer (FCO) to operate in the affected region.[32] This individual has historically reported to the head of FEMA, who in turn reports to the President and assumes overall operational control of the federal government's incident response. The NRF, and the NRP before it, established the role of Principal Federal Official (PFO), a different individual who reports directly to the Secretary of Homeland Security during an incident response. Confusion about the respective roles and authorities of these individuals was identified following Hurricane Katrina, and has remained a matter of concern to Congress.[33] It is reported that in December 2006, the Secretary of Homeland Security predesignated, in the event of a response to a flu pandemic, one national and five regional FCOs, *and* one national and five regional PFOs.[34] The respective roles of these individuals — all of whom would presumably be involved in response activities if a Stafford Act declaration were made — have not been clarified in any publicly available pandemic planning document.[35]

NRF EMERGENCY SUPPORT FUNCTION 8: ROLES AND CHALLENGES

Overview

The Hurricane Katrina response, and planning for a flu pandemic, each demonstrate the scope of *public health* and *medical* activities needed in response to a large-scale catastrophe. A flu pandemic would not likely impose the mass dislocations and destruction of health care infrastructure seen following Hurricane Katrina. But, as a pandemic would affect all areas of the nation simultaneously, responders could not necessarily count on the state-to-state mutual aid that was critical to the hurricane response.

A successful *public health response* involves such things as monitoring and assurance of the safety of food and water, prevention of injury, control of infectious diseases, and a host of other activities, and is carried out by a variety of entities, primarily government and not-for-profit agencies. A successful *medical response* is perhaps more complicated, requiring the coordination of several elements, which are variously based in federal, state or local authority, or in the private sector. These elements are (1) patients, who may require rescue or medical evacuation; (2) a treatment facility, which may be an existing hospital or a field tent with cots; (3) a competent health care workforce; (4) appropriate medical equipment and nonperishable medical supplies; (5) appropriate drugs, vaccines, tests and other perishable medical supplies; (6) a system of medical records; and (7) a health care financing mechanism.

According to the NRF (and the earlier NRP), the Secretary of HHS is tasked with coordinating *Emergency Support Function 8* (ESF-8), the public health and medical response to incidents.[36] (ESF-8 is one of 15 ESFs in the NRF. Other functions include public safety, energy supplies, and transportation, for example.) ESFs are coordinating mechanisms, not funding mechanisms. The response to a flu pandemic is likely to be primarily an ESF-8 response, in which public health and medical needs could be substantial. Less onerous burdens might be expected on other ESFs such as transportation, public works, and energy, compared to those imposed following hurricanes and other weather-related disasters. Nonetheless, planners note that a severe pandemic could still constitute a multi-sector incident. Staffing shortages and supply chain disruptions could affect the continuity of services, and possibly the integrity of infrastructure, in the transportation, public works, and energy sectors, among others.

The Secretary of HHS is responsible for coordinating the following activities under ESF-8, and may request assistance from 14 designated support agencies and the American Red Cross as needed:

- assessment of public health and medical needs;
- health surveillance;
- medical care personnel;
- health/medical/veterinary equipment and supplies;
- patient evacuation;
- patient care;
- safety and security of human and veterinary drugs and medical devices, and human biologics;[37]
- blood and blood products;
- food safety and security;
- agriculture safety and security;all-hazard public health and medical consultation, technical assistance and support;
- behavioral health care;
- public health and medical information;
- vector control (e.g., control of disease-carrying insects and rodents);
- potable water, wastewater and solid waste disposal;
- mass fatality management, victim identification and decontaminating remains; and
- veterinary medical support.

Depending on the incident, HHS may need other agencies to carry out certain of their ESF activities (e.g., public safety, road clearing, and power restoration) before some ESF-8 activities could begin. Some specific concerns resulting from overlaps or gaps in defined ESF duties are discussed below.

Unclear Federal Leadership for Certain Response Functions

In the response to Hurricane Katrina, it became apparent that federal responsibility to coordinate certain support activities was not clear in the existing ESF assignments in the NRP. The NRF has addressed some of these concerns, left others unclear, and possibly raised some new concerns.

Some had questioned whether the NRP clearly defined federal ESF-8 leadership, or whether the respective roles of the Secretaries of Homeland Security and HHS could conflict during a response. Some, including congressional investigators, felt this conflict was in evidence during the response to Hurricane Katrina.[38] Others were concerned that the respective roles were insufficiently clear to guide a coordinated response to a flu pandemic. In October 2006, the President signed P.L. 109-295, the Post-Katrina Emergency Management Reform Act of 2006 (called the "Post-Katrina Act"; included in DHS appropriations for FY2007), which reauthorized and reorganized programs in FEMA.[39] Among other things, the law also codified the position of Chief Medical Officer (CMO) at DHS, the individual who coordinates all departmental activities regarding medical and public health aspects of disasters. The Post-Katrina Act provided that the CMO "shall have the primary responsibility *within the Department* for medical issues related to natural disasters, acts of terrorism, and other man-made disasters."[40] (Emphasis added.) Subsequently, in December 2006, the President signed P.L. 109-417, the Pandemic and All-Hazards Preparedness Act, which provided that "The Secretary of Health and Human Services shall lead all *Federal* public health and medical response to public health emergencies and incidents covered by the National Response Plan...."[41] (Emphasis added.) The Government Accountability Office (GAO) has recommended, in the context of pandemic flu planning, that the two departments (DHS and HHS) conduct rigorous testing, training and exercises to ensure that these roles are clearly defined.[42]

Responsibility for the health and safety of disaster response workers was a matter of concern in the NRP, and remains so in the NRF. The Government Accountability Office (GAO) found that OSHA's efforts during the response to Hurricane Katrina were hampered by confusion about the agency's role. GAO noted in particular that disagreements between FEMA and OSHA regarding OSHA's role delayed FEMA's authorization of mission assignments to fund OSHA's response activities.[43] Some Members of Congress and others sought to have worker health and safety elevated to an Emergency Support Function in the NRF, which would give OSHA more autonomy in commencing its response activities.[44] Instead, the NRF contains a revised Worker Safety and Health Support Annex.[45]

Although both the NRP and the NRF address mass fatality management, the NRP did not, and the NRF does not, clearly delegate responsibility for the *retrieval* of human remains in mass fatality events. HHS is responsible for the ESF-8 function of coordinating federal assistance to identify victims and determine causes of death. Federal Disaster Mortuary Assistance Teams (DMORTs) comprise medical examiners, pathologists, dental technicians and other medical personnel.[46] These teams are not skilled in the safe retrieval of remains from hazardous sites such as waterways or collapsed buildings. Other responders, including Urban Search and Rescue teams and the U.S. Coast Guard, are trained to work safely in such dangerous conditions, but their mission is to rescue the living, not recover the dead.[47] The matter of mass fatality management is of considerable concern to pandemic planners, and this gap could be problematic during such an incident.

At times the distinction between ESF-6 and ESF-8 may be blurred. Emergency Support Function 6 (ESF-6), *Mass Care*, under the leadership of FEMA, lays out the coordination of emergency shelter, feeding, and related activities for affected populations. As was evident in the response to Hurricane Katrina, the ESF functions overlapped when evacuees in Red Cross shelters required medical care, or when large numbers of hospital patients evacuated to ESF-8 field hospitals required food and water. The revised ESF-6 and ESF-8 annexes accompanying the NRF provide substantially more detail regarding the coordination of these functions than did the corresponding NRP annexes. Also, this problem was reportedly considered by FEMA, HHS, and the American Red Cross in their reviews of the hurricane response, and in their subsequent preparedness planning.

In the NRF, as with the NRP, leadership for the federal coordination of mental and behavioral health services following a disaster appears to be split between ESF-6 and ESF-8. "Crisis counseling" is among the responsibilities delegated in ESF-6, while federal coordination of "behavioral health care" — including assessing mental health and substance abuse needs, and providing disaster mental health training for workers — is delegated in ESF-8. Hence, federal leadership for disaster mental health in the NRP is delegated to both FEMA and to HHS.[48] (When the disaster involves terrorism or other forms of violence, the Department of Justice may also become a key federal partner, as was seen following the Oklahoma City bombing.[49])

Finally, the NRF resolves a gap in the NRP regarding federal responsibility for pets during disasters. It is well established that some people are reluctant to abandon their pets and will remain at home, despite an evacuation order, if they cannot take pets with them. Hence, the absence of coordinated mechanisms to assure the safety of pets in disasters may jeopardize human safety as well. In the Post-Katrina Act, Congress required DHS, in developing standards for state and local emergency plans, to account for the needs of individuals with household pets and service animals before, during, and after a major disaster or emergency, in particular with regard to evacuation planning and planning for the needs of individuals with disabilities. In addition, the act authorized the President to make Stafford Act assistance available to states and localities to carry out pet rescue and sheltering activities in the immediate response to a major disaster.[50] Congress passed similar provisions in P.L. 109-308, the Pets Evacuation and Transportation Standards Act of 2006, though neither act addressed the matter of federal leadership for the needs of pets in disasters. The NRF, however, clearly assigns this responsibility under ESF-6 (Mass Care) and ESF-11 (Agriculture and Natural Resources). FEMA, when coordinating federal efforts to provide human sheltering services per ESF-6, is to ensure that the needs of pets can also be accommodated (various approaches to this are often referred to as "co-sheltering"), while USDA's Animal and Plant Health Inspection Service, per ESF-11, is to ensure that the sheltering needs of the pets are met.

FEDERAL FUNDING TO SUPPORT AN ESF-8 RESPONSE

Hurricane Katrina was the greatest test of ESF-8 since the establishment of DHS and the publication of the NRP. A variety of public health and medical activities were undertaken in the hurricane response. The costs of these activities were borne by agencies at the federal, state and local levels, not-for-profit groups, businesses, health care providers, insurers, families, and individuals. Private insurance covered some of the property damage, health care and other costs resulting from the disaster. Congress provided additional assistance through emergency appropriations to cover expanded federal agency activities and a portion of uninsured health care costs. Some other costs, such as the costs of rebuilding the devastated health care infrastructure in New Orleans, have not been fully met at this time, either through existing assistance mechanisms or mechanisms developed since the storm.[51] The response to Hurricane Katrina, and ongoing pandemic preparedness efforts, each offer a glimpse of the complexity of the challenge, and the adequacy of existing mechanisms to fund the costs of an ESF-8 response.

Funding Sources and Authorities

The Disaster Relief Fund

Activities undertaken pursuant to the Stafford Act are funded through appropriations to the Disaster Relief Fund (DRF), administered by FEMA. Federal assistance supported by the DRF is used by states, localities, and certain non-profit organizations to provide mass feeding and shelter, restore damaged or destroyed facilities, clear debris, and aid individuals and families with uninsured needs, among other activities. Federal agencies also receive *mission assignments* from FEMA to provide assistance pursuant to the NRF, and are reimbursed through funds appropriated to the DRF. Through mission assignments, the DRF supported a variety of federal public health activities in the response to Hurricane Katrina, including activities to assure the safety of food and water, monitor population health status (including mental health), control infectious diseases and mosquitoes, and evaluate potential health threats associated with chemical releases. However, the DRF is not generally available to pay or reimburse the costs of health care for affected individuals, though it may pay such costs to a limited extent. (See "Federal Assistance for Disaster-Related Health Care Costs," below.)

The DRF is a no-year account in which appropriated funds remain available until expended. Supplemental appropriations legislation is generally required each fiscal year to replenish the DRF to meet the urgent needs of particularly catastrophic disasters.[52]

The Public Health Emergency Fund

In 1983, Congress established authority for a no-year Public Health Emergency Fund (PHEF) to be available to the HHS Secretary.[53] In 2000, Congress reauthorized the fund, clarifying that it could only be used when the Secretary had made a determination of a public health emergency, pursuant to Section 319 of the Public Health Service Act (PHS Act),[54] as follows:

> (1) In general. There is established in the Treasury a fund to be designated as the "Public Health Emergency Fund" to be made available to the Secretary without fiscal year limitation to carry out subsection (a) only if a public health emergency has been declared by the Secretary under such subsection. There is authorized to be appropriated to the Fund such sums as may be necessary.
>
> (2) Report. Not later than 90 days after the end of each fiscal year, the Secretary shall prepare and submit to the Committee on Health, Education, Labor, and Pensions and the

Committee on Appropriations of the Senate and the Committee on Commerce and the Committee on Appropriations of the House of Representatives a report describing — (A) the expenditures made from the Public Health Emergency Fund in such fiscal year; and (B) each public health emergency for which the expenditures were made and the activities undertaken with respect to each emergency which was conducted or supported by expenditures from the Fund.[55]

Between 1988 and 2000, the fund was authorized for annual appropriations sufficient to have a balance of $45 million at the beginning of each fiscal year.[56] Despite this prior authorization of annual appropriations, the fund received appropriations only in response to a few public health threats (e.g., the emergence of hantavirus in the Southwest in 1993-1994), but did not receive an appropriation for its intended use as a reserve fund for unanticipated events. The fund has not received an appropriation since it was explicitly linked to the public health emergency authority in the PHS Act in 2000. As a consequence, the fund was not available for the response to four public health emergency determinations made subsequently: (1) nationwide, in response to the terrorist attacks on September 11, 2001; (2) in several states affected by Hurricane Katrina in August and September 2005 (including states that were directly affected, and a number of states that hosted evacuees); (3) in Texas and Louisiana, affected by Hurricane Rita in September 2005; and (4) in Iowa and Indiana, affected by severe flooding in June 2008.[57]

In 2002, Congress reauthorized the National Disaster Medical System (NDMS) in language suggesting that the emergency fund could be used to support additional activities of the HHS Secretary, including NDMS deployments, as follows:

> ... For the purpose of providing for the Assistant Secretary for Public Health Emergency Preparedness and the operations of the National Disaster Medical System, other than purposes for which amounts in the Public Health Emergency Fund under Section 319 are available, there are authorized to be appropriated such sums as may be necessary for each of the fiscal years 2002 through 2006.[58]

Depending on the availability of funds, this mechanism could be used to fund NDMS deployments that occurred in the absence of Stafford Act declarations.

Legislation introduced in the 110th Congress (H.R. 6569/S. 3312) would authorize the Secretary, when he or she has determined there to be a public health emergency pursuant to Section 319 of the PHS Act, to use the PHEF to provide temporary emergency health care coverage for uninsured individuals affected by the emergency.[59]

The Public Health and Social Services Emergency Fund

The Public Health and Social Services Emergency Fund (PHSSEF) is an account at HHS that has been used to provide annual or emergency supplemental appropriations for one-time or short-term public health activities in a variety of agencies and offices. Providing funding to the PHSSEF, which does not have an explicit authority in law, separates these amounts from an agency's annual "base" funding. Recent activities funded through the PHSSEF include preparedness activities for a flu pandemic, one-time purchases for the Strategic National Stockpile (SNS), and grants for state public health and hospital preparedness. Amounts appropriated to the PHSSEF may or may not be designated as emergency spending. Because the PHSSEF has been used only to fund certain planned activities, it is not a reserve fund for unanticipated events.

In FY2006, Congress appropriated certain amounts that had previously been provided through the PHSSEF directly to the various agencies overseeing the programs. These included funding for the SNS and grants for upgrading state and local public health capacity, amounts now appropriated in CDC's "Terrorism and Public Health Preparedness" budget line,[60] and grants to states for hospital preparedness, previously administered by the Health Resources and Services Administration (HRSA, an agency in HHS), and transferred to the HHS Assistant Secretary for Preparedness and Response (ASPR) in the Pandemic and All-Hazards Preparedness Act.[61]

Funding the ESF-8 Response to Hurricane Katrina

In response to the widespread destruction caused by Hurricane Katrina, the 109th Congress enacted two FY2005 emergency supplemental appropriations bills (P.L. 109-61 and P.L. 109-62), which together provided $62.3 billion for emergency response and recovery needs. The FY2006 appropriations legislation for the Department of Defense (P.L. 109-148) subsequently reallocated $23.4 billion in funds appropriated in the two emergency supplemental statutes, and an additional amount from a government-wide rescission, primarily to pay for the restoration of damaged federal facilities. In June 2006, Congress provided an additional $6 billion to the DRF in P.L. 109-234, the Emergency Supplemental Appropriations Act for Defense, the Global War on Terror, and Hurricane Recovery, 2006.[62]

A portion of supplemental appropriations to the DRF supported federal ESF-8 response activities. FEMA reports to Congress on expenditures for mission assignments to both HHS, and separately to CDC, for the responses to Hurricanes Katrina, Rita and Wilma.[63] A number of HHS agencies in addition to CDC were involved in the response to the hurricanes, and their activities, when requested by FEMA, were presumably reimbursed through the DRF.[64]

There were likely other HHS activities carried out in response to the hurricanes that would not fall within the scope of activities reimbursable by the DRF. For example, on September 16, 2005, CDC issued guidance to state grantees permitting them to redirect funds from a number of grant programs to their hurricane relief efforts as needed.[65] According to CDC, funds could be used for alternate activities within the state, or to support state-to-state mutual aid pursuant to the Emergency Management Assistance Compact (EMAC).[66] States were permitted to redirect funds from the following federal grant programs: infectious diseases (including immunization, sexually transmitted disease prevention, tuberculosis, West Nile virus, hepatitis, HIV, emerging infections and laboratory programs); environmental health; injury prevention; and, terrorism and emergency preparedness. CDC noted at the time that "No supplemental appropriations have been provided to CDC for Katrina relief, so any existing CDC funds used for relief will reduce the overall amount available to work non-relief grant issues."[67] HRSA also advised state grantees that some redirection of funds provided by the National Bioterrorism Hospital Preparedness Program (which HRSA administered at the time) was also permissible to support the hurricane response.[68]

Information regarding the overall amount of funds that may have been redirected by HHS agencies to support Hurricane Katrina response activities, and, for those expenditures that were not reimbursable by the DRF, whether there were alternate mechanisms to "backfill" the accounts, is not publicly available. HHS received limited direct supplemental appropriations for its response to Hurricane Katrina, namely $8 million to CDC for mosquito abatement and other pest control activities, and $4 million to HRSA to re-establish communications capability in health departments, community health centers, major medical centers, and other entities that would continue to provide health care in areas affected by Hurricane Katrina.[69]

Federal Assistance for Disaster-Related Health Care Costs

Overview

When Stafford major disaster assistance is available, as it was following Hurricane Katrina, it can be invaluable in supporting public health response activities under ESF-8. Typically, these activities are inherently governmental, and are generally reimbursable from the DRF. But even when a Stafford major disaster declaration applies, it does little to meet the uninsured or uncompensated costs of health care for disaster victims, or to reimburse institutions and providers who may have provided care without compensation. There is no federal assistance program designed purposely to cover the uninsured or uncompensated costs of individual health care that may be needed as a consequence of a disaster.

In a typical year, there are dozens of Stafford Act major disaster declarations (most resulting from weather-related events), potentially affecting millions of people. Given that some U.S. uninsured health care needs go unmet under normal circumstances, there is not consensus that the costs of health care for these disaster victims should be a federal responsibility. However, policy debates following two recent disasters, and concerns about pandemic flu, suggest that some Members of Congress and others are interested in exploring possible mechanisms to provide such assistance, at least in certain situations.

Following Hurricane Katrina, Congress provided $2.1 billion through the Medicaid program to assist states in providing for the health care needs of Katrina evacuees for five months following the storm. Katrina's victims continue to experience mental health problems in disproportionate numbers, however. These problems, and possibly others resulting from the storm and its aftermath, may linger beyond the duration of assistance programs that may be available to the storm's victims.

While there is not consensus that the costs of health care for disaster victims should be borne by the federal government, there has nonetheless been considerable discussion about the needs of victims of the terrorist attack of September 11, 2001, and whether terrorism should place upon the federal government a different responsibility for its victims than for victims of non-terrorist disasters.

Existing Mechanisms

Several federal assistance mechanisms are available to provide *limited* coverage for the costs of health care services that are rendered during, or required as a result of, a catastrophe. These programs provide a patchwork of coverage that in some cases fails to optimally match services with need (e.g., the Crisis Counseling Program), or in other cases fails to meet the magnitude of need (e.g., the FEMA Individuals and Households program). Furthermore, these programs are not generally coordinated with each other at the federal level, though programs that support state activities to finance or deliver health care services may be coordinated at that level. These programs include:

- Services provided by the National Disaster Medical System (NDMS) or other federalized employees while carrying out mission assignments requested by FEMA, pursuant to a Stafford Act declaration, may be reimbursed by the DRF, though efforts may be made to seek reimbursement from patients' insurers when possible. This assistance may be provided under both major disaster and emergency declarations that involve the provision of health and safety measures and the reduction of threats to public health and safety.[70]

- The FEMA Individuals and Households Program (IHP) provides, pursuant to a Stafford Act declaration and reimbursed from the DRF, cash assistance that may be used for uninsured medical expenses. Recipients might have to use the funds to meet other needs concurrently, such as rent and other costs of living. The amount available is the same for an individual or a household, and is capped in statute, with an annual adjustment based on the Consumer Price Index. The maximum amount available for Hurricane Katrina relief was $26,200, and the current ceiling (for FY2008) is $28,800.[71]

- Certain medications and supplies may be provided to patients from pre-paid stockpiles for which reimbursement is not expected. Examples may include supplies used in first aid stations or distributed to states from the CDC's Strategic National Stockpile. Agencies' costs may be reimbursed from the DRF if the incident resulted in a Stafford Act declaration.

- The Stafford Act authorizes the President, pursuant to a *major disaster* declaration, to provide financial assistance to state and qualified tribal mental health agencies for professional counseling services, or training of disaster workers, to relieve disaster victims' mental health problems caused or aggravated by the disaster or its aftermath. FEMA and the Substance Abuse and Mental Health Services Administration (SAMHSA) in HHS jointly administer the Crisis Counseling Assistance and Training Program (CCP). Financing for this assistance is drawn from the DRF.[72]

- Public Health Service agencies in HHS may provide support to states and other entities through existing non-emergency mechanisms to assist in managing surges in health care needs for specific populations.[73] In some cases, agencies have received supplemental appropriations to support these activities. Examples include SAMHSA Emergency Response Grants (SERG) to states, territories, and federally recognized tribal authorities for crisis mental health and substance abuse services,[74] and expanded federal support, including personnel, for health centers in disaster-affected areas.[75]

- Certain federal compensation programs may cover some or all health care costs for certain disaster victims, though these programs generally flow from the individual's employment status rather than from their status as disaster victims. Such programs include workers' compensation programs, for federal workers whose injuries are related to employment,[76] and benefits for federal, state, and local public safety officers (including police officers and firefighters) who are killed or permanently disabled while performing their duties.[77]

- For victims of disasters resulting from terrorism, certain forms of assistance to crime victims may be available to help defray health care costs.[78]

Health Care Needs of 9/11 Responders

Within two weeks of the terrorist attack on the World Trade Center (WTC) in New York City, Congress established the September 11th Victim Compensation Fund (VCF).[79] The program provided compensation for physical injury or death, from any cause, that resulted from an individual's presence at the sites at the time of the crashes or in their immediate aftermath.[80] The deadline for filing a claim was December 22, 2003.

Thousands of responders worked on the site in a rescue, recovery, and cleanup operation that lasted more than a year. Many of these workers and some residents in the area are experiencing, many years later, various respiratory, psychological, gastrointestinal and other problems felt to be related to their exposures at the site.[81] Physical hazards to which these individuals were potentially exposed include asbestos and other particulates, heavy metals, volatile organic compounds, and dioxin.

Congress provided funding to the CDC to establish the World Trade Center Health Registry, an effort to identify and periodically survey people who were exposed at the site or in the general vicinity, to track their health status over a 20-year period.[82] In addition, several medical monitoring programs were established to develop and deliver initial, and sometimes follow-up, health examinations to groups of individuals potentially at risk of future illness. While recruitment for both activities continues, the monitoring programs have identified a number of people with serious health problems presumably related to their WTC exposures, some of whom have died. Congress has provided intermittent appropriations to support the costs of medical treatment for some of these individuals, through treatment programs established after the terrorist attack.[83]

The VCF is not available to assist individuals whose symptoms arose after the fund's closing date. Routine sources of health care coverage may also elude these individuals. Some may have lost employer-based health insurance coverage, if they have become too sick to work. For some with health insurance, the plan may not cover needed prescription drugs or specialty care, or coverage may be denied if an insurer asserts that an illness is work-related and should be covered by workers' compensation. Some workers, such as volunteers or immigrants, may lack workers' compensation coverage. Others who have this coverage may still find that employers and insurers contest their claims on the basis that an illness is not work-related.[84]

Congressional interest in this issue has focused on matters of short- and long-term financing and accountability for the registry, monitoring, and treatment programs, and whether or how financial responsibility for the long-term needs of affected individuals should be shared, if at all, among the federal government, local governments, private insurers, and others. Bills introduced in the 110th Congress have proposed establishing programs to pay health care or other costs for workers and others who may be ill as a result of their exposures following the WTC incident, or providing eligibility for these individuals in existing programs.[85] None of these bills has advanced.

Financing Health Care Needs Following Hurricane Katrina

Hurricane Katrina was the largest mass casualty incident in recent times. Many of the storm's victims were dislocated to different states, separated from their documentation of health insurance, or both. Others lost employer-based health insurance due to the destruction or closure of businesses. In many cases, care was rendered without definitive financing mechanisms, while federal, state and private entities worked to retrofit these mechanisms in the disaster's aftermath. In response, HHS expanded a number of existing programs to assist state and local agencies, health care providers and the storms' victims with a variety of health and public health needs.[86] Information regarding the overall cost of these expansions is not publicly available.

In 2002, Congress gave the Secretary of HHS authority to waive certain administrative requirements for provider participation in Medicare, Medicaid and the State Children's Health Insurance Program (SCHIP) when there are in effect, concurrently, a Stafford Act declaration and a determination of public health emergency pursuant to Section 319 of the Public Health Service Act.[87] This authority was exercised in a number of affected and host states following Hurricane Katrina. While this authority may improve access to health care services in affected areas, it does not directly address the financing of these services.

A significant challenge following Hurricane Katrina involved setting up or reestablishing health care financing mechanisms for displaced individuals. Ultimately, the Medicaid program became the mechanism by which affected and host states financed certain health care costs that were not compensated through other public or private insurance sources. After several months of debate, Congress provided, in the Deficit Reduction Act of 2005, authority and funding to cover, for certain states through January 31, 2006, the Medicaid and SCHIP matching requirements for individuals enrolled in these programs, and the total cost of uncompensated care for the uninsured, for eligible individuals who had been displaced from declared major disaster areas.[88] Congress provided up to $2 billion for these activities.[89] This was in addition to $100 million earlier provided in supplemental appropriations to NDMS to cover expenses related to the response to Hurricane Katrina.[90] (Through an interagency agreement, most of the $100 million was transferred from FEMA to the HHS Centers for Medicare and Medicaid Services (CMS), which is also administering the $2 billion amount.[91]) According to HHS, as a result of this mechanism, eight states were able to reimburse providers that incurred uncompensated care costs as a result of serving an estimated 325,000 evacuees, and 32 states were able to provide continuity of coverage for up to five months for displaced low-income individuals by temporarily enrolling them in a host state's Medicaid program through a simplified enrollment process.[92]

Individuals, institutions, providers, and others affected by Hurricane Katrina continue to face challenges that are beyond the scope of the nation's disaster assistance mechanisms. The Louisiana Health Care Redesign Collaborative was established in 2006 to develop a health care system that would integrate Gulf Coast and greater New Orleans rebuilding into a broader statewide plan.[93] A key funding strategy for the Collaborative is the development and approval by CMS of a comprehensive Medicaid waiver and Medicare demonstration proposal.[94]

ESF-8 Funding Needs during a Flu Pandemic

While a severe flu pandemic may constitute a national catastrophe, requiring a robust ESF-8 public health and medical response, funding needs may not be readily addressed through existing assistance mechanisms pursuant to the Stafford Act (to the extent that they apply), and could outstrip existing government and private resources. While the need for public health and medical services could be considerable, extensive damage to public or private infrastructure is not anticipated. Costs associated with workforce surge capacity (e.g., overtime pay) and consumption of certain supplies (e.g., for public health laboratory tests) could increase substantially. Presuming a surge of patients in the health care system, non-urgent procedures (which are often more lucrative) could be postponed for weeks or months at a time. This has raised questions regarding whether there would be shifts in overall revenue to providers for services rendered during a pandemic, and how such shifts could affect providers and insurers. Finally, the cost of providing health care services during a pandemic, when about 47 million Americans currently lack health insurance, is of concern to many. Some are concerned that disease control efforts could suffer if some subgroups of the population were unwilling, because of their insurance status or for other reasons, to seek care or otherwise interact with disease control authorities during a pandemic.

In March 2007, FEMA issued a Disaster Assistance Policy for pandemic flu, outlining, among other types of assistance, the types of health care services that would be reimbursable through the Disaster Relief Fund, presuming that a Stafford major disaster declaration were made.[95] Assistance would be provided to eligible entities (including state and local government agencies) to support a number of ESF8 activities, including establishing temporary medical facilities, public communication, and mass fatality management. With respect to the costs of medical care provided to individuals, the policy states that the following services may be eligible for reimbursement, for a period of time to be determined by the Secretary of Homeland Security or his designee: "Emergency medical care (non-deferrable medical treatment of disaster victims in a shelter or temporary medical facility and related medical facility services and supplies, including emergency medical transport, X-rays, laboratory and pathology services, and machine diagnostic tests....)"[96] Neither "emergency medical care" nor "non-deferrable medical treatment" are defined. Given the potential for there to be many casualties of a flu pandemic who require extended critical medical care, the extent to which the Disaster Relief Fund could be tapped to support the costs of such care is not entirely clear.

As previously noted, following Hurricane Katrina, Congress provided $2.1 billion to states to cover the states' usual share of Medicaid and SCHIP costs for storm victims for a defined time period, and the cost of uncompensated care for the uninsured. This federal assistance mechanism required legislative action and took nearly six months to enact, in the absence of a pre-existing mechanism to provide such federal assistance. Whether this could serve as a model for federal assistance during a flu pandemic is unclear. An important element of the discussion regarding the Katrina assistance was the desire to help both states that had been directly affected, and states that had assumed fiscal liability by accepting evacuees. While the element of victim displacement would not likely be seen during a pandemic, Congress may nonetheless debate the merits of expanding federal assistance for health care costs during a flu pandemic, and the model developed following Hurricane Katrina may serve as a useful starting point for discussion.

Health Care Financing Proposals for Future Emergencies

Legislation introduced in the 110th Congress (H.R. 6569/S. 3312) would require the Secretary to establish a program to provide temporary emergency health care coverage for uninsured or underinsured individuals affected by public health emergencies. The Secretary would be authorized to provide such coverage when he or she has determined there to be a public health emergency pursuant to Section 319 of the Public Health Service Act, after considering the extent to which the situation may overwhelm health care providers in the affected area, and the potential financial burdens those providers may face as a result. The program would apply certain administrative approaches used in other federal health care programs (e.g., Medicare payment rates), but would be financed solely through appropriations to the Public Health Emergency Fund. The proposals would authorize the appropriation of $7 million for each fiscal year, beginning with FY2009, for program planning, and for an outreach and education campaign for providers and the public about the potential availability of this assistance in a public health emergency. The proposals would require that if the Secretary activates the program of emergency health care coverage, he or she shall also establish a program for medical monitoring and reporting on the health care needs of the affected population over time.

CONCLUSION

Both the Secretaries of Homeland Security and HHS have statutory authority to provide additional assistance to state and local governments, and others, in response to catastrophes. Following Hurricane Katrina, Congress defined in statute the roles of the two Secretaries with respect to the public health and medical response to catastrophes. Numerous aspects of these relationships are yet to be sorted out, through specific planning, exercises, and other approaches. In carrying out the federal response to public health and medical emergencies and disasters, the Secretary of HHS has broad authority and considerable discretion in providing assistance, but lacks a sound funding source to support the response to these unanticipated events. In contrast, the President, acting pursuant to the Stafford Act, has, in the Disaster Relief Fund (DRF), a ready source of funds to support an immediate response to emergencies and disasters. Stafford Act assistance is, however, not especially well-tailored for the response to public health and medical threats. Indeed, some of these threats (e.g., bioterrorism) may not even trigger Stafford Act major disaster assistance.

APPENDIX. FEDERAL PUBLIC HEALTH EMERGENCY AUTHORITIES[97]

Broad Authority in Section 319 of the Public Health Service Act

The Secretary of HHS[98] has broad authority to determine that a public health emergency exists. Congress reauthorized this authority in 2000, as follows:

> If the Secretary determines, after consultation with such public health officials as may be necessary, that — (1) a disease or disorder presents a public health emergency; or (2) a public

health emergency, including significant outbreaks of infectious diseases or bioterrorist attacks, otherwise exists, the Secretary may take such action as may be appropriate to respond to the public health emergency, including making grants, providing awards for expenses, and entering into contracts and conducting and supporting investigations into the cause, treatment, or prevention of a disease or disorder as described in paragraphs (1) and (2).[99]

This authority, found in Section 319 of the Public Health Service Act and codified at 42 U.S.C. § 247d, is the basis for much, but not all of, the Secretary's authority to waive or streamline administrative requirements and certain statutory requirements, and to take certain other actions, when needed, to prepare for or respond to non- routine threats to public health.

Also in 2000, Congress reauthorized a no-year public health emergency fund that is available to the HHS Secretary for use during a public health emergency, determined pursuant to the authority above, as follows:

> There is established in the Treasury a fund to be designated as the 'Public Health Emergency Fund' to be made available to the Secretary without fiscal year limitation to carry out subsection (a) only if a public health emergency has been declared by the Secretary under such subsection. There is authorized to be appropriated to the Fund such sums as may be necessary. ... Not later than 90 days after the end of each fiscal year, the Secretary shall prepare and submit to the Committee on Health, Education, Labor, and Pensions and the Committee on Appropriations of the Senate and the Committee on Commerce and the Committee on Appropriations of the House of Representatives a report describing — (A) the expenditures made from the Public Health Emergency Fund in such fiscal year; and (B) each public health emergency for which the expenditures were made and the activities undertaken with respect to each emergency which was conducted or supported by expenditures from the Fund.[100]

Subsequent to the 2000 reauthorization, Congress expanded or clarified the Section 319 emergency authority, as follows:

- **Duration of emergency, notification of Congress:** "Any such determination of a public health emergency terminates upon the Secretary declaring that the emergency no longer exists, or upon the expiration of the 90-day period beginning on the date on which the determination is made by the Secretary, whichever occurs first. Determinations that terminate under the preceding sentence may be renewed by the Secretary (on the basis of the same or additional facts), and the preceding sentence applies to each such renewal. Not later than 48 hours after making a determination under this subsection of a public health emergency (including a renewal), the Secretary shall submit to the Congress written notification of the determination."[101]

- **Data submittal and reporting deadlines:** "In any case in which the Secretary determines that, wholly or partially as a result of a public health emergency that has been determined pursuant to subsection (a), individuals or public or private entities are unable to comply with deadlines for the submission to the Secretary of data or reports required under any law administered by the Secretary, the Secretary may, notwithstanding any other provision of law, grant such extensions of such deadlines as the circumstances reasonably require, and may waive, wholly or partially, any sanctions otherwise applicable to such failure to comply. Before or promptly after granting such an extension or waiver, the Secretary shall notify the Congress of such action and publish in the Federal Register a notice of the extension or waiver."[102]

- **Requirement for notification:** During the period in which the Secretary of HHS has determined the existence of a public health emergency under 42 U.S.C. § 247d, the Secretary "shall keep relevant agencies, including the Department of Homeland Security, the Department of Justice, and the Federal Bureau of Investigation, fully and currently informed."[103]

- **Emergency use of countermeasures:** The Secretary may declare an emergency justifying expedited use of certain medical countermeasures on the basis of: (1) a determination by the Secretary of Homeland Security that there is a domestic emergency, or a significant potential for a domestic emergency; or (2) on the basis of a determination by the Secretary of Defense that there is a military emergency, or a significant potential for a military emergency; or (3) on the basis of a "determination by the Secretary of a public health emergency under Section 247d of Title 42 that affects, or has a significant potential to affect, national security, and that involves a specified biological, chemical, radiological, or nuclear agent or agents, or a specified disease or condition that may be attributable to such agent or agents."[104] This provision in the Federal Food, Drug and Cosmetic Act is referred to as the *Emergency Use Authorization.*

- **Waiver of certain requirements:** In order to assure "that sufficient health care items and services are available to meet the needs of individuals in ... (an emergency, and) ... that health care providers ... that furnish such items and services in good faith, but that are unable to comply with one or more requirements ... may be reimbursed for such items and services and exempted from sanctions for such noncompliance, absent any determination of fraud or abuse," the Secretary may modify or waive certain statutory or regulatory requirements following a determination of public health emergency pursuant to 42 U.S.C. § 247d *and* an emergency or disaster declaration by the President pursuant to the National Emergencies Act (50 U.S.C. § 1601 *et seq.*) or the Stafford Act (42 U.S.C. § 5121 *et seq.*).[105] Requirements that may be waived or modified pursuant to this section include (1) conditions of participation and certain other requirements in the Medicare, Medicaid and SCHIP programs;[106] (2) federal requirements for state licensure of health professionals; (3) certain provisions of the Emergency Medical Treatment and Active Labor Act of 1985 (EMTALA); (4) certain sanctions prohibiting physician self-referral (so-called "Stark" provisions); (5) modification, but not waiver, of deadlines and timetables for performance of required activities; (6) limitations on certain payments for health care items and services furnished to individuals enrolled in a Medicare + Choice plan; and (7) sanctions and penalties that arise from noncompliance with certain patient privacy requirements of the Health Insurance Portability and Accountability Act of 1996.

- **Alternate Medicare drug reimbursement method:** In situations where a public health emergency has been determined to exist under 42 U.S.C. § 247d, and "there is a documented inability to access drugs and biologicals," the Secretary may, under certain circumstances, use an alternative methodology for determining payments of certain drugs under the Medicare program.[107]

- **Deployment of the Public Health Service Commissioned Corps:** The Secretary may deploy officers in the Commissioned Corps of the U.S. Public Health Service to respond to an "urgent or emergency public health care need," as determined by the Secretary, arising as the result of (1) a national emergency declared by the President under the National Emergencies Act (50 U.S.C. § 1601 *et seq.*); (2) an emergency or major disaster declared by the President under the Stafford Act (42 U. S.C. § 5121 *et seq.*); (3) a public health emergency declared by the Secretary pursuant to 42 U.S.C. § 247d; or (4) any emergency that, in the judgment of the Secretary, is appropriate for the deployment of members of the Corps.[108]

Pursuant to the authority in Section 319, the Secretary of HHS has determined that a public health emergency exists on four recent occasions: (1) nationwide, in response to the terrorist attacks on September 11, 2001; (2) in several states affected by Hurricane Katrina in August and September 2005; (3) in several states affected by Hurricane Rita in September 2005; and (4) in Iowa and Indiana as a result of severe flooding in June 2008.[109]

Other Public Health Emergency Authorities of the HHS Secretary

The following is a list of statutory authorities or requirements of the Secretary or others within HHS to take certain additional actions during public health emergencies that are not explicitly defined or linked to an emergency determination pursuant to Section 319 authority. In some cases these actions flow from federal emergency or major disaster declarations pursuant to the Stafford Act. In other cases reference is made to a situation of public health emergency, but such emergency is not defined.

- **Assistance to states:** Pursuant to Section 311 of the Public Health Service Act, the Secretary of HHS has broad authority to assist state and local governments in their disease control efforts, upon their request, as follows: "The Secretary may, at the request of the appropriate State or local authority, extend temporary (not in excess of six months) assistance to States or localities in meeting health emergencies of such a nature as to warrant Federal assistance. The Secretary may require such reimbursement of the United States for assistance provided under this paragraph as he may determine to be reasonable under the circumstances. Any reimbursement so paid shall be credited to the applicable appropriation for the Service for the year in which such reimbursement is received."[110] The term "health emergencies" is not defined in this context, but this authority underpins a variety of unanticipated activities which are undertaken each year such as CDC's deployment of Epidemic Intelligence Service officers to assist states affected by an ongoing mumps outbreak.

- **National Health Security Strategy:** "Preparedness and response regarding public health emergencies: Beginning in 2009 and every four years thereafter, the Secretary shall prepare and submit to the relevant committees of Congress a coordinated strategy (to be known as the National Health Security Strategy) and any revisions thereof, and an accompanying implementation plan for public health emergency preparedness and response. Such National Health Security Strategy shall identify the process for achieving the preparedness goals described in subsection (b) and shall be consistent with the National Preparedness Goal, the National Incident Management System, and the National Response Plan developed pursuant to section 502(6) of the Homeland Security Act of 2002 [6 U.S.C. § 3 14(6)], or any successor plan."[111]

- **HHS exemption from "Select Agent" regulation:** The Secretary maintains regulatory control over certain biological agents and toxins which have the potential to pose a severe threat to public health and safety. The Secretary may temporarily exempt a person from the regulatory requirements of this section if "the Secretary determines that such exemption is necessary to provide for the timely participation of the person in a response to a domestic or foreign public health emergency (whether determined under Section 247d(a) of this Title *or otherwise*)." (Emphasis added).[112]

- **USDA exemption from "Select Agent" regulation:** The Secretary, after granting an exemption under 42 U.S.C. § 262a(g) (relating to regulation of certain biological agents and toxins) pursuant to "a finding that there is a public health emergency" may request the Secretary of Agriculture to "temporarily exempt a person from the applicability of the requirements of this section with respect to an overlap agent or toxin, in whole or in part, to provide for the timely participation of the person in a response to the public health emergency."[113]

- **Activation of NDMS:** The Secretary may activate the National Disaster Medical System (NDMS) to "provide health services, health-related social services, other appropriate human services, and appropriate auxiliary services to respond to the needs of victims of a public health emergency (*whether or not determined to be a public health emergency* under Section 247d of this Title)" (emphasis added).[114]

- **Authority for the Strategic National Stockpile:** "The Secretary, in coordination with the Secretary of Homeland Security, shall maintain a stockpile or stockpiles of drugs, vaccines and other biological products, medical devices, and other supplies in such numbers, types, and amounts as are determined by the Secretary to be appropriate and practicable, taking into account other available sources, to provide for the emergency health security of the United States, including the emergency health security of children and other vulnerable populations, in the event of a bioterrorist attack or other public health emergency."[115]

- **Authority for the Emergency System for Advance Registration of Volunteer Health Professionals (ESAR-VHP):** "Not later than 12 months after the date of enactment of the Pandemic and All-Hazards Preparedness Act, the Secretary shall link existing State verification systems to maintain a single national interoperable network of systems, each system being maintained by a State or group of States, for the purpose of verifying the credentials and licenses of health care professionals who volunteer to provide health services during a public health emergency."[116] "Public health emergency" is not defined.

- **Federal quarantine authority:** The Secretary has the authority to "make and enforce such regulations as in his judgment are necessary to prevent the introduction, transmission, or spread of communicable diseases from foreign countries into the States or possessions, or from one State or possession into any other State or possession." These regulations may "provide for the apprehension and examination of any individual reasonably believed to be infected with a communicable disease in a qualifying stage." The term "qualifying stage" means that the disease is "in a communicable stage" or is "in a precommunicable stage, if the disease would be likely to cause a public health emergency if transmitted to other individuals."[117]

- **Authority for the administration of smallpox countermeasures:** The Secretary may issue a declaration "concluding that an actual or potential bioterrorist incident or other actual or potential public health emergency makes advisable the administration of" certain countermeasures against smallpox for Public Health Service employees.[118]

- **Liability protection for certain countermeasures:** If the Secretary "makes a determination that a disease or other health condition or other threat to health constitutes a public health emergency, or that there is a credible risk that the disease, condition, or threat may in the future constitute such an emergency, the Secretary may make a declaration, through publication in the Federal Register, recommending, under conditions as the Secretary may specify, the manufacture, testing, development, distribution, administration, or use of one of more covered countermeasures...." Liability protection is provided for certain persons with respect to claims resulting from the administration of covered countermeasures following a declaration of a public health emergency under this authority.[119]

- **Disaster relief for aging services organizations:** The Assistant Secretary for Aging, in HHS, "may provide reimbursements to any State (or to any tribal organization receiving a grant under Title VI [42 U.S.C. §§ 3057 et seq.]), upon application for such reimbursement, for funds such State makes available to area agencies on aging in such State (or funds used by such tribal organization) for the delivery of supportive services (and related supplies) during any major disaster declared by the President in accordance with the Robert T. Stafford Disaster Relief and Emergency Assistance Act."[120]

- **Authority to expedite research:** If the Secretary "determines, after consultation with the Director of NIH, the Commissioner of the Food and Drug Administration, or the Director of the Centers for Disease Control and Prevention, that a disease or disorder constitutes a public health emergency, the Secretary, acting through the Director of NIH," shall expedite certain review procedures for applications for research grants on diseases relevant to the disease or disorder involved in the emergency and take other specified administrative measures to assist relevant grants or contracts. (NIH is the National Institutes of Health.)[121]

- **Fisheries management:** The Secretary of Commerce may take certain measures relating to the national fishery management program in case of an emergency. If the emergency is a public health emergency, then the Secretary of HHS is to "concur" with the "emergency regulation or interim measure promulgated" by the Secretary of Commerce.[122]

- **ATSDR assistance for exposure to toxic substances:** The Administrator of the Agency for Toxic Substances and Disease Registry (ATSDR, an agency within HHS) shall, "in cases of public health emergencies caused or believed to be caused by exposure to toxic substances, provide medical care and testing to exposed individuals."[123]

- **Mosquito-borne diseases:** The Secretary has enhanced budget authority for the response to public health emergencies related to mosquito-borne diseases as follows: "In the case of any control programs carried out in response to a mosquito-borne disease that constitutes a public health emergency, the authorization of appropriations (in this provision) is in addition to applicable authorizations of appropriations under the Public Health Security and Bioterrorism Preparedness and Response Act of 2002."[124]

Additional Public Health Emergency Authorities

The following are public health emergency authorities of individuals other than the HHS Secretary.

- **Authority of the Attending Physician to Congress:** "The Attending Physician to Congress shall have the authority and responsibility for overseeing and coordinating the use of medical assets in response to a bioterrorism event and other medical contingencies or public health emergencies occurring within the Capitol Buildings or the United States Capitol Grounds. This shall include the authority to enact quarantine and to declare death. These actions will be carried out in close cooperation and communication with the Commissioner of Public Health, Chief Medical Examiner, and other Public Health Officials of the District of Columbia government."[125]

- **Health and medical monitoring following a disaster**: The President, acting through the Secretary of HHS, is authorized to carry out a program for the coordination, protection, assessment, monitoring, and study of the health and safety of individuals (including but not limited to responders) who may have had hazardous exposures as a result of a disaster declared pursuant to the Stafford Act (42 U.S.C. § 5121 *et seq.*).

If the President carries out such a program, it must be commenced in a timely manner to ensure the highest level of public health protection and effective monitoring.[126]

- **Crisis counseling assistance and training during a disaster:** "The President is authorized to provide professional counseling services, including financial assistance to State or local agencies or private mental health organizations to provide such services or training of disaster workers, to victims of major disasters in order to relieve mental health problems caused or aggravated by such major disaster or its aftermath."[127] This provision in the Stafford Act is administered by the Substance Abuse and Mental Health Services Administration in HHS.[128]

- **Authority of the Secretary of DHS to deploy the Strategic National Stockpile:** "The [DHS] Secretary [Secretary's responsibilities] ... shall include ... coordinating other Federal response resources, including requiring deployment of the Strategic National Stockpile, in the event of a terrorist attack or major disaster"....[129]

- **Authority of the Secretary of Veterans Affairs to provide care:** The Secretary of Veterans Affairs is authorized to furnish hospital care and medical services to individuals, including non-veterans, affected by (1) a major disaster or emergency declared by the President under Stafford Act (42 U.S.C. § 5121 *et seq.*) or (2) a disaster or emergency in which NDMS is activated.[130]

- **Notification during potential public health emergencies:** "In cases involving, or potentially involving, a public health emergency, but in which no determination of an emergency by the Secretary of Health and Human Services under Section 319(a) of the Public Health Service Act (42 U.S.C. 247d(a)), has been made, all relevant agencies, including the Department of Homeland Security, the Department of Justice, and the Federal Bureau of Investigation, shall keep the Secretary of Health and Human Services and the Director of the Centers for Disease Control and Prevention fully and currently informed."[131]

Methodology

The above listing of federal public health emergency authorities was developed by reviewing the results of a search of the U.S. Code for the terms "public health emergency," "health threat," or "disaster," or for citations to the public health emergency authority at 42 U.S.C. § 247d. Not included in the listing are references to the suspension of certain routine activities in the event of a disaster, requirements for disaster planning in health care facilities, or other provisions not directly related to the declaration or determination of a federal public health emergency or the activities authorized or required when such a declaration or determination is made.

End Notes

[1] The terms *emergency* and *major disaster* have specific meanings in the Stafford Act. To avoid confusion, in this chapter the terms *event, incident*, and *catastrophe* will be used in general reference to events, whether or not Stafford Act assistance applies. The term *public health emergency* is also commonly used in both a generic manner and to describe one or more specific authorities in law. This is discussed further in the Appendix.

[2] Information on the Stafford Act is provided, in part, by Keith Bea of the Government and Finance Division of the Congressional Research Service (CRS). For background on the Stafford Act, see CRS Report RL33053, *Federal Stafford Act Disaster Assistance: Presidential Declarations, Eligible Activities, and Funding*, by Keith Bea, and CRS Report RL34 146, *FEMA 's Disaster Declaration Process: A Primer*, by Francis X. McCarthy.

[3] 42 U.S.C. §§ 5170(a)-5189. For more information, see CRS Report RL33053, *Federal Stafford Act Disaster Assistance: Presidential Declarations, Eligible Activities, and Funding*, by Keith Bea, under the section titled "Types of Assistance and Eligibility."

[4] 42 U.S.C. § 5122(2).

[5] 42 U.S.C. § 5170.

[6] Ibid.

[7] 42 U.S.C. §§ 5192-5193. For more information, see CRS Report RL33053, *Federal Stafford Act Disaster Assistance: Presidential Declarations, Eligible Activities, and Funding*, by Keith Bea, under the section titled "Emergency Declaration Assistance."

[8] 42 U.S.C. § 5122(1).

[9] 42 U.S.C. § 5191. Examples of emergencies involving Federal primary responsibility include the 1995 bombing of the Alfred P. Murrah Federal Building in Oklahoma City, and the 2001 attack on the Pentagon, both federally owned facilities.

[10] For background, see Federal Emergency Management Agency (FEMA) notices at [http://www.fema.gov/news/disasters.fema?year=2000#em].

[11] 42 U.S.C. § 247d(a).

[12] For more information regarding the National Emergencies Act, see CRS Report 98-5 05, *National Emergency Powers*, by Harold C. Relyea.

[13] 42 U.S.C. § 243c.

[14] The 2001 determination applied to the September 11 attacks, and not to the subsequent anthrax attack (66 *Federal Register* 54998, October 31, 2001). More information about the 2005 hurricane determinations is available in CRS Report RL33096, *2005 Gulf Coast Hurricanes: The Public Health and Medical Response*, by Sarah A. Lister. More information about the 2008 flood determinations is available on the website of the HHS Centers for Medicare and Medicaid Services (CMS), at [http://www.cms.hhs.gov/emergency/20_midwestflooding.asp]. Stafford major disaster and emergency declarations may be found on FEMA's website at [http://www.fema.gov/hazard/index.shtm].

[15] See the subsequent section "Federal Funding to Support an ESF-8 Response."

[16] FEMA's administration of the Disaster Relief Fund (DRF), which supports the response to Stafford Act emergency and major disaster declarations, may offer an instructive comparison. The DRF is discussed further in a subsequent section of this chapter. See also CRS Report RL34146, *FEMA 's Disaster Declaration Process: A Primer*, by Francis X. McCarthy.

[17] Applicable waiver authorities are described in "Waiver of certain requirements" in the Appendix. For more information about waivers applied in response to the Midwest floods of 2008, see HHS, "HHS Takes Action to Help Medicare Beneficiaries and Providers in Iowa and Indiana," press release, June 16, 2008.

[18] For more information, see the subsequent section "Health Care Financing Proposals for Future Emergencies."

[19] For example, as Hurricane Katrina approached, Louisiana received an emergency declaration on August 27, 2006, prior to landfall. This was superceded by a major disaster declaration on August 29, 2006, the day of landfall. The Secretary of HHS also determined that a public health emergency existed in Louisiana, effective August 29, 2006. To further complicate matters, at least two types of assistance to Louisiana citizens — Medicaid and Crisis Counseling Program grants — were based on their evacuation status *from* Stafford major disaster areas, and were available to them in host areas (including other states), some of which were not themselves subject to major disaster declarations.

[20] 6 U.S.C. § 312(6). Department of Homeland Security (DHS), National Response Plan, December 2004. The NRP was mandated in the Homeland Security Act, P.L. 107-296, and superceded the earlier Federal Response Plan.

[21] DHS, *National Response Framework*, (NRF) January 2008, hereinafter referred to as NRF, at [http://www.fema.gov/emergency/nrf/].

[22] See the subsequent section"The Disaster Relief Fund" for an explanation of how activities authorized by the Stafford Act may be funded.

[23] Implementation of the NRF represents a departure from the earlier NRP, which required certain triggers. In contrast, the NRF "is always in effect, and elements can be implemented at any level at any time." (NRF, p. 7)

As a result, while the NRF serves as the blueprint for coordinated national response actions following Stafford Act declarations, such declarations are not required in order for the NRF to be in effect. Consequently, the NRF serves also to guide and coordinate homeland security activities during special events such as the Super Bowl and political conventions.

[24] See [http://www.pandemicflu.gov/].

[25] For more information, see CRS Report RL34 190, *Pandemic Influenza: An Analysis of State Preparedness and Response Plans,* by Sarah A. Lister and Holly Stockdale.

[26] NRF, p. 73.

[27] See the subsequent section on "The Disaster Relief Fund" for an explanation of how activities authorized by the Stafford Act may be funded.

[28] See DHS, Office of the Inspector General, *A Review of the Top Officials 3 Exercise,* Office of Inspections and Special Reviews, OIG-06-07, November 2005, p. 30, at [http://www.dhs.gov/xoig/rpts/mgmt/editorial_0334.shtm]. Also, the anthrax attack in 2001 did not result in a Stafford Act declaration.

[29] Pandemic Implementation Plan, Appendix C, "Authorities and References," p. 212.

[30] FEMA, "Emergency Assistance for Human Influenza Pandemic," Disaster Assistance Policy 9523.17, March 31, 2007, at [http://www.fema.gov/pdf/government/grant/pa/ policy.pdf].

[31] Even so, the types of activities for which assistance is authorized pursuant to a Stafford major disaster declaration are not necessarily well aligned to the types of activities that would be needed during a pandemic response, or during an incident with a substantial public health and medical response component in general. This is discussed further in a subsequent section on "Federal Funding to Support an ESF-8 Response."

[32] 42 U.S.C. § 5143.

[33] In FY2008 appropriations for DHS, Congress prohibited the use of appropriated funds for "any position designated as a Principal Federal Official" for any disasters or emergencies declared pursuant to the Stafford Act. P.L. 110-161, the Consolidated Appropriations Act, 2008, § 541, 121 Stat. 2079, December 26, 2007. See also, DHS Office of Inspector General, "FEMA's Preparedness for the Next Catastrophic Disaster," OIG-08-34, March 2008, at [http://www.dhs.gov/xoig/].

[34] See Government Accountability Office (GAO), "Influenza Pandemic: Further Efforts Are Needed to Ensure Clearer Federal Leadership Roles and an Effective National Strategy," GAO-07-781, p. 18, August 14, 2007.

[35] Ibid. GAO reported that DHS was developing a "Federal Concept Plan for Pandemic Influenza," which would clarify these roles, but such plan has not been published.

[36] NRF, Annex ESF #8, at [http://www.fema.gov/emergency/nrf/]. See also HHS, "HHS Maintains Lead Federal Role for Emergency Public Health and Medical Response," press release, January 6, 2005. Many ESF-8 responsibilities and activities are delegated to the HHS Assistant Secretary for Preparedness and Response (ASPR, formerly called the Assistant Secretary for Public Health Emergency Preparedness). See HHS, Office of the Secretary, Office of Public Health Emergency Preparedness, "Statement of Organization, Functions, and Delegations of Authority," 71 *Federal Register* 38403, July 6, 2006.

[37] These are products regulated by HHS's Food and Drug Administration (FDA).

[38] See U.S. Senate, Committee on Homeland Security and Governmental Affairs, *Hurricane Katrina: A Nation Still Unprepared,* chap. 24, p. 28ff, May 2006, at [http://hsgac.senate.gov/], hereafter called *A Nation Still Unprepared*; and the White House, *The Federal Response to Hurricane Katrina: Lessons Learned,* p. 47, February 2006, at [http://www.whitehouse.gov/reports/katrina-lessons-learned/].

[39] See CRS Report RL33729, *Federal Emergency Management Policy Changes After Hurricane Katrina: A Summary of Statutory Provisions,* by Keith Bea, Barbara L. Schwemle, L. Elaine Halchin, Francis X. McCarthy, Frederick M. Kaiser, Henry B. Hogue, Natalie Paris Love and Shawn Reese.

[40] P.L. 109-295, 120 Stat. 1409.

[41] P.L. 109-417, § 101.

[42] GAO, "Influenza Pandemic: Further Efforts Are Needed to Ensure Clearer Federal Leadership Roles and an Effective National Strategy," GAO-07-78 1, August 14, 2007.

[43] GAO, "Disaster Preparedness: Better Planning Would Improve OSHA' s Efforts to Protect Workers' Safety and Health in Disasters," GAO-07-193, March 28, 2007.

[44] Katherine Torres, "DHS Denies OSHA Power to Invoke Emergency Response Plan, Official Says," *Occupational Hazards,* vol. 70, March 1, 2008; and Anon., "Despite Lawmakers' Concerns, OSHA's Role in NRF Remains Unchanged," *Inside OSHA,* vol. 15, February 4, 2008.

[45] NRF, ESF-8 Annex and Worker Safety and Health Support Annex, at [http://www.fema.gov/emergency/nrf/].

[46] DMORTs are a component of the National Disaster Medical System (NDMS), which comprises teams of medical professionals who are pretrained, and are "federalized" to deploy and provide medical services in the immediate aftermath of a disaster before other federal assets arrive. NDMS is administered by the HHS ASPR. For more information, see [http://www.hhs.gov/aspr/opeo/ndms/index.html].

[47] Further discussion of the difficulties in coordinating body retrieval following Hurricane Katrina is available in *A Failure of Initiative,* p. 299.

[48] For more information, see CRS Report RL33738, *Gulf Coast Hurricanes: Addressing Survivors' Mental Health and Substance Abuse Treatment Needs,* by Ramya Sundararaman, Sarah A. Lister, and Erin D. Williams.

[49] The Department of Justice shares leadership responsibilities with DHS for ESF-13, *Public Safety and Security.* ESF-13 does not explicitly mention mental health.

[50] P.L. 109-295, §§ 536, 653 and 689.

[51] See Government Accountability Office (GAO), "Status of the Health Care System in New Orleans," GAO-06-576R, March 28, 2006; the Louisiana Health Care Redesign Collaborative, at [http://www.hhs.gov/louisianahealth/]; and Bruce Alpert, "GAO Says Hospitals not Worth Salvaging," Times-Picayune, March 30, 2006.

[52] For more information, see CRS Report RL33053, *Federal Stafford Act Disaster Assistance: Presidential Declarations, Eligible Activities, and Funding,* by Keith Bea.

[53] P.L. 98-49.

[54] 42 U.S.C. § 247d(a).

[55] 42 U.S.C. § 247d(b), as amended by P.L. 106-505.

[56] P.L. 100-607, § 256(a).

[57] The 2001 determination applied to the September 11 attacks, and not to the subsequent anthrax attack (66 *Federal Register* 54998, October 31, 2001). More information about the 2005 hurricane determinations is available in CRS Report RL33096, *2005 Gulf Coast Hurricanes: The Public Health and Medical Response,* by Sarah A. Lister. More information about the 2008 flood determinations is available on the website of the HHS Centers for Medicare and Medicaid Services (CMS), at [http://www.cms.hhs.gov/ emergency/20_midwestflooding. asp]. Stafford major disaster and emergency declarations may be found on FEMA's website at [http://www.fema.gov/hazard/index.shtm].

[58] 42 U.S.C. § 300hh-1 1, as amended by P.L. 107-188. Pursuant to P.L. 109-417, the HHS Assistant Secretary for Public Health Emergency Preparedness is now designated as the HHS Assistant Secretary for Preparedness and Response (ASPR).

[59] For more information, see the subsequent section "Health Care Financing Proposals for Future Emergencies."

[60] More information on CDC's budget is available at [http://www.cdc.gov/fmo/ fmofybudget.htm].

[61] See HHS, the Hospital Preparedness Program, at [http://www.hhs.gov/aspr/opeo/hpp/ index.html].

[62] For more information, see CRS Report RS22239, *Emergency Supplemental Appropriations for Hurricane Katrina Relief,* by Keith Bea; and CRS Report RL33298, *FY2006 Supplemental Appropriations: Iraq and Other International Activities; Additional Hurricane Katrina Relief,* coordinated by Paul M. Irwin and Larry Nowels.

[63] DHS, FEMA, "Disaster Relief Fund (DRF) Report," Congressional Monthly Report, as of June 1, 2008.

[64] For information regarding the activities of HHS agencies in response to the 2005 hurricanes, see CRS Report RL33 096, *2005 Gulf Coast Hurricanes: The Public Health and Medical Response,* by Sarah A. Lister; and HHS, Centers for Medicare and Medicaid Services (CMS), "Summary of Federal Payments Available for Providing Health Care Services to Hurricane Evacuees and Rebuilding Health Care Infrastructure," January 25, 2006, at [http://www.hhs.gov/katrina/#hhs].

[65] CDC, letter from William P. Nichols, Director, CDC Procurement and Grants Office, to CDC directors and grants management personnel, regarding "Treatment of Grants under Emergency Conditions due to Hurricane Katrina," September 16, 2005, hereafter referred to as the Nichols letter.

[66] The Emergency Management Assistance Compact is a congressionally approved interstate mutual aid agreement that provides a legal structure by which states affected by a catastrophe may request emergency assistance from other states. For more information, see CRS Report RS2 1227, *The Emergency Management Assistance Compact (EMAC): An Overview,* by Keith Bea.

[67] Nichols letter.

[68] See notice posted by the Association of State and Territorial Health Officials at [http://www.astho.org/templates/display_pub .php?pub _id=1 681 &admin=1].

[69] P.L. 109-234, the Emergency Supplemental Appropriations Act for Defense, the Global War on Terror, and Hurricane Recovery, 120 Stat. 463. See also CRS Report RS22239, *Emergency Supplemental Appropriations for Hurricane Katrina Relief,* by Keith Bea.

[70] 42 U.S.C. § 5170b (major disaster) and 42 U.S.C. § 5192 (emergency).

[71] 72 *Federal Register* 57341, October 9, 2007. For more information on the FEMA Individuals and Households Program, see DHS, Office of Inspector General, "A Performance Review of FEMA's Disaster Management Activities in Response to Hurricane Katrina," OIG-06-32, Appendix B, pp. 149 ff., March 2006, at [http://www.dhs.gov/ xoig/rpts/mgmt/OIG_mgmtrpts_FY06.shtm].

[72] 42 U.S.C. § 5183. For more information, see CRS Report RL33738, *Gulf Coast Hurricanes: Addressing Survivors' Mental Health and Substance Abuse Treatment Needs,* by Ramya Sundararaman, Sarah A. Lister, and Erin D. Williams.

[73] For more information on Public Health Service agencies and their functions, see CRS Report RL34098, *Public Health Service (PHS) Agencies: Background and Funding,* Pamela W. Smith, Coordinator.

[74] For more information, see CRS Report RL33738, *Gulf Coast Hurricanes: Addressing Survivors' Mental Health and Substance Abuse Treatment Needs*, by Ramya Sundararaman, Sarah A. Lister, and Erin D. Williams.

[75] Health centers provide health care services regardless of ability to pay. For more information, see HRSA, Bureau of Primary Health Care, Health Center Program, at [http://bphc.hrsa.gov/].

[76] State and private workers' compensation programs generally provide similar benefits.

[77] For more information on these programs, see CRS Report RL33927, *Selected Federal Compensation Programs for Physical Injury or Death*, by Sarah A. Lister and C. Stephen Redhead, hereinafter referred to as CRS Report RL33927.

[78] See CRS Report RL32579, *Victims of Crime Compensation and Assistance: Background and Funding*, by Celinda Franco.

[79] P.L. 107-42, signed into law on September 22, 2001.

[80] For more information, see CRS Report RL33927, the section "September 11th Victim Compensation Fund."

[81] See CDC/National Institute for Occupational Safety and Health (NIOSH), "World Trade Center Response," at [http://www.cdc.gov/niosh/topics/wtc/].

[82] For more information, see New York City Department of Health and Mental Hygiene, World Trade Center Health Registry site, at [http://www.nyc.gov/html/doh/html/ wtc/index.html].

[83] See CRS Report RL33927, section on "World Trade Center Medical Monitoring and Treatment Program."

[84] See, for example, the House Committee on Energy and Commerce, Subcommittee on Health, hearing on, "Answering the Call: Medical Monitoring and Treatment of 9/11 Health Effects," September 18, 2007, 110th Cong., 1st Sess., Washington, DC.

[85] See, for example, H.R. 1247, H.R. 1414/S. 201, and H.R. 6594.

[86] HHS, Centers for Medicare and Medicaid Services (CMS), "Summary of Federal Payments Available for Providing Health Care Services to Hurricane Evacuees and Rebuilding Health Care Infrastructure," January 25, 2006, at [http://www.hhs.gov/katrina/#hhs].

[87] 42 U.S.C. § 1320b-5, enacted in P.L. 107-188.

[88] P.L. 109-171, the Deficit Reduction Act of 2005, § 6201, enacted February 8, 2006. This arrangement was designated for those states covered under a Medicaid and SCHIP waiver developed specifically for Hurricane Katrina relief. See CRS Report RL33083: *Hurricane Katrina: Medicaid Issues*, by Evelyne P. Baumrucker, April Grady, Jean Hearne, Elicia J. Herz, Richard Rimkunas, Julie Stone, and Karen Tritz. FEMA had previously determined, regarding a Medicaid waiver proposed by New York state in response to the terror attack of September 11, 2001, that the DRF may not be used to reimburse a state for a federal matching requirement. FEMA cited its grant regulations at 44 CFR § 13.24(b)(1), which say that "Except as provided by Federal statute, a cost sharing or matching requirement may not be met by costs borne by another Federal grant." (Letter from Joseph F. Picciano, Acting Regional Director, FEMA Region II, to Edward F. Jacoby, Jr., Director, New York State Emergency Management Office, January 13, 2003.)

[89] See GAO, "Hurricane Katrina: Allocation and Use of $2 Billion for Medicaid and Other Health Care Needs," GAO-07-67, February 28, 2007.

[90] P.L. 109-62, 119 Stat. 1991, September 8, 2005.

[91] HHS, Centers for Medicare and Medicaid Services, *Justification of Estimates for Appropriations Committees*, FY2007, p. 192.

[92] HHS, "HHS Participation in the Recovery of the Gulf Coast," at [http://www.hhs.gov/ louisianahealth/background/].

[93] Louisiana Health Care Redesign Collaborative, at [http://www.dhh.state.la.us/offices/?ID=288].

[94] Ibid. See also the House Committee on Energy and Commerce, Subcommittee on Oversight and Investigations, hearing on "Post Katrina Health Care: Progress and Continuing Concerns — Part II," August 1, 2007, 110th Cong., 1st Sess., Washington, DC.

[95] See the earlier section of this chapter, "Would the Stafford Act Apply in a Flu Pandemic?"

[96] FEMA, "Emergency Assistance for Human Influenza Pandemic," Disaster Assistance Policy 9523.17, March 31, 2007, at [http://www.fema.gov/pdf/government/grant/pa/policy.pdf].

[97] Kathleen S. Swendiman, legislative attorney in the American Law Division of CRS, contributed to this section. Federal law contains numerous authorities relating to instances of public health emergency. In some cases the term "public health emergency" is defined in statute, such as for the HHS Secretary's key emergency authority in Section 319 of the Public Health Service Act, though definitions vary. In other cases the term is not defined, or does not refer explicitly to related authorities.

[98] In this appendix, unless otherwise stated, "the Secretary" refers to the Secretary of HHS.

[99] 42 U.S.C. § 247d, as amended by P.L. 106-505, the Public Health Improvement Act.

[100] 42 U.S.C. § 247d, as amended by P.L. 106-505. This fund has not received a recent appropriation.

[101] 42 U.S.C. § 247d, as amended by P.L. 107-188, the Public Health Security and Bioterrorism Preparedness and Response Act of 2002.

[102] Ibid.

[103] 6 U.S.C. § 467, authorized in P.L. 107-296, the Homeland Security Act of 2002.

[104] 21 U.S.C. § 360bbb-3, authorized in P.L. 108-276, the Project BioShield Act of 2004.

[105] 42 U.S.C. § 1320b-5, as amended by P.L. 107-188, P.L. 108-276, and P.L. 109-417.

[106] For more information on the use of these waivers following Hurricane Katrina, see CRS Report RL33083, *Hurricane Katrina: Medicaid Issues*, by Evelyne P. Baumrucker, April Grady, Jean Hearne, Elicia J. Herz, Richard Rimkunas, Julie Stone, and Karen Tritz.

[107] 42 U.S.C. § 1395w-3a(e), authorized in P.L. 108-173, the Medicare Prescription Drug, Improvement, and Modernization Act of 2003.

[108] 42 U.S.C. § 204a, as amended by P.L. 109-417, the Pandemic and All-Hazards Preparedness Act.

[109] The 2001 determination applied to the September 11 attacks, and not to the subsequent anthrax attack (66 *Federal Register* 54998, October 31, 2001). More information about the 2005 hurricane determinations is available in CRS Report RL33096, *2005 Gulf Coast Hurricanes: The Public Health and Medical Response*, by Sarah A. Lister. More information about the 2008 flood determinations is available on the website of the HHS Centers for Medicare and Medicaid Services (CMS), at [http://www.cms.hhs.gov/emergency/20_midwestflooding. asp]. Stafford major disaster and emergency declarations may be found on FEMA's website at [http://www.fema.gov/hazard/index.shtm].

[110] 42 U.S.C. § 243c.

[111] 42 U.S.C. § 300hh-1, as established in P.L. 109-417.

[112] 42 U.S.C. § 262a, as amended by P.L. 107-188. Additional information regarding the regulation of so-called "Select Agents" may be found at [http://www.cdc.gov/od/sap/ index.htm] and CRS Report RL3 1719: *An Overview of the U.S. Public Health System in the Context of Emergency Preparedness*, by Sarah A. Lister.

[113] 7 U.S.C. § 8401, as amended by P.L. 107-188.

[114] 42 U.S.C. § 300hh-11, as amended by P.L. 107-188.

[115] 42 U.S.C. § 247d-6b, as amended by P.L. 108-276, the Project BioShield Act of 2004.

[116] 42 U.S.C. § 247d-7b, as amended by P.L. 109-417.

[117] 42 U.S.C. § 264. There are other sections dealing with quarantines such as 42 U.S.C. § 243, assistance to States in the enforcement of quarantine regulations and public health plans; § 249, medical care for quarantined persons; and § 267, dealing with quarantine stations. For more information, see CRS Report RL3320 1, *Federal and State Quarantine and Isolation Authority*, by Kathleen S. Swendiman and Jennifer K. Elsea.

[118] 42 U.S.C. § 233(p). See also sections immediately following this section, including 42 U.S.C. §§ 239 et seq.

[119] 42 U.S.C. § 247d-6d. Additional information regarding this authority is available in CRS Report RS22327, *Pandemic Flu and Medical Biodefense Countermeasure Liability Limitation*, by Henry Cohen and Vanessa K. Burrows.

[120] 42 U.S.C. § 3030.

[121] 42 U.S.C. § 289c.

[122] 16 U.S.C. § 1855(c).

[123] 42 U.S.C. § 9604.

[124] 42 U.S.C. § 247b-21.

[125] 2 U.S.C. § 121g, first authorized in P.L. 108-199, the Consolidated Appropriations Act, 2004.

[126] 42 U.S.C. § 300hh-14, as amended by P.L. 109-347, the SAFE Port Act.

[127] 42 U.S.C. § 5183, Section 416 of the Stafford Act.

[128] For more information, see CRS Report RL33738, *Gulf Coast Hurricanes: Addressing Survivors' Mental Health and Substance Abuse Treatment Needs,* by Ramya Sundararaman, Sarah A. Lister, and Erin D. Williams.

[129] Under current law, both the Secretary of Homeland Security and the Secretary of HHS have authority to deploy the SNS, as well as certain joint authorities regarding procurement. The deployment authority of the Secretary of DHS is codified at 6 U.S.C. § 314. The authority of the Secretary of HHS to deploy the SNS is codified at 42 U.S.C. § 247d-6b, as are certain procurement authorities provided jointly to the two secretaries.

[130] 38 U.S.C. § 1785, as established in P.L. 107-287, the Department of Veterans Affairs Emergency Preparedness Act of 2002. Activation of NDMS may be done at the discretion of the Secretary of HHS, and does not require any type of federal emergency or disaster declaration. The VA has proposed regulations to implement this authority at 72 *Federal Register* 38042-38045, July 12, 2007.

[131] 6 U.S.C. § 467, authorized in P.L. 107-296, the Homeland Security Act of 2002.

In: Influenza Pandemic - Preparedness and Response to …   ISBN: 978-1-60692-953-7
Editor: Emma S. Brouwer pp.35-66   © 2010 Nova Science Publishers, Inc.

Chapter 2

PANDEMIC INFLUENZA: DOMESTIC PREPAREDNESS EFFORTS

Sarah A. Lister

SUMMARY

In 1997, a new avian influenza ("flu") virus emerged in Asia and jumped directly from birds to humans, killing six people. The virus has since spread to more than 50 countries in Asia, Europe and Africa, where it has killed millions of birds and infected more than 270 people, killing more than 160 of them. The virus bears some similarity to the deadly 1918 Spanish flu, which caused a global pandemic estimated to have killed more than 50 million people worldwide. The current spread of avian flu raises concerns about another human flu pandemic.

Global pandemic preparedness and response efforts are coordinated by the World Health Organization (WHO). Domestic preparedness efforts are led by the White House Homeland Security Council, with the U.S. Department of Health and Human Services (HHS) playing a major role. Domestic response efforts would be carried out under the all-hazards blueprint for a coordinated federal, state and local response laid out in the National Response Plan, overseen by the Department of Homeland Security (DHS). HHS officials would have the lead in the public health and medical aspects of a response. The federal government has released several pandemic flu plans to govern federal, state, local and private preparedness activities.

There are concerns about how a domestic public health and medical response would be managed during a flu pandemic. There is precedent, under the Stafford Act, for the President to declare an infectious disease threat an emergency (which provides a lower level of assistance), but no similar precedent for a major disaster declaration (which provides a higher level of assistance). In any case, many of the needs likely to result from a flu pandemic could not be met with the types of assistance provided pursuant to the Stafford Act, even if a major disaster declaration applied.

Vaccination is the best flu prevention measure. But because of continuous changes in the genes of flu viruses, vaccines must be "matched" to specific strains to provide good protection. A pandemic flu strain would, by definition, be novel. Stockpiled vaccine would not match, so stockpiling in anticipation of a pandemic is of limited value. In addition, global and domestic capacity to produce flu vaccine is limited. The U.S. government, primarily through HHS, has launched an aggressive effort to expand domestic vaccine production capacity, and to develop technologies to support more rapid production of a matched vaccine at the onset of a pandemic.

Since matched vaccine would not be available at the outset of a flu pandemic that occurred within the next several years, planning efforts focus on measures to slow the spread of disease, and mitigate its effects. These include stockpiling of antiviral drugs to prevent or treat flu infection, planning for medical surge capacity, and continuity planning for businesses and utilities.

This chapter discusses pandemic flu in general, WHO and U.S. preparedness and response plans, and a number of relevant policy issues. The focus of this chapter is U.S. domestic public health preparedness and response planning, and the projected impacts of an influenza pandemic on Americans.

> *Between pathogens and humans it is a race of their genes against our wits.*
> — Joshua Lederberg, winner of the 1958 Nobel Prize in Medicine for his work on genetic
> recombination in bacteria

INTRODUCTION

The U.S. Department of Health and Human Services (HHS) defines the following influenza (flu) terms:

- *Seasonal (or common) flu* is a respiratory illness that can be transmitted person to person. Most people have some immunity, and a vaccine is available.

- *Avian (or bird) flu* is caused by flu viruses that occur naturally in wild birds. The H5N1 strain of current concern is highly pathogenic in birds, deadly to domestic fowl, and can be transmitted from birds to humans. There is no human immunity, and no human vaccine is available.

- *Pandemic flu* is virulent human flu that causes a global outbreak, or pandemic, of serious illness. Because there is little natural immunity, the disease can spread easily from person to person. Currently, there is no pandemic flu.[1]

In this chapter, unless otherwise noted, the term *pandemic* will be used to refer to pandemic influenza.

In 1997 a new strain of *avian flu* jumped from poultry directly to humans in Hong Kong, causing several human deaths. This was the first documented occurrence of direct transmission of an avian flu virus from birds to people. Despite efforts to contain the virus through culling of poultry flocks, the virus (designated as H5N1 for specific proteins on its surface) re-emerged in 2003. It has since been reported in domestic poultry and/or wild birds in more than 50 countries in Asia, Europe and Africa.[2] Also since 2003, it has infected more than 270 people (and killed more than 160 deaths) in ten countries.[3] As of yet the virus has not developed the ability to transmit efficiently from person to person. Were that to occur, a global influenza pandemic could ensue.

The high lethality of the H5N1 strain and its tendency to affect healthy young people remind health authorities of the deadly 1918 Spanish flu, which is estimated to have killed up to 2% of the world's population, and was a substantial cause of mortality in U.S. military personnel in World War I. The World Health Organization (WHO) says, "If an influenza pandemic virus were to appear again similar to the one that struck in 1918, even taking into account the advances in medicine since then, unparalleled tolls of illness and death could be expected."[4]

U.S. and world health authorities believe that while periodic influenza pandemics are inevitable, their progress may be slowed, and their impacts blunted, by rapid detection and local control efforts. The added time would allow affected countries to better manage the situation, and countries not yet affected to better prepare. To realize these benefits, countries affected by avian flu must be able to track the spread of the virus in birds, and quickly detect and investigate suspected human cases. Hence, a country's capabilities in epidemiology, laboratory detection and other public health services affect the welfare of the global community as well as the country itself. This presents developed nations with novel policy challenges. For example, should they reserve scarce health resources such as antiviral drugs for themselves, or deploy them to other countries at the center of an emerging pandemic?

WHO released an updated pandemic preparedness plan in early 2005. The United States released a draft pandemic plan in August 2004, and has since released a number of documents addressing government-wide planning, public health and medical preparedness, planning for critical infrastructure readiness, and others. (See the subsequent section, "Pandemic Influenza Planning," for plans and descriptions.) States were required to prepare pandemic plans as a condition of their federal bioterrorism preparedness grants. The Administration has created a government-wide public website to disseminate information on pandemic flu preparedness and response activities.[5]

A recurring theme in planning documents and consultations is the need to engage sectors beyond healthcare and public health in planning. The Secretary of HHS, Michael Leavitt, has said, "If a pandemic hits our shores, it will affect almost every sector of our society, not just health care, but transportation systems, workplaces, schools, public safety and more. It will require a coordinated government-wide response, including federal, state and local governments, and it will require the private sector and all of us as individuals to be ready."[6] A 1918-style pandemic could be so severe that non-health-related essential services would be impaired by high absenteeism or supply chain disruptions, and health services could be in such short supply that law enforcement protection might be required for them. Though WHO does not recommend it, except in some narrow circumstances for pre-pandemic control, countries might seal their borders or take similar measures, with impacts on trade and commerce.[7]

If a flu pandemic were to occur in the next several years, the U.S. response would be affected by the limited availability of a vaccine (the best preventive measure for flu), as well as by limited availability of certain drugs used to treat severe flu infections, and by the general lack of surge capacity within our healthcare system. The U.S. healthcare system is largely private, while the public health system is largely based in state, rather than federal, authority. This structure creates numerous challenges in assuring the needed response capacity, and coordinating the various response elements. Planning is further complicated by the fact that while periodic influenza pandemics have been seen over the years, their timing and severity have been unpredictable.

Domestic planning efforts presume that the National Response Plan (NRP), an *all-hazards* plan developed by the Department of Homeland Security (DHS), would be activated if needed to streamline the federal response to a pandemic. Pandemic flu is unlike most other threats, though. Since flu is communicable, there is no scene to secure, and all states might be affected nearly simultaneously. Thus, while a pandemic could cause catastrophic levels of illness and death, the nation's traditional disaster response mechanisms — using geographical declarations of emergency and disaster, and state-to-state mutual aid — may be ill-suited for this threat.[8]

This chapter discusses pandemic influenza in general, previous pandemics and their global and domestic impacts, and the possible impacts of another pandemic caused by the H5N1 avian flu strain. It also discusses WHO and U.S. preparedness plans and their context in broader emergency preparedness efforts. Finally, the report looks at a number of policy issues in pandemic influenza preparedness and response. While reference is made when relevant to global preparedness efforts and to animal health impacts, this chapter focuses on U.S. domestic public health preparedness and response planning, and the projected impacts of an influenza pandemic on Americans.

For more information on avian, pandemic and seasonal flu preparedness, see the following CRS Reports:

- RL33219, *U.S. and International Responses to the Global Spread of Avian Flu: Issues for Congress*, by Tiaji Salaam-Blyther;
- RL3 3795, *Avian Influenza in Poultry and Wild Birds*, by Jim Monke and M. Lynne Corn;
- RL33871, *Foreign Countries' Response to the Avian Influenza (H5N1) Virus: Current Status*, Emma Chanlett-Avery, coordinator;
- RS22576, *Pandemic Influenza: Appropriations for Public Health Preparedness and Response*, by Sarah A. Lister.
- RL32655, *Influenza Vaccine Shortages and Implications*, by Sarah A. Lister and Erin D. Williams.

UNDERSTANDING PANDEMIC INFLUENZA

What Is Pandemic Influenza?

A *pandemic* (from the Greek, for "all of the people") is an epidemic of human disease occurring over a very wide area, crossing international boundaries and affecting a large number of people. Though it does so with some regularity, influenza is not the only pathogen that can cause pandemics. A pandemic of the "Black Death," which affected most of Europe in the 14th century, is generally attributed to plague (technically *Yersinia pestis)*. The global spread of HIV/AIDS is often referred to as a pandemic. Literature offers numerous examples of such episodes of widespread contagion.

Influenza is a virus that causes respiratory disease in humans, with typical symptoms of fever, cough, and muscle aches, and, rarely, pneumonia and death. Though primarily a human pathogen, influenza viruses also circulate and cause illness in swine, horses, mink, seals, and domestic poultry, and may be carried without apparent illness in these species as well as a number of species of waterfowl. Influenza is highly contagious in humans, spreading through direct contact and airborne exposure. The virus can also persist for several hours on inanimate objects such as toys or doorknobs. In addition, influenza is infectious before symptoms appear in its victims, which also enhances its spread.[9]

Influenza viruses have a genome composed of eight segments of RNA. In addition to random mutation, flu viruses also undergo change by shuffling or *reassorting* these gene segments among different strains. Human flu viruses are of two types: Influenza A and B. Influenza A strains are further identified by two important surface antigens (proteins) that are responsible for virulence: hemagglutinin (H) and neuraminidase (N). Fifteen different H antigens and nine different N antigens have been identified in birds and mammals. Not all possible combinations of H and N antigens have been documented, and very few combinations have been shown to cause human illness. The avian flu strain causing great concern at this time is designated as H5N1 for its surface antigens.

New influenza strains typically circle the globe within three to six months of emergence. New strains circulate each year, changing slightly from prior strains (called *antigenic drift*). Each year the virus, its genome in constant flux, typically makes healthy people sick, but is generally not deadly. Healthy adults typically have partial immunity to new strains, but a newly formulated vaccine is required each year to provide full immunity. Now and then, often several times in a century, the virus changes enough through mutation or reassortment (called *antigenic shift*) that there is no partial immunity in the population. This event, an influenza pandemic, results in severe illness and death, even in healthy people. The extent and severity of illness, and the disabling impact on healthy young people, could cause serious disruptions in services and social order.

Pandemic Phases

According to WHO, the hallmarks of an influenza pandemic are: (1) the emergence of a novel influenza virus strain; (2) the finding that the strain can cause human disease; and (3) sustained person-to-person transmission of the strain. Novel influenza viruses typically acquire these characteristics in phases. **Table 1** shows the phases of an influenza pandemic as described by WHO. In the *interpandemic period*, there is no human circulation of novel viruses. During this period, there is annual circulation of common influenza viruses, which cause outbreaks each winter. In the *pandemic alert period*, a new strain is present, with increasing ability for human-tohuman spread. During a *pandemic period* there is sustained human-to-human transmission of the new strain. **Table 1** also shows the public health goals WHO recommends to slow the development and spread of novel virus strains as much as possible. WHO reports the current global status at "Pandemic Alert Level 3:" a new virus is causing human cases of illness, but with no or very limited human-to-human transmission.[10]

Influenza Pandemics in the 20th Century[11]

Historical records suggest that influenza pandemics have occurred periodically for at least four centuries. In the 20th century there were three influenza pandemics, and several "pandemic threats."

The **1918 Spanish Flu** (H1N1) pandemic is estimated to have killed more than 50 million people worldwide, and at least 675,000 in the United States.[12] Illness and death rates were highest among adults 20-50 years old. HHS notes that "the severity of that virus has not been seen again." Similarities between the 1918 pandemic and the current H5N1 avian flu situation have the global public health community on edge.

Table 1. WHO Pandemic Phases

Phase	Description	Overarching public health goals
Interpandemic period		
Phase 1	No new influenza virus strains have been detected in humans. A virus strain that has caused human infection may be present in animals. If so, the risk of human infection is considered to be low.	Strengthen global influenza pandemic preparedness at the global, regional and national levels.
Phase 2	No new influenza virus strains have been detected in humans. However, a circulating animal influenza virus strain poses a substantial risk of human disease.	Minimize the risk of transmission to humans; detect and report such transmission rapidly if it occurs.
Pandemic alert period		
Phase 3	Human infection(s) with a new strain, but no human-to-human spread, or at most rare instances of spread to a close contact.	Ensure rapid characterization of the new virus strain, and early detection, notification and response to additional cases.
Phase 4	Small cluster(s) with limited human-to-human transmission, but spread is highly localized, suggesting that the virus is not well adapted to humans.	Contain the new virus within limited foci or delay spread to gain time to implement preparedness measures, including vaccine development.
Phase 5	Larger cluster(s), but human-to- human spread still localized, suggesting that the virus is becoming increasingly better adapted to humans, but may not yet be fully transmissible (substantial pandemic risk).	Maximize efforts to contain or delay spread, to possibly avert a pandemic, and to gain time to implement pandemic response measures.
Pandemic period		
Phase 6	Pandemic: increased and sustained transmission in the general population	Minimize the impact of the pandemic.

Source: WHO Global Influenza Preparedness Plan, 2005, at [http://www.who.int/csr/disease/influenza/pandemic/en/index.html].

The **1957 Asian Flu** (H2N2) was first identified in Asia in February 1957 and spread to the United States during the summer. Health officials responded quickly and vaccine was available in limited supply by August. This pandemic killed about 69,800 people in the United States.

The **1968 Hong Kong Flu** (H3N2) became widespread in the United States in December of that year. It is estimated that 33,800 people died from this pandemic in the United States, (affecting those over the age of 65 disproportionately), making it the mildest pandemic of the 20th century.

The **1976 Swine Flu Scare**[13] (H1N1) began when a novel virus, identified in New Jersey, was thought to be related to the Spanish flu virus of 1918 and to have pandemic potential. Federal officials mounted a vaccination campaign, and Congress provided liability protection for the manufacturer and federal injury compensation for those harmed by the vaccine. Ultimately, the virus did not spread, but the vaccine was linked with a rare neurological condition that affected more than 500 people and killed 32. The episode damaged confidence in public health officials.

The **1977 Russian Flu Scare** (H1N1) involved a virus strain that had been in circulation prior to 1957. As a result, severe illness was generally limited to those without prior immunity (i.e., children and young adults). The epidemic is not, therefore, considered a true pandemic.

In **1997, H5N1 Avian Flu,** emerged in Hong Kong and appeared to have been stamped out by mass culling of poultry. The virus re-emerged in 2003 and has spread to three continents. Global containment efforts continue.

In **1999, an H9N2** flu strain was found to have caused human illness in Hong Kong. This strain continues to circulate in birds and remains of concern to public health officials, but has not as yet shown the same lethal potential as the H5N1 strain. In August, 2004, the National Institutes of Health (NIH) awarded a contract to the Chiron corporation to produce up to 40,000 doses of an investigational vaccine against this strain, should it develop the capacity for human-to-human transmission.[14]

Current Situation

H5N1 Avian Influenza

WHO maintains a Web page with a cumulative count of human H5N1 cases.[15] As of February 19, 2007, WHO reported 274 cases, 167 of them fatal, in 11 countries: Azerbaijan, Cambodia, China, Djibouti, Egypt, Indonesia, Iraq, Nigeria, Thailand, Turkey and Vietnam. The WHO describes pandemic influenza and the situation with H5N1 as follows:[16]

> ... outbreaks ... caused by H5N1 are of particular concern because of their association with severe illness and a high case fatality. Of even greater concern is the uniqueness of the present H5N1 situation in Asia. Never before has an avian influenza virus with a documented ability to infect humans caused such widespread outbreaks in birds in so many countries. This unprecedented situation has significantly increased the risk for the emergence of an influenza pandemic.

> ... The risk (of a pandemic) ... remains so long as H5N1 is present in an animal reservoir, thus allowing continuing opportunities for human exposure and infection. ... Most experts agree that control of the present outbreaks in poultry will take several months or even years. ...

The recent detection of highly pathogenic avian influenza in wild birds adds another layer of complexity to control.

... The world may therefore remain on the verge of a pandemic for some time to come. At the same time, the unpredictability of influenza viruses and the speed with which transmissibility can improve means that the time for preparedness planning is right now. Such a task takes on added urgency because of the prospects opened by recent research: good planning and preparedness might mitigate the enormous consequences of a pandemic, and this opportunity must not be missed.

The H5N1 strain now circulating has been especially virulent in both human and avian hosts. Studies suggest that the virus prompts an over-reaction of the inflammatory response in some human victims, causing rapid and severe damage to the lungs.[17] This primary damage cannot be remedied with antibiotics or antiviral drugs. Victims may require mechanical ventilation, and may succumb despite swift and capable care. In 2004, scientists published the results of research in which they sequenced several genes from the 1918 pandemic strain. These genes, when inserted into flu viruses and used to infect mice, were found to have a similar property.[18] Recently, scientists re-created and published the entire genome of the 1918 strain, reinforcing this finding.[19] This property may explain the high lethality of both the 1918 and H5N1 strains in apparently healthy young people.

The H5N1 avian flu may never slip its moorings as a bird pathogen and become a serious human threat. But that possibility is a worst-case scenario for the world's public health experts. Should H5N1 become a pandemic strain, scientists are concerned that it may retain much of its virulence as it changes to a more transmissible form. In the face of such a deadly pathogen, miracles of modern medicine, unavailable in much of the developing world, may not be of much help in developed countries either. Such a scenario would challenge governments around the globe.

Other Flu Strains with Pandemic Potential

While H5N1 is the most worrisome, it is not the only recent flu strain with pandemic potential. Several novel strains of avian influenza associated with human transmission have resulted in pandemic alert status in the past several years. For example, in 2003 an H7N7 strain affecting commercial poultry flocks in the Netherlands resulted in 89 cases of human illness.[20] Most illnesses were mild, but there was one death. In 2004 in the Canadian province of British Columbia, an H7N3 avian influenza strain in commercial poultry was found to have infected at least two people. While both recovered, WHO issued a pandemic alert for the Canadian outbreak.[21] A government worker who became ill while involved in culling flocks of poultry during a 2002 outbreak of H7N2 avian flu in Virginia was later shown to have antibodies to that strain, providing suggestive but not conclusive evidence of infection.[22]

These cases demonstrate a newer understanding of the potential for direct birdto-human transmission of avian flu viruses, and the fact that while the H5N1 strain is of special concern, public health officials can not neglect other strains. The Centers for Disease Control and Prevention (CDC) has noted several outbreaks of various strains of avian flu in North American poultry flocks in 2003 and 2004, and publishes guidance and recommendations for the protection of persons potentially exposed during such outbreaks.[23]

Potential Impacts of an Influenza Pandemic

Deaths and Hospitalizations

In its pandemic flu plan, HHS estimates that about 209,000 U.S. deaths could result from a moderate pandemic, similar to those in 1957 and 1968, while 1.9 million deaths could result from a severe pandemic like that in 1918.[24] (CDC estimates that on average, about 36,000 die of influenza during an annual flu season.)

Estimates of impacts of a future pandemic are generally based on experience from past pandemics, which varied considerably in their severity. Trust for America's Health (TFAH), a non-profit public health advocacy group, published a report estimating deaths and hospitalizations in the United States based on mild, moderate and severe pandemic scenarios. The report presents death estimates that range from 180,000 to more than 1 million.[25] The report also contains estimated state-by-state health impacts.

Predicted hospitalization rates provide an idea of the potential burden on the U.S. healthcare system, but they are prone to the same degree of uncertainty. In its final pandemic plan, HHS estimates of hospitalizations range from 865,000 to 9.9 million. TFAH estimates that U.S. hospitalizations would range from almost 800,000 to more than 4.7 million, and cites a statistic from the American Hospital Association that in 2003 there were 965,256 staffed hospital beds in registered hospitals. These projected impacts would occur over a compressed time frame of several weeks or a few months, rather than spread over a full year.

Simple extrapolations of health effects from events in 1918 do not account for advances in medical care that have occurred since then. Antibiotics are now available to treat bacterial pneumonia that often results from influenza infection, and sophisticated respiratory care is now available to treat those with severe pneumonia.

Experts caution, though, that the H5N1 avian flu virus can cause severe primary damage to the lungs. If this strain were to launch a pandemic and retain this trait, large numbers of victims may require intensive care and ventilatory support, likely exceeding national capacity to provide this level of care. In any event, such specialized care is not available in most developing countries, and access to it is uneven within the United States.

Economic Impacts

An analysis published by CDC in 1999, based on the relatively mild 1968 pandemic, estimated the cost of a pandemic in the United States at between $71.3 and $166.5 billion.[26] The study modeled direct healthcare costs, lost productivity for those affected, and lost expected future lifetime earnings for those who died. Loss of life accounted for the majority of economic impact. The model did not include the potential effect of disruptions in commerce.

In December 2005, the Congressional Budget Office (CBO) prepared an assessment of the possible macroeconomic effects of a mild flu pandemic, such as those in 1957 and 1968, and a severe pandemic, such as the one in 1918. CBO estimated from the severe pandemic scenario that real Gross Domestic Product (GDP) would be about 4-1/4 percent lower over the subsequent year than it would have been had the pandemic not taken place, similar to a typical U.S. recession. From the mild pandemic scenario, CBO estimated about a 1 percent reduction in GDP, which might not be distinguishable from normal economic variation.[27]

In November 2005, the World Bank estimated the overall U.S. economic impacts of a potential pandemic of moderate severity at $100 to $200 billion, and global impacts at around $800 billion, if certain impacts were to last for a full year.[28] Subsequently, the International Monetary Fund commented that while the global economic and financial impacts of a severe pandemic were likely to be significant, economic activity would likely recover quickly once the pandemic had run its course.[29] CBO provided a synopsis of several recent studies of the macroeconomic effects of a possible pandemic, noting that the estimates span a wide range of effects, reflecting the considerable uncertainties involved.[30]

There have been several studies of the economic impacts of Severe Acute Respiratory Syndrome (SARS) in 2003. One analysis showed significant short- and long-term decreases in Gross Domestic Product (GDP) in China and Hong Kong, attributing most of the losses to "the behavior of consumers and investors" rather than to actual medical costs.[31] The World Bank economic analysis of a possible flu pandemic discusses the likely interplay between government actions, public behavior, and economic effects. Similarly, CBO notes in its assessment that government actions could either amplify or mitigate economic impacts, saying that attempts to quarantine people would probably amplify the reductions in trade, travel and tourism, but that rapid disease detection, vaccine development and deployment, and other actions, including quarantine, if effective in controlling the spread of disease, could blunt adverse economic impacts as a pandemic progressed.[32]

PANDEMIC INFLUENZA PLANNING

The United States has engaged in pandemic flu planning activities for several decades, with heightened activity in recent years in response to the threat posed by H5N1 avian flu. In addition to response efforts in the public health and medical sectors, a serious pandemic would trigger the National Response Plan (NRP) , developed by the Department of Homeland Security (DHS) as a blueprint for the coordination of federal agencies during an emergency. The NRP, discussed in greater detail in later sections of this chapter, is an *all-hazards* plan for emergencies ranging from hurricanes to wildfires to terrorist attacks.

Described below are a number of preparedness and response plans to assist U.S. federal, state and local agencies in specific preparedness and response for a flu pandemic. U.S. plans reflect the timelines, goals and international capabilities described by the WHO in its pandemic plan. In addition, U.S. federal, state and local plans for this specific threat are intended to be consistent with the all-hazards principles in the NRP.

WHO Global Influenza Preparedness Plan

In order to guide country planning efforts, the WHO released a revised pandemic preparedness plan in early 2005.[33] The plan lays out goals and actions to be taken by WHO, as well as recommended actions for individual nations, at each of the pandemic phases (shown in **Table 1**). For each phase, actions are grouped into five categories: (1) planning and coordination; (2) situation monitoring and assessment; (3) prevention and containment; (4) health system response; and (5) communications. In addition, recommended actions for individual nations are grouped according to whether the country is affected or not at a particular phase. For Phase 6 (Pandemic Phase), when it is assumed that all countries will inevitably be affected, there are recommended immediate actions for all countries, and specific actions for those affected, those not yet affected, and those for which the pandemic has subsided, noting that subsequent pandemic waves may follow the first one.

The WHO pandemic plan contains an annex of recommendations to nations for "nonpharmaceutical public health interventions," actions such as isolation, quarantine and travel restrictions. The annex stresses the use of voluntary rather than compulsory measures, noting the lack of demonstrated utility of certain practices, or that enforcement is considered impractical for others. The annex also notes that certain practices used to control SARS, such as temperature screening at airports, are not necessarily recommended for control of pandemic influenza, depending on pandemic phase. The plan and annex also stress avoiding stigmatization of persons affected by pandemic influenza or its control measures.

U.S. Federal Pandemic Plans

In November 2005, the Administration unveiled a central federal website, run by HHS, containing interagency pandemic preparedness and response information.[34] The following section describes a number of government pandemic flu planning documents. Unless otherwise noted, plans discussed in this section are available on the central website, along with other information about national pandemic preparedness efforts.

National Pandemic Plans

In November 2005, the White House Homeland Security Council released the **National Strategy for Pandemic Influenza** (the National Strategy). The strategy lays out three goals: (1) stopping, slowing or otherwise limiting the spread of a pandemic to the United States; (2) limiting the domestic spread of a pandemic, and mitigating disease, suffering and death; and (3) sustaining infrastructure and mitigating impact to the economy and the functioning of society. In order to meet those goals, the strategy lays out three "pillars" of implementation activities:

- Preparedness and Communication: Activities that should be undertaken before a pandemic to ensure preparedness, and the communication of roles and responsibilities to all levels of government, segments of society and individuals.
- Surveillance and Detection: Domestic and international systems that provide continuous "situational awareness," to ensure the earliest warning possible to protect the population.
- Response and Containment: Actions to limit the spread of the outbreak and to mitigate the health, social and economic impacts of a pandemic.

Finally, roles and responsibilities are laid out for the federal government, state and local governments, the private sector, individuals and families, and international partners.[35]

In May 2006, the White House Homeland Security Council released the **National Strategy for Pandemic Influenza: Implementation Plan** (the Implementation Plan), containing more than 300 required actions — with timelines and performance measures — to be taken by federal departments and agencies, state and local governments, communities, and the private sector, to prepare for a possible pandemic. Required actions span six functional areas, as follows:

- International Efforts: Prevent and contain outbreaks abroad;
- Transportation and Borders: Slow the arrival and spread of a pandemic;
- Protecting Human Health: Limit spread and mitigate illness;
- Protecting Animal Health: Control influenza with human pandemic potential in animals;
- Law Enforcement, Public Safety, and Security: Ensure civil order during a pandemic;
- Planning by Institutions: Protect personnel and ensure continuity of operations.

The White House released a six-month status report in December 2006, stating that 92% of all actions due within six months of release of the Implementation Plan in May 2006 had been completed.

Health Sector Pandemic Plans

In August 2004, HHS released the **Draft Pandemic Influenza Preparedness and Response Plan**. The draft plan articulated steps to be taken by HHS agencies and offices, and by state and local public health authorities, in preparing for and responding to a pandemic. Specific activities discussed included surveillance, vaccine development and use, antiviral drug use, and communications. The draft plan was criticized by some as being vague, and for delegating certain critical activities — such as designating priority groups for rationing of vaccine and antiviral drugs — to states.

The draft plan was superceded by the **HHS Pandemic Influenza Plan** (the HHS Pandemic Plan), published in November 2005. The final plan built on elements in the draft plan, and has three parts: (1) a Strategic Plan, which outlines key planning assumptions and HHS agency roles; (2) a Public Health Guidance for State and Local Partners, which lays out activities on such matters as surveillance, laboratory testing, and quarantine at the borders; and (3) a part currently under development, to consist of detailed operational plans for HHS agencies involved in pandemic response. According to the plan, the HHS Secretary would direct, and the Assistant Secretary for Public Health Emergency Preparedness[36] would coordinate, all HHS pandemic response activities.

The final plan addressed some of the gaps in the draft plan, such as the designation of priority groups to receive limited vaccine and antiviral drugs.[37] Other elements of the final plan received immediate criticism. For example, the section on healthcare planning focuses on individual healthcare facilities and refers to plans for surge capacity. Some experts have commented that there is little surge capacity in the healthcare sector under normal circumstances, and that officials might have to resort to the use of alternate facilities (e.g., convention centers) to care for large numbers of flu patients. The HHS Pandemic Plan does not address that contingency.

Department of Defense Planning

Shortly after the release of the HHS draft pandemic plan in August 2004, the Assistant Secretary of Defense for Health Affairs released the Department of Defense (DOD) **Pandemic Influenza Preparation and Response Planning Guidance.**[38] The DOD guidance follows many of the assumptions used in civilian planning, modifying them to protect a highly mobile military force during wartime. Frequent mention is made of the extremely high mortality suffered by U.S. troops during World War I as a result of the 1918 pandemic. The guidance notes that 43,000 uniformed soldiers, more than one third of all U.S. military casualties in the war, died of pandemic influenza, most of them during one 10-week period in 1918.

The DOD guidance notes that the military will use the same vaccine formulation as that developed for civilian use, though DOD will be responsible for securing its own supplies of vaccine and antiviral drugs. Priority for countermeasures in limited supply would be given to forward-deployed troops. The guidance does not set out strict tiers of priority recipients. The guidance discusses the limited utility of individual control measures such as isolation and quarantine, and suggests that larger-scale adjustments (such as extending the tour of ships at sea) could slow disease transmission. The guidance also mentions the consideration of coalition forces from other nations, and the possibility that countermeasures such as vaccine and antiviral drugs may be provided to them under certain conditions.

Department of Veterans Affairs Planning

The Department of Veterans Affairs (VA) released a comprehensive pandemic flu plan in March 2006. The plan notes that the VA owns a supply of approximately 500,000 treatment courses of the antiviral drug Tamiflu.

State Pandemic Plans

All states were required to have submitted plans for pandemic flu preparedness to HHS (through CDC) by July 2005, as a condition of receipt of public health preparedness funding for FY2005.[39] This deadline pre-dated the publication of the National Strategy and the HHS Pandemic Plan. The plans of all 50 states and the District of Columbia are available on the central federal pandemic flu website. Many states continue to update their plans.

Private Sector Planning

In September 2006, the Department of Homeland Security released the **Pandemic Influenza Preparedness, Response, and Recovery Guide for Critical Infrastructure and Key Resources.** The guide provides business planners with guidance to assure continuity, during a pandemic, for facilities comprising critical infrastructure sectors (e.g., energy and telecommunications) and key resources (e.g., dams and nuclear power plants).

Domestic and global corporations have adopted specific pandemic flu plans to varying degrees. In July 2006, the Conference Board, a global business membership and research organization, reported the findings of its survey of pandemic preparedness in 553 global companies. The Board found that nearly three-fourths of respondents reported either having a pandemic plan, or being well along in developing one. But the Board commented that "... the effectiveness of business plans and the quality of relationships necessary for their successful implementation in times of extreme public, private and social stress remains open to question."[40] According to the report, "the most significant disadvantage in not conducting formal pandemic preparedness planning may be the virtually total absence of coordination with the public sector. An overwhelming 94% of participating companies report that they have not had discussions with any level of government officials about their organization's ability to provide essential services or access to facilities, equipment, or staff during a pandemic."[41]

ISSUES IN PANDEMIC INFLUENZA PLANNING

Could an Influenza Pandemic Be Stopped?

Public health experts note that vaccine, the primary measure for influenza prevention, will be available in very limited supply at the start of a pandemic. Antiviral drugs are also likely to be available in a limited supply. For both, there is limited global surge capacity for production during a pandemic. Conventional wisdom once held that there was an inevitability to the global wave of disease that a pandemic would bring, but lately this notion has been challenged. WHO and many national experts believe that scientific advances in studying and detecting flu viruses may make it possible to detect the spread of the virus early, and rein in localized clusters of infection. While not suggesting that a pandemic could necessarily be averted, they posit that if progression were slowed enough, a vaccine could be available by the time worldwide infection ensued. While there still might not be enough vaccine for everyone, if countries had at least enough for essential personnel, it would soften the impact somewhat.

Realizing this hope rests on two conditions: first, exceptional "pandemic intelligence" in countries at the epicenter of a developing pandemic; and second, an effective response in these epicenter countries. In hopes of having the best possible information in real time, WHO, along with the U.S. State Department, CDC, DOD, other U.S. federal agencies, and health officials from many other nations, are building epidemiology and lab capacity in Southeast Asia and other regions affected by H5N1 avian flu, when countries have requested assistance. The U.S. government has also participated in global pandemic response planning, through the International Partnership on Avian and Pandemic Influenza.[42]

Who's in Charge?

A serious flu pandemic would affect many sectors of society, not just the public health and medical communities. As such, it is useful to consider federal efforts to meet this threat across sectors, and to consider those efforts in the contexts of *preparedness* and *response.* Federal leadership may be somewhat different for each of these phases, but the nature of the threat may blur the line between them.

WHO monitors the spread of H5N1 avian flu and other novel flu viruses, and will make formal announcements of changes in pandemic threat status including, were it to occur, the onset of pandemic, defined as sustained human-to-human transmission of a novel flu virus. At that point, global response activities would ensue. However, since this threat can be anticipated, the federal government has launched a specific, comprehensive, long-term preparedness strategy. Of the more than 300 tasks in the Implementation Plan, 27 were to have been completed within three months of the plan's publication in May 2006, while others, such as establishing domestic capacity for rapid, large-scale pandemic vaccine production, may take many years to achieve.[43] If a pandemic were to occur before then, unfinished preparedness activities would be completed, if appropriate, as part of the pandemic response.

WHO urges that countries plan for a pandemic as a multi-sector threat, not merely a health challenge. However, federal relationships that support state and local jurisdictions traditionally operate sector-by-sector (e.g., HHS with health services, and the Department of Transportation with transit agencies). While HHS had been the lead federal agency for pandemic planning prior to 2005, the White House Homeland Security Council appears now to be the hub through which federal preparedness activities are coordinated.

Following release of the National Strategy and the HHS Pandemic Plan in November 2005, HHS Secretary Michael Leavitt and other federal officials hosted pandemic planning summits in all 50 states, to support states' multi-sector planning activities. Nonetheless, state plans were required as a condition of CDC grants to state health departments, and many of them remain predominantly focused on health sector preparedness. For example, many plans don't mention a possible role for the National Guard during a pandemic. Since the National Guard is a state response asset under the control of the Governor, and since a flu pandemic could be catastrophic, there has been considerable discussion of the possible role of law enforcement in pandemic response. Hence, it could be helpful if state plans specifically described how the National Guard might be used during a pandemic.

The National Response Plan (NRP), published by DHS, is a blueprint for the coordinated efforts of federal agencies during disasters.[44] In the event of a significant influenza pandemic, the NRP may be activated to coordinate federal agency activities. Responsibilities for specified activities (e.g., transportation, energy, and public works) are set out in 15 *Emergency Support Functions* (ESFs). When the NRP is activated, the Secretary of Homeland Security serves as the overall lead for a coordinated federal response, while the Secretary of HHS serves as the lead for ESF-8, Public Health and Medical Services.[45] While public health and medical activities may comprise the bulk of the federal response to a pandemic, other ESF authorities may be involved to sustain infrastructure affected by absenteeism or supply chain disruptions, requiring the coordination of other federal departments.

The National Strategy notes the federal departments designated as the lead for various aspects of a pandemic response: HHS for the medical response, the U.S. Department of Agriculture (USDA) for the veterinary response, the Department of State for international activities, and DHS for overall domestic incident management. In addition, DHS is responsible for coordinating the preparedness of privately owned critical infrastructures such as banking and telecommunications.

While pandemic influenza scenarios have been used to exercise specific elements of response, such as distribution of stockpiled medications, there has been no national exercise to test a multi-sector, multi-jurisdictional response. As a condition of receipt of $350 million in FY2006 supplemental appropriations, Congress called on states to conduct pandemic flu exercises that would "enable public health and law enforcement officials to establish procedures and locations for quarantine, surge capacity, diagnostics, and communication."[46] The funds, awarded by CDC, are to be used by states to test three aspects of response: control of community gatherings (e.g., school closings); medical surge capacity; and mass vaccination / mass prophylaxis.[47] While no doubt useful, these exercises will be carried out state-by-state, retaining a health-sector focus. The only national multi- sector pandemic exercise to date has been a table-top simulation conducted by members of the Cabinet.[48]

Emergency Declarations and Federal Assistance

In the United States, public health authority rests principally with the states as an exercise of their *police powers*.[49] States play a leading role in preparing for and responding to public health threats, with HHS (primarily CDC) providing support through funding, training, technical assistance, advanced laboratory support, data analysis and other activities. The Public Health Service Act grants the Secretary of HHS the authority to declare a situation a public health emergency, which triggers an expansion of certain federal authorities.[50] Though states already have considerable power in responding to public health events, most can also declare public health emergencies and expand their powers further. In an influenza pandemic, response measures such as quarantine or prohibitions against administration of vaccine to non-priority individuals would likely be carried out, at least initially, by state rather than federal authorities.[51]

An influenza pandemic may disrupt services beyond the health sector. Each of the pandemic influenza plans listed earlier is written with the premise that the NRP could be triggered by a flu pandemic, thereby guiding a coordinated federal response to problems within the health sector and other affected sectors through routine, non- emergency, federal assistance mechanisms.[52] According to the Implementation Plan, the Secretary of Homeland Security may declare a pandemic an *Incident of National Significance,* triggering the NRP, early in the event, perhaps while foreign countries were affected, but before the disease had reached the United States.[53]

States may require additional federal assistance to maintain essential services during an influenza pandemic. Typically, such assistance is triggered by presidential emergency or disaster declarations pursuant to the Robert T. Stafford Disaster Relief and Emergency Assistance Act (the Stafford Act).[54] Disaster assistance authorized by the Stafford Act includes the provision of emergency funds and supplies to stricken households, as well as aid in clearing and rebuilding damaged infrastructure. While a virus would not cause infrastructure damage directly, certain sectors may nonetheless be affected as a result of widespread absenteeism or supply chain disruptions. For example, water treatment facilities may be damaged, or may have to be shut down, if they are not adequately maintained, or if replacement parts are unavailable. Sectors that depend heavily on continuous computer support (e.g., banking) may be disrupted by absenteeism.

It is unclear whether Stafford Act major disaster assistance could be provided in response to a pandemic. Emergency declarations pursuant to the Stafford Act were made in response to West Nile virus in 2000, so there is precedent for a presidential emergency declaration, (providing a lower level of federal assistance) in response to an infectious disease threat. The matter of presidential authority to declare a major disaster (providing a higher level of federal assistance) in response to an infectious disease threat generally, and a flu pandemic specifically, is less clear. In the past, FEMA has, in the context of the national TOPOFF exercises, interpreted biological disasters as ineligible for major disaster assistance pursuant to the Stafford Act.[55] However, the Administration view is that the President's authority to declare a major disaster pursuant to the Stafford Act could be applied to an influenza pandemic.[56]

Limited Surveillance and Testing Capability

The CDC coordinates domestic surveillance for seasonal flu in humans.[57] Monitoring for pandemic flu is integrated into these existing systems. Key challenges in the rapid detection of novel flu viruses in humans are the vagueness of flu symptoms, which can be seen with many other diseases, and the difficulty in distinguishing specific flu strains of interest from the background of other strains commonly in circulation.

The routine CDC system for domestic flu surveillance has seven reporting components: (1) more than 120 laboratories; (2) more than 1,000 sentinel healthcare providers; (3) death records from 122 cities; (4) reports from health departments in the states, territories, New York City and the District of Columbia; (5) influenza- associated deaths in children; (6) Emerging Infections Program sites in 10 states; and (7) laboratory-confirmed hospitalizations for influenza in young children in three sentinel counties.[58] Reporting to these systems at CDC by state and local health departments and healthcare providers is voluntary. Information is gathered and analyzed weekly during the winter flu season.

CDC has issued recommendations to public health and medical professionals for the investigation of possible human cases of avian or pandemic flu in individuals who have a history of recent travel to a region affected by H5N1 avian flu, and who exhibit symptoms of severe respiratory disease.[59] Between February 2003 and May 2006, 59 such case reports were made to CDC by clinicians or health departments. Investigations showed no evidence of H5N1 virus infections.[60]

There is not, at this time, a rapid point-of-care (bedside) test that healthcare workers or epidemiologists can use to screen a person for H5N1 flu, or any other *specific* strain of influenza. CDC recommends the use of commercial flu screening tests for initial patient evaluation. The agency cautions that commercially available screening tests cannot reliably distinguish H5N1 flu from other influenza A strains; therefore, specimens that test positive on screening should be followed up with specimens sent to the state's public health laboratory to determine which flu strain is involved. At this time, public health labs in all 50 states have the capability to test for H5N1 influenza, though there is a lag time in shipping the samples, and in test turnaround.[61] The Implementation Plan calls on HHS, in coordination with DOD, VA and DHS, to support the private-sector development of reliable, rapid, point-ofcare diagnostic tests for specific flu strains. CDC awarded contracts for this purpose to four companies in December 2006.[62]

Isolation and Quarantine

Isolation and quarantine have been used for hundreds of years to prevent the spread of communicable diseases. Both methods restrict the movement of those affected, but they differ depending on whether an individual has been exposed to a disease (*quarantine*), or is actually infected (*isolation*). Persons in isolation may be significantly ill, so isolation often occurs in a healthcare setting. Persons under quarantine are, by definition, not ill from the disease in question, though they may have other health conditions that complicate the quarantine process.

In the United States, quarantine authority is generally based in state rather than federal law.[63] The federal government has the responsibility to prevent the introduction, transmission, and spread of communicable diseases from foreign countries, and the authority to impose quarantine on incoming travelers suspected to be infected with or exposed to certain diseases on a list of quarantinable communicable diseases. Diseases are listed by an executive order of the President, in consultation with the Secretary of HHS. On April 1, 2005, President Bush added to the list "influenza caused by novel or re-emergent influenza viruses that are causing, or have the potential to cause, a pandemic."[64] Federal quarantine is carried out by CDC's Division of Global Migration and Quarantine, which operates quarantine stations at major ports, and also works closely with states to carry out quarantine activities.[65] CDC has noted that having pandemic influenza on the list assures the agency of this option for disease control, should it be felt to be worthwhile.

On October 4, 2005, in response to a question at a press conference, President Bush suggested the use of the military to enforce quarantines during a flu pandemic.[66] The comment prompted questions on two issues: the role of quarantine in controlling pandemic flu, and the role of the military in responding to domestic disasters.

While isolation and quarantine were crucial in the worldwide response to SARS, these methods are less likely to be successful in controlling influenza. Influenza has a shorter incubation period than SARS, and is often contagious in the absence of symptoms or before symptoms appear, making it difficult to identify persons who should be quarantined.[67]

There has been considerable interest in recent years in studying or predicting the effects of a variety of so-called "non-pharmaceutical interventions" (NPI), including isolation and quarantine, on the potential spread of pandemic flu.[68] The Implementation Plan discusses CDC's readiness to implement quarantines for incoming travelers, and strategies for school closures and other "social distancing" measures that may be used by local governments to slow disease spread. The Plan also notes the need for continued study of the potential impacts, both good and bad, of various approaches. The Plan makes specific reference to the practice of *geographic quarantine* (also known as *cordon sanitaire*), the "isolation, by force if necessary, of localities with documented disease transmission from localities still free of infection,"[69] saying, "The implementation of conventional geographic quarantine imposes significant opportunity costs and may result in the diversion of significant resources and assets that might be used to better effect supporting less draconian disease containment measures."[70] In February 2007, CDC released a planning guide for the graded use of NPI — including school closures, liberal work leave policies, and teleworking strategies — matched to pandemic severity.[71] The guide does not propose the use of compulsory isolation or quarantine measures, recommending that such actions be voluntary.

Following the terror attacks of 2001, DOD activated a new combatant command, Northern Command or NORTHCOM, to, among other functions, provide military assistance to civil authorities in response to terrorist attacks.[72] The NRP also articulates this role for the military in response to terrorist attacks, major disasters, and other emergencies.[73] There has, however, long been a prohibition against the use of federal military personnel for domestic law enforcement, except in extraordinary circumstances.[74] There were no instances in the 20th century in which federal troops were used to enforce a domestic quarantine for any disease, though there are earlier examples.[75]

Medical Surge Capacity

An influenza pandemic of even limited magnitude has the potential to disrupt the normal workings of the healthcare system in a variety of ways. These may include deferral of elective medical procedures; diversion of patients away from overwhelmed hospital emergency departments and tertiary care facilities; protective quarantines of susceptible populations such as residents of long-term care facilities; and hoarding, theft or black-marketeering of scarce resources such as vaccines or antiviral drugs.

Several additional factors complicate the healthcare burden posed by pandemic flu. First, it is thought that a pandemic would spread across the United States in a compressed timeframe similar to seasonal flu, that is, over a six- to eight-week period. Second, while it is desirable that affected patients be kept in isolation, domestic isolation capacity is limited. Third, the healthcare workforce is likely to be affected by pandemic flu. Even if they are protected directly by limited vaccines or antiviral drugs, their family members may be affected and require additional care at home. Fourth, supplies of healthcare consumables such as gloves, masks and antibiotics would be stressed by a surge in global demand.[76] Even a mild flu pandemic would likely place a significant and near-simultaneous strain on the nation's healthcare system.

Table 2. NVAC and ACIP Recommendations for Pandemic Vaccine Priority Groups (Persons in Thousands)

Group and Tier		Group total	Cumulative total
1A	Healthcare workers with direct patient contact	9,000	9,000
	Vaccine and antivirals manufacturing personnel	40	9,040
1B	Highest risk of serious flu complications	25,840	34,880
1C	Pregnant women, immunocompromised individuals, and household contacts of infants	10,700	45,580
1D	Key government leaders and responders	151	45,731
2A	Rest of high risk individuals	59,100	104,831
2B	Most critical infrastructure and public health emergency responders	8,500	113,331
3	Other key government health decision makers, mortuary services personnel	500	113,831
4	Healthy 2- to 64-year-olds not in other groups	179,260	293,091

Rationing Scarce Resources

The WHO recommends that countries identify priority groups for vaccination and antiviral drugs, as these measures become available, and recommends that countries make these decisions before a pandemic occurs. The National Vaccine Advisory Committee (NVAC, which reports to the director of the National Vaccine Program in HHS) and the Advisory Committee on Immunization Practices (ACIP, which reports to the HHS Secretary and CDC) met in joint session in July 2005 to report to HHS Secretary Leavitt their recommendations for prioritizing vaccine and antiviral drugs for the U.S. civilian population during a pandemic.[77] The two committees put forth unanimous recommendations for prioritizing pandemic flu vaccine. Their recommendations were incorporated into the HHS Pandemic Plan, and are displayed in **Table 2**.

Healthcare workers with direct patient contact and those involved in making the vaccine were given top priority by the committees. Next were those at highest risk of serious complications from flu. During seasonal flu, and during the 1957 and 1968 pandemics, those at highest risk were the very old, the very young, and individuals with certain serious chronic diseases. The committees noted that during a pandemic other groups may be shown to be at higher risk, and that tiers could be redefined according to the specific epidemiologic findings. For example, during the 1918 pandemic, healthy young people were found to be at increased risk of death when they became infected. According to the committees' estimates, more than 60% of the U.S. population, including most children, would not fall into any of the designated priority groups.

The proposed scheme comports with a tradition in public health practice to prioritize the most vulnerable, in this case those most vulnerable to severe complications from flu. Such a strategy does not necessarily save the most lives, though. To accomplish that when resources are scarce, resources would be given to those most likely to survive or to have better outcomes as a result, to the extent that one could determine who those people were. Conversely, treatment would be withheld from those who were unlikely to benefit, so that others may. The HHS proposal has prompted considerable debate about strategies for withholding resources during a pandemic, and shown that rationing schemes to optimize one goal (e.g., equity and fairness) may conflict with schemes to optimize another (e.g., slowing disease transmission). These are ethically complex decisions with which the civilian medical community has little experience.[78]

Although HHS included recommendations for vaccine priorities in its pandemic plan, these recommendations may change. On December 14, 2006, HHS published a request for information (RFI) in the Federal Register asking for "input on pandemic influenza vaccine prioritization considerations from all interested and affected parties...."[79] The Implementation Plan requires HHS, in coordination with DHS, to make priority recommendations for access to pre-pandemic and pandemic influenza vaccines. The recommendations are to reflect the pandemic response goals that were described in the National Strategy,[80] as well as maintaining national security. A federal interagency working group has been established to recommend priority groups, and the RFI will provide information for the working group. The working group's draft guidance and recommendations will be published in the Federal Register for comment. HHS noted that it was particularly interested in responses to several questions concerning priorities for vaccines, including, "How can fairness, equity, efficiency and related principles be reflected in the determination of priority groupings for receipt of pre-pandemic or pandemic vaccine?" The initial deadline for responses to HHS was January 18, 2007; it was subsequently extended to February 5, 2007.[81]

Influenza Vaccine Supply and Use

Overview

Vaccination is considered the best preventive measure for influenza. But, because of continuous changes in the genes of flu viruses, vaccines must be "matched" to specific strains to provide good protection. Flu vaccine is currently produced in chicken eggs, using a time-consuming process with a six-month lead time. Since a vaccine could not be mass produced against a pandemic flu strain until that strain emerged, planning assumes that a matched flu vaccine would not be available for initial global pandemic control. Health officials are working to increase the speed of flu vaccine production, to increase global flu vaccine production capacity, to develop and create limited stockpiles of prototype vaccines for H5N1 and other novel flu strains, and to develop "universal" flu vaccines that don't require strain matching for effectiveness.

On November 1, 2005, the Administration requested $7.1 billion in emergency funding for pandemic preparedness. Congress provided FY2006 emergency supplemental appropriations of $3.8 billion in December 2005, of which $3.3 billion was provided to HHS. A second FY2006 supplemental appropriation in June 2006 provided HHS with an additional $2.3 billion.[82] The bulk of this funding has gone to support flu vaccine related activities. The Administration has established two primary vaccine goals: (1) establishment and maintenance of stockpiles of pre- pandemic vaccine adequate to immunize 20 million persons against influenza strains that present a pandemic threat; and (2) expansion of domestic influenza vaccine manufacturing surge capacity for the production of pandemic vaccines for the entire domestic population within six months of a pandemic declaration.[83]

Limited Vaccine Production Capacity

In 2005, there was worldwide capacity to produce at most 300 million doses of injectable *trivalent* flu vaccine, the annual vaccine that contains three different strains of influenza.[84] Only one (sanofi pasteur[85]) of nine manufacturers was located in the United States. WHO reports that in 2006, worldwide capacity had expanded to 400 million doses.[86] Though production capacity can, in theory, be tripled by converting to single-strain production for a pandemic vaccine, two doses (vs. the single dose given each year) may be required to afford protection, because there is no prior immunity to be "boosted." Furthermore, in initial trials of an H5N1 prototype vaccine, immunity was produced only by very high doses of viral antigen, which means that more capacity would be needed to make a given number of doses.

One means to increase domestic vaccine production capacity is to expand manufacturing infrastructure. In July 2006, HHS issued a solicitation for proposals to retrofit existing domestic manufacturing facilities to enable the emergency production of pandemic vaccine. HHS plans to award these contracts in February 2007. HHS plans to issue a request for proposals later in 2007 to assist in building new domestic manufacturing plants to produce of seasonal and pandemic influenza vaccines using new cell-based technologies, which may have several advantages over egg-based production.[87]

Vaccine Research and Development

In addition to expanding bricksand-mortar vaccine capacity, HHS has also used emergency supplemental appropriations to award contracts for research on improved methods of flu vaccine production. Research efforts, generally overseen by the NIH, include cell-based (rather than egg-based) production, recombinant and DNA vaccines, and so-called "antigen-sparing" approaches to boost the immune response to lower doses of virus. NIH also supports intramural and extramural research to enhance understanding of the basic nature of human immunity to influenza, and efforts to develop a universal vaccine that would provide durable immunity against diverse flu strains, eliminating the need for annual vaccination and protecting against pandemic flu strains that have yet to emerge.[88]

Global Vaccine Availability

Some have been critical of the U.S. approach to pandemic flu vaccine development, which sets the goal of universal vaccine availability for Americans, but does not address the provision of vaccine to other countries.[89] In early February 2007, officials in Indonesia announced that they would no longer provide WHO with samples of H5N1 avian flu affecting their country, samples that are used by manufacturers to develop pandemic vaccines that would not likely be available to developing countries during a pandemic. On February 16, Indonesian officials and the WHO jointly announced an agreement whereby Indonesia would resume sending avian flu virus samples to the WHO as soon as it is guaranteed access to affordable vaccines against the disease.[90] The episode foreshadows the types of international tensions that may arise during a pandemic.[91]

Regulatory Issues

From a regulatory standpoint, the Food and Drug Administration (FDA) considers that a pandemic flu vaccine produced using currently-approved processes would merely represent a strain change (as with seasonal flu vaccine), not a new product.[92] This would allow for a streamlined approval process in which a licensed manufacturer would submit additional information as a supplement to its current product license. The agency considers that virus derived by reverse genetics or grown using cell culture methods does not pose additional regulatory obstacles.[93] Prototype human vaccines ideally should undergo clinical trials to establish efficacy, dosage and scheduling protocols. The FDA recommends that these trials be carried out before a pandemic occurs, to the extent possible.

The HHS final plan notes that if a pandemic were to spread swiftly, pandemic vaccine may be pressed into service before standard safety and efficacy tests could be completed. Such unlicensed vaccine could be used under FDA's Investigational New Drug (IND) provisions. These include strict inventory control, record keeping, and informed consent requirements, which would pose an additional challenge for public health officials during a vaccination campaign.

Congress provided an additional mechanism, permitting the use of unapproved drugs and vaccines in an emergency, in the Project BioShield Act of 2004 (P.L. 108- 276). This *Emergency Use Authorization* (EUA) permits the use of unapproved products during a declared public health emergency when alternatives are not available.[94] In early 2005, when FDA issued an EUA for an anthrax vaccine for the military, the agency noted that the statute is self-executing, and that implementing regulations were not required.[95]

Intellectual Property Issues

To produce a vaccine against H5N1 or another pandemic flu strain, scientists start with a virus in circulation, and modify it for mass production. Flu virus for vaccine is grown in fertilized chicken eggs. Avian flu strains must first be weakened, or *attenuated*, or they would kill the chicken embryos, making it impossible to produce vaccine. Traditionally, flu viruses were attenuated using a cumbersome trial-and-error gene-swapping process. In developing prototype H5N1 vaccines, the virus was attenuated using a process called *reverse genetics* (RG). RG is a more efficient and reliable means of genetic modification, which removes unwanted genes and substitutes others.

RG is a patented invention. One of the patent holders, Medimmune, Inc., has waived compensation for production of prototype pandemic flu vaccines and clinical trials, saying that it had:

> notified the World Health Organization in December 2003 that it would grant free access to its intellectual property to government organizations and companies developing pandemic influenza vaccines gratis for public health purposes. In addition, MedImmune, Inc., has given similar notification to NIH and (other officials) in the United States, and the National Institute for Biological Standards and Control (NIBSC) in the United Kingdom. For corporate manufacturers considering the commercial sale of pandemic influenza vaccines produced by reverse genetics, MedImmune, Inc., has sent out letters to all such manufacturers offering licenses to its intellectual property under reasonable terms.[96]

In the United States, the federal government may use patented processes without consent, as long as the patent holder is appropriately compensated.[97] The situation is more complicated in other countries with vaccine plants (mainly in Europe), and would require that certain agreements among RG patent holders and governments be ironed out before mass production could begin.

Vaccine Tracking and Distribution

The sudden shortage of seasonal flu vaccine in the United States for the 2004-2005 season offered an unplanned exercise for pandemic preparedness, highlighting the implications of limited production capacity for vaccines and antiviral drugs, and the absence of a coordinated national system for their distribution.

In December 2006, Congress passed **P.L. 109-417**, the Pandemic and All- Hazards Preparedness Act. The act authorizes the Secretary of HHS, with the voluntary cooperation of manufacturers, wholesalers, and distributors, to track the initial distribution of federally purchased flu vaccine during a pandemic. The act also requires the Secretary to improve the effective distribution of seasonal flu vaccine, by promoting communication between state, local, and tribal public health officials and those manufacturers, wholesalers, and distributors who agree to participate in the tracking program. Vaccine distribution information submitted to the Secretary shall remain confidential in accordance with the exception to the Freedom of Information Act (FOIA) governing trade secrets and commercial or financial information, and be subject to the privacy regulations promulgated under the Health Insurance Portability and Accountability Act of 1996 (P.L. 104-191).

Antiviral Drug Supply and Use

Since pandemic flu vaccine would be unavailable in the early stages of a pandemic, governments and private parties have been interested in drugs that could treat or prevent serious illness from flu. Because influenza is a virus, antibiotics, which treat bacterial infections, are not effective in treating the direct effects of flu. Two types of antiviral drugs have been developed to treat flu: *adamantanes* and *neuraminidase inhibitors* (NIs).[98] Though both types are used to treat serious infections of seasonal influenza, the H5N1 flu strain has been shown to be resistant to adamantanes. Hence, planning efforts for a possible H5N1 pandemic have focused on NIs. Two NIs are available, and both are licensed by the FDA: oseltamivir (Tamiflu®) and zanamivir (Relenza®). The drugs can be used either for treatment when someone is severely ill with flu, or for prevention in those at risk of severe illness. When used for prevention, also called *prophylaxis*, the drug must be given for weeks (rather than the five-day treatment regime), as long the flu virus is in circulation. This has implications for stockpiling, and for the potential development of viral resistance to the drugs.

WHO has recommended that countries create stockpiles of NIs to prepare for a pandemic. Initially, the availability and cost of Tamiflu, a patented drug, were of concern to government officials seeking to acquire the drug in large amounts for their citizens. The patent holder, the Swiss pharmaceutical company Roche, Inc., has since signed agreements to manufacture the drug with more than 15 external contractors in 10 different countries.[99] Several countries have stockpiled enough Tamiflu to treat one-fifth or more of their populations.

The federal government has established two primary goals for stockpiling existing antiviral medications: (1) establishment and maintenance of stockpiles adequate to treat 75 million persons (one-fourth of the population), divided between federal and state stockpiles; and (2) establishment and maintenance of a federal stockpile of 6 million treatment courses reserved for domestic containment efforts.[100] States were expected to procure 31 million of the 75 million treatment courses, for which HHS would reimburse 25% of the cost. Some public health officials and Members of Congress protested the 75% state matching requirement.[101] In an October 2006 survey of state health officials, 29 reported that they had not yet identified and put in place state funds to purchase antiviral drugs, though all but 10 of them reported that they planned, ultimately, to purchase the full amount allotted to them under the federal subsidy program.[102]

Priority groups for antiviral drugs are laid out in the HHS Pandemic Plan, beginning with treatment for those who are admitted to hospitals with severe illness from flu. Priority categories are otherwise fairly similar to those for vaccine (See **Table 2.**), encompassing certain groups of high risk individuals as well as healthcare workers and other responders.

In June 2005, it was reported that farmers in China were using the flu antiviral drug amantadine (an adamantane) to treat poultry flocks to prevent avian flu, and that this may have caused the H5N1 strain to become resistant to the drug.[103] Health officials in China and elsewhere denounced the practice. Tamiflu, the more widely available of the two NIs, is generally effective against H5N1 flu, but resistance to the drug has been documented in strains of seasonal flu that circle the globe each year, and in at least four cases of H5N1 avian flu in humans. Scientists caution that resistance to Tamiflu could become a problem if the drug were pressed into service during an influenza pandemic, especially if it were used for prolonged periods for prophylaxis.[104] In March 2006, the FDA issued an order prohibiting the extra-label use, in poultry, of all approved human anti-influenza drugs, to help prevent the emergence of resistance, preserving the effectiveness of these drugs for treating or preventing influenza infections in humans.[105]

Public health officials have cautioned against an over-reliance on antiviral drugs in pandemic planning. There would likely be limited availability, and drug resistance could emerge as a serious problem. Also, it has not been clearly shown that treatment with Tamiflu, for example, would actually improve survival rates in clinical settings during a potential H5N1 pandemic.[106] Nonetheless, given that the best pandemic response tool — vaccine — will be largely unavailable in the early going, governments can offer antiviral drug stockpiling as a tangible effort to protect their citizens.

Liability and Compensation for Pandemic Countermeasures

Status of Current Planning Efforts

Certain vaccines are covered under the National Vaccine Injury Compensation Program (VICP). Under VICP, an excise tax applied to vaccine sales pays for a public compensation fund. Congress enacted the program in 1986 as a no-fault alternative to the tort system for resolving personal injury claims resulting from adverse reactions to selected childhood vaccines (i.e., those that CDC has recommended be routinely administered to children.) Individuals of any age alleging injury from any covered vaccine must seek compensation through the program first, though they may decline a proposed award and then sue in court.[107] In the American Jobs Creation Act of 2004 (P.L.108-357), Congress added *trivalent* flu vaccine — the annual vaccine that contains three flu strains — to the Vaccine Injury Table, a list of vaccines covered under VICP. Since the law explicitly covered trivalent vaccine, *monovalent* (or single-strain) pandemic vaccines would not be covered under this mechanism.

In December 2005, Congress passed P.L. 109-148, the Department of Defense, Emergency Supplemental Appropriations to Address Hurricanes in the Gulf of Mexico, and Pandemic Influenza Act, 2006. Division C of the act limits liability with respect to countermeasures (including vaccine) for pandemic flu and other public health emergencies. Specifically, upon a declaration by the Secretary of HHS of a public health emergency, or the credible risk of such emergency, the act would, with respect to a "covered countermeasure," eliminate liability (except in the case of willful misconduct) for the United States, and for manufacturers, distributors, program planners, persons who prescribe, administer or dispense the countermeasure, and employees of any of the above.

On February 1, 2007, HHS Secretary Leavitt made a declaration of emergency pursuant to P.L. 109-148, saying he had "determined there is a credible risk that the spread of avian influenza viruses and resulting disease could in the future constitute a public health emergency," triggering liability protections solely for "pandemic countermeasure influenza A (H5N1) vaccine...."[108] The declaration is effective from December 1, 2006 through February 28, 2010.

P.L. 109-148 also called for the establishment in the Treasury of the "Covered Countermeasure Process Fund" to provide compensation to eligible individuals for covered injuries (i.e., serious physical injury or death) directly caused by the administration or use of a covered countermeasure during a declared public health emergency, depending upon an appropriation to the fund. The act does not establish appropriations authority for the fund, however.[109]

The Implementation Plan tasked HHS with developing a protocol and decision tools for medical countermeasures, to implement the act's liability protections and compensation mechanism. HHS published its protocol and decision tool in December 2006.[110]

Smallpox Vaccine Injury Compensation

During implementation of the smallpox vaccination program in 2003, Congress grappled with waiving liability in order to protect the manufacturer, public officials, health providers and others who would make, recommend and deliver the product, while assuring that those who suffered adverse events resulting from the vaccine could be appropriately compensated.[111] The smallpox vaccine used for the 2003 campaign carries an unusually high risk of adverse events, and most scientists do not believe that a pandemic flu vaccine would carry a comparable risk.

The 1976 Swine Flu Affair

A 1976 vaccination campaign that was intended to protect Americans from the threat of a swine flu pandemic in 1976 is often referred to as a debacle.[112] In January 1976, a novel influenza strain ("swine flu") emerged in New Jersey. In March, the Ford Administration announced a campaign to vaccinate the U.S. population by December. On August 18, Congress passed P.L. 94-380, the National Swine Flu Immunization Program of 1976. Among other provisions, the law shielded manufacturers, distributors, and public or private organizations that would administer the vaccine, from claims of injury or death that might result, and established that all such claims would be asserted directly against the United States. More than 40 million civilians were vaccinated against swine flu between October 1 and December 16. The campaign was suspended at that time due to several cases of Guillain-Barré syndrome, a potentially serious neurological condition causing paralysis and sometimes death, suspected to have been caused by the vaccine. Meanwhile, a flu pandemic never emerged. The worrisome virus from New Jersey never led to a global pandemic, or even to localized outbreaks. The federal government ultimately paid out $93 million to individuals injured by the vaccine.[113]

Analysts have commented that delays in indemnifying manufacturers threatened the availability of swine flu vaccine in 1976, while delays in providing for injury compensation compromised voluntary participation in the civilian smallpox vaccine campaign in 2003. A successful emergency vaccination campaign may depend on resolving both policy concerns expediently.

Influenza as a Weapon

In the late 1990s, Congress authorized the Select Agent program to track the movement of certain bacteria and viruses that could potentially be used as biological weapons.[114] The program, which is administered by CDC and the U.S. Department of Agriculture, was expanded in statute following the anthrax attacks of 2001. An interagency working group determines which pathogens to place on the list of Select Agents. Once an organism is listed, those individuals and facilities working with it must be registered, undergo background investigations, and follow various guidelines in facility maintenance and management, shipping, recordkeeping and other practices. The list does not include common human strains of influenza, though it does include highly pathogenic strains of avian influenza, i.e., strains which are shown to cause disease in commercial poultry. As such, H5N1 influenza is a listed pathogen. When scientists from the CDC and the Armed Forces Institute of Pathology recently re-created the 1918 pandemic flu virus, since it was a human influenza virus, it was not on the Select Agent list. It was subsequently added by HHS Secretary Leavitt on October 20, 2005.[115] Other flu strains that typically affect humans (rather than birds) remain unregulated at this time.

When asked about the possibility that influenza viruses could be used deliberately as biological weapons, CDC Director Julie Gerberding replied, "... we recognize that influenza has some of the important characteristics of an excellent threat agent. It's easily transmissible, it's relatively easy to produce and it's very easy to modify or engineer. So it does have characteristics that if a person was intent on modifying ..., it is not beyond our imagination to consider that beyond our preparedness efforts."[116] Dr. Gerberding also noted the natural behavior of the virus, which constantly shuffles its genes to produce new combinations, saying that "mother nature herself is a very effective terrorist."

If H5N1 avian flu were to cause a human pandemic, it would be reasonable to assume it was a natural event. Nonetheless, since influenza viruses are amenable to intentional manipulation, the Implementation Plan states that in the event of a pandemic, "The Federal Bureau of Investigation (FBI) will closely monitor events through coordination with the [CDC] and take appropriate action in the event that it is suspected that there was deliberate human intervention in the spread of the pandemic."[117]

End Notes

[1] Adapted from HHS, "Flu Terms Defined," at [http://www.pandemicflu.gov].

[2] World Organization for Animal Health (known by its French acronym, OIE), "Update on Avian Influenza in Animals in Asia (Type H5)," at [http://www.oie.int/downld/AVIAN% 20INFLUENZA/A_AI-Asia.htm]. OIE is an intergovernmental organization of 167 nations and is not part of the United Nations system.

[3] World Health Organization, "Confirmed Human Cases of Avian Influenza A/(H5N1)," as of Feb 19, 2007, at [http://www.who.int/csr/disease/avian_influenza/country/en/].

[4] WHO, "Global Influenza Preparedness Plan: The Role of WHO and Recommendations for National Measures before and during Pandemics," 2005, (hereafter called the WHO pandemic plan), p. 3, at [http://www.who.int/csr/disease/influenza/pandemic/en/].

[5] See [http://www.pandemicflu.gov/].

[6] Remarks of HHS Secretary Michael Leavitt on "Avian Flu," National Press Club, Oct. 27, 2005, CQ Transcriptions.

[7] See CRS Report RS22453, *Avian Flu Pandemic: Potential Impact of Trade Disruptions*, by Danielle Langton.

[8] For more information, see CRS Report RL33 579, *The Public Health and Medical Response to Disasters: Federal Authority and Funding*, by Sarah A. Lister.

[9] David L. Heymann, *Control of Communicable Diseases Manual*, 18th ed., an official report of the American Public Health Association, 2004; and the Centers for Disease Control and Prevention (CDC) influenza home page, at [http://www.cdc.gov/flu/].

[10] WHO, Current WHO Phase of Pandemic Alert, as of February 20, 2007, at [http://www.who.int/csr/disease/avian_influenza/phase/en/index.html].

[11] Unless otherwise noted, information for this section is found on the U.S. federal government pandemic flu website, at [http://www.pandemicflu.gov/].

[12] The U.S. population in 1918 was about one-third its current size, based on decennial census reports of more than 92 million in 1910, and more than 106 million in 1920. The U.S. population is currently slightly more than 300 million. See [http://www.census.gov].

[13] Sources for this section are: Richard E. Neustadt and Harvey V. Fineberg, *The Swine Flu Affair,* a report to the Secretary of Health, Education and Welfare, June, 1978; and HHS Draft Pandemic Influenza Preparedness and Response Plan, Annex 11: "Lessons Learned from 1976 Swine Influenza Program," Aug. 2004. This incident is discussed further in a later section on vaccine liability and compensation issues.

[14] NIH, National Institute for Allergy and Infectious Diseases (NIAID), "H9N2 Avian Flu Vaccine Paired with Adjuvant Provokes Strong Human Immune Response at Low Doses," Sept. 25, 2006, at [http://www.nih.gov/news/].

[15] WHO, "Confirmed Human Cases of Avian Influenza A (H5N1)," at [http://www.who.int/csr/disease/avian _influenza/country/en/].

[16] WHO pandemic plan, p. 3.

[17] This phenomenon is often called a "cytokine storm," named after molecules in the immune system that are produced in excess. See Zhou, J, et al., "Differential Expression of Chemokines and their Receptors in Adult and Neonatal Macrophages Infected with Human or Avian Influenza Viruses," *Journal of Infectious Diseases,* vol. 194(1), pp. 61-70, July, 2006; and De Jong MD, et al., "Fatal Outcome of Human Influenza A (H5N1) is Associated with High Viral Load and Hypercytokinemia (letter), *Nature Medicine,* vol. 12, pp. 1203-1207, Nov. 2006.

[18] D. Kobasa, et al., "Enhanced Virulence of Influenza A Viruses with the Haemagglutinin of the 1918 Pandemic Virus," *Nature* vol. 431, Oct. 7, 2004, pp. 703-707.

[19] See Jeffery K. Taubenberger, et al., "Characterization of the 1918 Influenza Virus Polymerase Genes," *Nature,* vol. 437, pp. 889-893, Oct. 6, 2005; and Terrence M. Tumpey, et al., "Characterization of the Reconstructed 1918 Spanish Influenza Pandemic Virus," *Science,* vol. 310, Oct. 2005, pp. 77-80.

[20] Bosman, et al., "Final Analysis of Netherlands Avian Influenza Outbreaks Reveals Much Higher Levels of Transmission to Humans than Previously Thought," *Eurosurveillance Weekly,* vol. 10(1), Jan. 6, 2005, at [http://www.eurosurveillance.org/index-02.asp].

[21] WHO, "Avian Influenza A(H7) Human Infections in Canada," Apr. 5, 2004, at [http://www.who.int/c sr/don/en/]; and CDC, "Avian Influenza Infections in Humans," Oct. 17, 2005, at [http://www.cdc.gov/flu/avian/gen-info/avian-flu-humans.htm].

[22] A.J. Hostetler and Calvin Trice, "Va. Worker May Have Caught Avian Flu," *Richmond Times-Dispatch,* Feb. 28, 2004.

[23] See CDC website on avian flu outbreaks in North America at [http://www.cdc.gov/ flu/avian/outbreaks/past.htm#nahumans].

[24] HHS "Pandemic Influenza Plan," Part 1: Strategic Plan, p. 18, Nov. 2005, at [http://www.pandemicflu.gov].

[25] Trust for America's Health (TFAH), *A Killer Flu?,* June 2005, at [http://healthyamericans.org/reports/flu/], applies a set of assumptions and ranges of severity to a CDC-developed computer model, FluAid 2.0, to generate death, hospitalization and outpatient rates based on populations with different age distributions.

[26] M. I. Meltzer et al., "The Economic Impact of Pandemic Influenza in the United States: Priorities for Intervention," *Emerging Infectious Diseases,* vol. 5(5), Sept.-Oct. 1999.

[27] Congressional Budget Office, "A Potential Influenza Pandemic: Possible Macroeconomic Effects and Policy Issues," Dec. 8, 2005, revised July 27, 2006.

[28] The World Bank Group, "Avian Flu: Economic Losses Could Top US$800 Billion," Nov. 8, 2005, at [http://www.worldbank.org/].

[29] International Monetary Fund, "The Global Economic and Financial Impact of an Avian Flu Pandemic and the Role of the IMF," Feb. 28, 2006, at [http://www.imf.org/external/ pubs/ft/afp/2006/eng/022806.htm].

[30] CBO, "A Potential Influenza Pandemic: An Update on Possible Macroeconomic Effects and Policy Issues," p. 1, May 22, 2006, revised July 27, 2006.

[31] Warwick J. McKibben, "SARS: Estimating the Economic Impacts," Institute of Medicine, Forum on Microbial Threats, Workshop, "Learning from SARS: Preparing for the Next Disease Outbreak," Sept. 30, 2003, at [http://www.iom.edu/event.asp?id=14647].

[32] CBO, "A Potential Influenza Pandemic: Possible Macroeconomic Effects and Policy Issues," p. 11, Dec. 8, 2005, revised July 27, 2006.

[33] WHO pandemic plan, at [http://www.who.int/csr/disease/influenza/pandemic/en/].

[34] See [http://www.pandemicflu.gov/].

[35] With the release of the strategic plan, President Bush sent a request to Congress for $7.1 billion in emergency spending for the departments of HHS, Agriculture, Defense, Homeland Security, Interior, State and Veterans Affairs, and the U.S. Agency for International Development. For more information, see CRS Report RS22576, *Pandemic Influenza: Appropriations for Public Health Preparedness and Response,* by Sarah A. Lister.

[36] This position has been redesignated as the Assistant Secretary for Preparedness and Response, pursuant to P.L. 109-417.

[37] Though the plan includes specific tiers of priority groups, and estimates of the number of people in each group, the designations may be modified in light of the actual behavior of a pandemic flu strain. For example, if atypical groups such as healthy young people were found to be at increased risk of severe illness, the tiers could be adjusted accordingly.

[38] Department of Defense, "Pandemic Influenza Preparation and Response Planning Guidance," Sept. 15, 2004, at [http://www.geis.fhp.osd.mil/GEIS/SurveillanceActivities/ Influenza/fluPolicy.asp].

[39] According to cooperative agreement guidance for FY2004 funds, states were required to submit pandemic plans along with their applications for FY2005 funds. See CDC, "Cooperative Agreement Guidance for Public Health Emergency Preparedness," Program Announcement AA 154, May 13, 2005, at [http://www.bt.cdc.gov/planning/guidance05/].

[40] The Conference Board, "Most Companies Planning for an Avian Flu Pandemic, but Outcomes Remain Uncertain," press release, July 6, 2006, at [http://www.conference-board. org/utilities/press. cfm].

[41] Ibid.

[42] For more information, see CRS Report RL33219, *U.S. and International Responses to the Global Spread of Avian Flu: Issues for Congress*, by Tiaji Salaam-Blyther. See also, Department of Defense Global Emerging Infections Surveillance and Response System (DoD-GEIS), at [http://www.geis.fhp.osd.mil/aboutGEIS.asp].

[43] HHS anticipates that its efforts to establish adequate domestic surge capacity for flu vaccine production will continue through 2013. See Testimony of Gerald W. Parker, Principal Deputy Assistant Secretary, Office of the Assistant Secretary for Preparedness and Response, HHS, hearing on "Pandemic Flu: Progress Made and Challenges Ahead," before the U.S. Senate Committee on Appropriations, Subcommittee on Labor, Health and Human Services, Education and Related Agencies, 110th Cong., 1st Sess., Jan. 24, 2007.

[44] See DHS, *National Response Plan*, Dec. 2004, hereafter called the NRP, at [http://www.dhs.gov/xprepresp/committees/editorial_0566.shtml], and CRS Report RL3 2803, *The National Preparedness System: Issues in the 109th Congress*, by Keith Bea.

[45] For more information on ESF-8, see CRS Report RL33579, *The Public Health and Medical Response to Disasters: Federal Authority and Funding*, by Sarah A. Lister.

[46] H.Rept. 109-359, to accompany H.R. 2863, Department of Defense, Emergency Supplemental Appropriations to Address Hurricanes in the Gulf of Mexico, and Pandemic Influenza Act, 2006, p. 523.

[47] CDC, "Pandemic Influenza Guidance Supplement: Phase 2," guidance for FY2006 funds, July 10, 2006, at [http://www.bt.cdc.gov/planning/coopagreement/].

[48] White House, "Press Gaggle after Avian Flu Tabletop Exercise with Homeland Security Advisor Fran Townsend, Secretary of Health and Human Services Michael Leavitt, and Secretary of Homeland Security Michael Chertoff," transcript, Dec. 10, 2005, at [http://www.whitehouse.gov/news/releases/2005/12/20051210-2.html.]

[49] The term *police powers* derives from the 10th Amendment to the Constitution, which reserves to the states those rights and powers not delegated to the United States. Historically these have been interpreted to include authority over public health and safety.

[50] For more information, see CRS Report RL33579, *The Public Health and Medical Response to Disasters: Federal Authority and Funding*, by Sarah A. Lister.

[51] For a discussion of the exercise of federal and state authorities in response to the shortage of influenza vaccine in 2004, see CRS Report RL32655, *Influenza Vaccine Shortages and Implications*, by Sarah A. Lister and Erin D. Williams. See also CRS Reports: RL3320 1, *Federal and State Quarantine and Isolation Authority*, by Kathleen S. Swendiman and Jennifer K. Elsea; RL33 609, *Quarantine and Isolation: Selected Legal Issues Relating to Employment*, by Nancy Lee Jones and Jon O. Shimabukuro; RS222 19, *The Americans with Disabilities Act (ADA) Coverage of Contagious Diseases*, by Nancy Lee Jones; and RS21414, *Mandatory Vaccinations: Precedent and Current Laws*, by Kathleen S. Swendiman.

[52] In addition, the NRP Biological Incident Annex notes that "Actions described in this annex take place with or without a presidential Stafford Act declaration or a public health emergency declaration" by the Secretary of HHS. See NRP, Biological Incident Annex, p. BIO-1. While this annex addresses intentional bioterrorism events, it also addresses naturally occurring biological threats, and explicitly mentions pandemic influenza. In contrast, the NRP Catastrophic Incident Annex does not explicitly mention pandemic influenza. While this annex is designed to address disasters with "extraordinary levels of mass casualties" such as could occur with a pandemic, it is also explicitly focused on "no-notice or short-notice incidents of catastrophic magnitude," a definition that would not likely apply to an influenza pandemic. See NRP, Catastrophic Incident Annex, p. CAT-1, and DHS, Notice of Change to the National Response Plan, May 25, 2006, pp. 9-10, at [http://www.dhs.gov/xprepresp/programs/].

[53] Implementation Plan, p. 37.

[54] See CRS Report RL33053, *Federal Stafford Act Disaster Assistance: Presidential Declarations, Eligible Activities, and Funding*, by Keith Bea.

[55] See DHS, Office of the Inspector General, *A Review of the Top Officials 3 Exercise*, Office of Inspections and Special Reviews, OIG-06-07, November 2005, p. 30, at [http://www.dhs.gov/xoig/rpts/mgmt/editorial_0334.shtml]. The anthrax attack in 2001 also did not result in a Stafford Act declaration.

[56] Implementation Plan, Appendix C, "Authorities and References," p. 212.

[57] Another key activity is the enhanced monitoring of avian flu in birds. The H5N1 strain of concern has not yet been detected in humans or birds in the United States. For more information on domestic monitoring in birds, see CRS Report RL33795, *Avian Influenza in Poultry and Wild Birds*, by Jim Monke and M. Lynne Corn.

[58] CDC, "Overview of Influenza Surveillance in the United States," June 26, 2006, at [http://www.cdc.gov/flu/weekly/pdf/flu-surveillance-overview.pdf].

[59] CDC, "Health Updates on Avian Influenza," June 7, 2006, and previous, at [http://www.cdc.gov/flu/avian/professional/updates.htm].

[60] J. R. Ortiz, et al., "No Evidence of Avian Influenza A (H5N1) among Returning U.S. Travelers," *Emerging Infectious Diseases*, vol. 13(2), Feb. 2007, at [http://www.cdc.gov/ EID/content/1 3/2/294.htm].

[61] An H5N1 influenza diagnostic test, developed by CDC, was approved by the Food and Drug Administration (FDA) and delivered to laboratories in the national Laboratory Response Network, which includes public health labs in all 50 states, many federal labs, and others, in February 2006. See [http://www.bt.cdc.gov/lrn/].

[62] CDC, "CDC Awards $11.4 Million to Develop New Rapid Diagnostic Tests for Avian Influenza," press release, Dec. 4, 2006.

[63] For more information, see CRS Report RL3320 1, *Federal and State Quarantine and Isolation Authority*, by Kathleen S. Swendiman and Jennifer K. Elsea. See also: CRS Reports RL33609, *Quarantine and Isolation: Selected Legal Issues Relating to Employment*, by Nancy Lee Jones and Jon O. Shimabukuro; and RS222 19, *The Americans with Disabilities Act (ADA) Coverage of Contagious Diseases*, by Nancy Lee Jones.

[64] See Executive Order: "Amendment to E.O. 13295 Relating to Certain Influenza Viruses and Quarantinable Communicable Diseases," Apr. 1, 2005, at [http://www.whitehouse.gov/ news/releases/2005/04/2005 0401 - 6.html]; and CDC, "Questions and Answers on the Executive Order Adding Potentially Pandemic Influenza Viruses to the List of Quarantinable Diseases," Apr. 11, 2005, at [http://www.cdc.gov/ncidod/dq/qa_influenza_ amendment_to_eo_1 3295 .htm].

[65] See CDC Division of Global Migration and Quarantine home page at [http://www.cdc. gov/ncidod/dq/index.htm].

[66] Press conference with President George Bush, Federal News Service transcript, Oct. 4, 2005.

[67] Christophe Fraser, et al., "Factors that Make an Infectious Disease Outbreak Controllable," *Proceedings of the National Academy of Sciences*, vol. 101(16), pp. 6146-6151, Apr. 20, 2004, at [http://www.pnas.org/cgi/reprint/1 01/16/6146].

[68] See, for example: the Models of Infectious Disease Agent Study (MIDAS), funded by the National Institutes of Health, at [http://www.nigms.nih.gov/Initiatives/MIDAS/]; and studies of the effectiveness of measures applied during the 1918 flu pandemic, conducted by Dr. Howard Markel with funding from the Defense Threat Reduction Agency, presented to the Institute of Medicine, workshop on "Ethical and Legal Considerations in Mitigating Pandemic Disease," Sept. 19, 2006, at [http://www.iom.edu/CMS/3783/3924/35857/ 37298.aspx].

[69] Implementation Plan, p. 108.

[70] Ibid, p. 109.

[71] CDC, "Interim Pre-pandemic Planning Guidance: Community Strategy for Pandemic Influenza Mitigation in the United States — Early Targeted Layered Use of Non-Pharmaceutical Interventions," Feb. 2007, at [http://www.pandemicflu.gov/].

[72] CRS Report RS2 1 322, *Homeland Security: Evolving Roles and Missions for United States Northern Command*, by Steve Bowman and James Crowhurst.

[73] NRP, "Defense Support of Civil Authorities," pp. 41 ff.

[74] CRS Report RS22266 , *The Use of Federal Troops for Disaster Assistance: Legal Issues*, by Jennifer K. Elsea.

[75] Information provided by Dr. Dale Smith, medical historian, Uniformed Services University of the Health Sciences, Bethesda, Maryland, Oct. 13, 2005.

[76] See CRS Report RS22453, *Avian Flu Pandemic: Potential Impact of Trade Disruptions*, by Danielle Langton.

[77] Charles M. Helms, NVAC Chairman, letter to HHS Acting Assistant Secretary for Health Cristina V. Beato, on NVAC recommendations regarding priority use of vaccine and antiviral drugs during an influenza pandemic, Aug. 10, 2005, at [http://www.hhs.gov/ nvpo/nvac/documents/chairletter.pdf].

[78] For further discussion, see CRS Report RL333 81, *The Americans with Disabilities Act (ADA): Allocation of Scarce Medical Resources During a Pandemic*, by Nancy Lee Jones, and the section on Strategies for Rationing in CRS Report RL32655, *Influenza Vaccine Shortages and Implications*, by Sarah A. Lister and Erin D. Williams.

[79] 71 *Federal Register* 75252, Dec. 14, 2006.

[80] These goals are: (1) stopping, slowing or otherwise limiting the spread of a pandemic to the United States; (2) limiting the domestic spread of a pandemic, and mitigating disease, suffering and death; and (3) sustaining infrastructure and mitigating impact to the economy and the functioning of society. National Strategy, p. 2.

[81] See HHS, "Request for Information (RFI): Guidance for Prioritization of Pre-pandemic and Pandemic Influenza Vaccine," at [http://aspe.hhs.gov/PIV/RFI/]; and CRS Report RL33381, *The Americans with Disabilities Act (ADA): Allocation of Scarce Medical Resources During a Pandemic*, by Nancy Lee Jones.

[82] Sec CRS Report RS22576, *Pandemic Influenza: Appropriations for Public Health Preparedness and Response*, by Sarah A. Lister.

[83] Implementation Plan," p. 9.

[84] David S. Fedson, "Preparing for Pandemic Vaccination: An International Policy Agenda for Vaccine Development," *Journal of Public Health Policy*, Vol. 26, pp. 4-29, 2005, (hereafter called Fedson article), at [http://www.palgrave-journals.com/jphp/fedson.pdf].

[85] The company does not use capital letters in its name.

[86] WHO, "WHO Reports Some Promising Results on Avian Influenza Vaccines," press release, Feb. 16, 2007, at [http://www.who.int/mediacentre/news/notes/2007/np07/en/ index.html].

[87] See testimony of Gerald W. Parker, Principal Deputy Assistant Secretary, Office of the Assistant Secretary for Preparedness and Response, HHS, hearing on "Pandemic Flu: Progress Made and Challenges Ahead," before the U.S. Senate Committee on Appropriations, Subcommittee on Labor, Health and Human Services, Education and Related Agencies, 110th Cong., 1st Sess., Jan. 24, 2007.

[88] Ibid. See, also, testimony of Anthony S. Fauci, Director, National Institute of Allergy and Infectious Diseases, National Institutes of Health, HHS, hearing on "Pandemic Flu: Progress Made and Challenges Ahead," before the U.S. Senate Committee on Appropriations, Subcommittee on Labor, Health and Human Services, Education and Related Agencies, 110th Cong., 1st Sess., Jan. 24, 2007; and CBO, "A Potential Influenza Pandemic: An Update on Possible Macroeconomic Effects and Policy Issues," p. 1, May 22, 2006, revised July 27, 2006.

[89] See, for example, the Fedson article.

[90] Donald G. McNeil Jr., "Indonesia and WHO in Accord on Flu Virus," *The International Herald Tribune*, Feb. 19, 2007.

[91] See "Global Solidarity Needed in Preparing for Pandemic Influenza," *The Lancet*, editorial, vol. 369, p. 532, Feb. 17, 2007; and WHO, "WHO Reports Some Promising Results on Avian Influenza Vaccines," press release, Feb. 16, 2007, at [http://www.who.int/ mediacentre/news/notes/2007/np07/en/index.html].

[92] Presentation of Jesse L. Goodman, Director, FDA Center for Biologics Evaluation and Research, "Meeting the Challenge of Pandemic Vaccine Preparedness: An FDA Perspective," at the Institute of Medicine Symposium on Pandemic Influenza Research, Apr. 5, 2005, at [http://www.iom.edu/project.asp?id=252 18]. See also Jennifer Corbett Dooren, "FDA Aims to Approve New Flu Treatments in Weeks," Dow Jones News Service, Nov. 4, 2005.

[93] Reverse genetics is a technique to modify viruses so they can be grown more easily for vaccine production. Cell culture is a streamlined method of growing large amounts of virus. Both techniques are explained in greater detail in CRS Report RL32655, *Influenza Vaccine Shortages and Implications*, by Sarah A Lister and Erin D. Williams.

[94] FDA, "Emergency Use Authorization of Medical Products," draft guidance, not for implementation, June 2005, at [http://www.fda.gov/oc/bioterrorism/emergency _use .html]. This emergency us e authority is somewhat broader than the Secretary's authority to declare a public health emergency. For more information, see the Appendix, "Federal Public Health Emergency Authorities," in CRS Report RL33579, *The Public Health and Medical Response to Disasters: Federal Authority and Funding*, by Sarah A. Lister.

[95] FDA, "Authorization of Emergency Use of Anthrax Vaccine Adsorbed for Prevention of Inhalation Anthrax by Individuals at Heightened Risk of Exposure Due to Attack With Anthrax; Availability," 70 *Federal Register* 5452, Feb. 2, 2005.

[96] See Statement from Medimmune, Inc., regarding reverse genetics technology, in "Reverse Genetics, Intellectual Property, and Influenza Vaccination," Institute of Medicine, *The Threat of Pandemic Influenza: Are We Ready? Workshop Summary*, p. 192 ff., Nov. 2004, at [http://www.iom.edu/CMS/3783/3924/23639.aspx].

[97] See CRS Report RL3 205 1: *Innovation and Intellectual Property Issues in Homeland Security*, by John R. Thomas. This authority is based in existing law and does not require an emergency declaration or other special circumstance.

[98] See CDC, antivirals for influenza, at [http://www.cdc.gov/flu/professionals/treatment/].

[99] See CRS Report RL33 159, *Influenza Antiviral Drugs and Patent Law Issues*, by Brian T. Yeh.

[100] National Strategy, p. 9.

[101] See Gardiner Harris, "Administration's Flu Plan Gets Mixed Reception in Congress," *The New York Times*, Nov. 3, 2005.

[102] Association of State and Territorial Health Officials, (ASTHO), "ASTHO Survey of State and Territorial Pandemic Influenza Antiviral Purchase and Stockpiling," Oct. 2006, at [http://www.astho.org/pubs/AntiviralSurvey121806.pdf]. Respondents included officials from all 50 states, the District of Columbia, and three territories.

[103] See, for example, Fu Jing, "Misuse of Antiviral on Poultry Must Stop," *China Daily*, June 21, 2005, at [http://www.chinadaily.com.cn/english/doc/2005-06/21/content_453023.htm].

[104] Q. Mai Le, "Avian Flu: Isolation of Drug-resistant H5N1 Virus," *Nature* 437, 1108 Oct. 20, 2005; and Luciana L. Borio and John G. Bartlett, "Isolation of H5N1 Influenza Virus Resistant to Oseltamivir," *Clinician's Biosecurity Network Weekly Bulletin*, Oct. 18, 2005.

[105] 71 *Federal Register* 14374-14377, Mar. 22, 2006.

[106] In addition, Tamiflu may, in some people, cause adverse effects that would require that it be discontinued. See CDC, "Antiviral Medications for Influenza," at [http://www.cdc.gov/ flu/professionals/treatment/].

[107] For more information, see the National Vaccine Injury Compensation Program Home Page at [http://www.hrsa.gov/vaccinecompensation/].

[108] 72 *Federal Register* 4710-4711, Feb. 1, 2007.

[109] For more information, see CRS Report RS22327, *Pandemic Flu and Medical Biodefense Countermeasure Liability Limitation,* by Henry Cohen.

[110] HHS, "Public Readiness and Emergency Preparedness Act (PREP Act) for Pandemic Influenza Medical Countermeasures Utilization Protocol & Decision Tools," Dec. 4, 2006, at [http://www.pandemicflu.gov/plan/federal/prep_act.html].

[111] See CRS Report RL3 1960, *Smallpox Vaccine Injury Compensation*, by Susan Thaul.

[112] Sources for this section are: Richard E. Neustadt and Harvey V. Fineberg, *The Swine Flu Affair*, a report to the Secretary of Health, Education and Welfare, June, 1978; and HHS Draft Pandemic Influenza Preparedness and Response Plan, Annex 11: "Lessons Learned from the 1976 Swine Influenza Program," Aug. 2004.

[113] U.S. Department of Justice, Civil Division, Torts Branch, "Swine Flu Statistics," Jan. 3, 1991. Overall, 4,179 claims were filed under the act. Not all claims were resolved administratively, and 1,604 claimants proceeded to file suit.

[114] For more information, see the CDC Select Agent program page at [http://www. cdc.gov/od/sap] and CRS Report RL3 1719, *An Overview of the U.S. Public Health System in the Context of Emergency Preparedness*, by Sarah A. Lister.

[115] CDC, "Possession, Use, and Transfer of Select Agents and Toxins - Reconstructed Replication Competent Forms of the 1918 Pandemic Influenza Virus Containing Any Portion of the Coding Regions of All Eight Gene Segments," 70 *Federal Register* 61047, Oct. 20, 2005.

[116] Testimony of CDC Director Julie Gerberding before the House Committee on Homeland Security, Subcommittee on Prevention of Nuclear and Biological Attacks, hearing on "National Biodefense Strategy," July 28, 2005, 109th Congress, 1st Sess.

[117] Implementation Plan, p. 156.

In: Influenza Pandemic - Preparedness and Response to ...   ISBN: 978-1-60692-953-7
Editor: Emma S. Brouwer pp.67-92   © 2010 Nova Science Publishers, Inc.

Chapter 3

PANDEMIC INFLUENZA: AN ANALYSIS OF STATE PREPAREDNESS AND RESPONSE PLANS

Sarah A. Lister and Holly Stockdale

SUMMARY

States are the seat of most authority for public health emergency response. Much of the actual work of response falls to local officials. However, the federal government can impose requirements upon states as a condition of federal funding. Since 2002, Congress has provided funding to all U.S. states, territories, and the District of Columbia, to enhance federal, state and local preparedness for public health threats in general, and an influenza ("flu") pandemic in particular. States were required to develop pandemic plans as a condition of this funding.

This chapter describes an approach to the analysis of state pandemic plans, and presents the findings of that analysis. State plans that were available in July 2006 were analyzed in eight topical areas: (1) leadership and coordination; (2) surveillance and laboratory activities; (3) vaccine management; (4) antiviral drug management; (5) other disease control activities; (6) communications; (7) healthcare services; and (8) other essential services. A history of federal funding and requirements for state pandemic planning is provided in an **Appendix**. This analysis is not intended to grade or rank individual state pandemic plans or capabilities. Rather, its findings indicate that a number of challenges remain in assuring pandemic preparedness, and suggest areas that may merit added emphasis in future planning efforts.

Generally, the plans analyzed here reflect their authorship by public health officials. They emphasize core public health functions such as disease detection and control. Other planning challenges, such as assuring surge capacity in the healthcare sector, the continuity of essential services, or the integrity of critical supply chains, may fall outside the authority of public health officials, and may require stronger engagement by emergency management officials and others in planning.

Since different threats — such as hurricanes, earthquakes or terrorism — are expected to affect states differently, many believe that states should have flexibility in emergency planning. This complicates federal oversight of homeland security grants to states, however. Which requirements should be imposed on all states? When is variability among states desirable, and when is it not? A flu pandemic is perhaps unique in that it would be likely to affect all states at nearly the same time, in ways that are fairly predictable. This may argue for a more directive federal role in setting pandemic preparedness requirements. But the matter of what the states should do to be prepared for a pandemic is not always clear. For example, uncertainties about the ways in which flu spreads, the lack of national consensus in matters of equity in rationing, and a long tradition of federal deference to states in matters of public health, all complicate efforts to set uniform planning requirements for states.

In addition to assuring the strength of planning efforts, readiness also depends on assuring that states can execute their plans. This assurance can be provided through analysis of the response during exercises, drills, and relevant real-world incidents. Such an analysis is not within the scope of this chapter.

BACKGROUND

In 1997, a new strain of avian influenza ("bird flu") — named H5N1 for its genetic makeup — emerged in Hong Kong and killed six people. It has since spread to other countries in Asia, Europe and Africa, where it has infected more than 300 people, killing more than half of them. The situation has raised concern about the possibility of a global human pandemic.[1] A flu pandemic of modest severity would strain public health and healthcare systems worldwide. And, although flu viruses do not directly harm physical infrastructure, a severe pandemic could nonetheless affect infrastructure and commerce through high absenteeism, supply chain disruptions, and other effects.

Public health functions in the United States are decentralized, with states in the lead for most public health authorities, such as disease surveillance and quarantine. In many states, local public health authority is also decentralized, not falling under the direct control of state health officials. The federal government provides funding, guidance and technical assistance to state and local planners, and can require that certain activities be carried out as a condition of funding. But the federal government has limited authority to precisely direct the planning efforts of states and localities.[2]

Because the states are the seat of most authority for public health and medical preparedness, national preparedness for public health threats depends, in part, on the preparedness of individual states. Pandemic planning at the federal, state and local levels is woven into broader "all-hazards" emergency planning, and the response to a pandemic would employ the same basic approaches to leadership, authority, coordination, assistance, and financing as with other incidents.[3] However, a flu pandemic would pose at least two challenges that may be unique to this threat, and that may merit specific attention in planning: the likelihood that all jurisdictions would be affected, at nearly the same time; and the potentially prolonged period — many months — during which a response posture would have to be maintained. The near-simultaneous nature of a pandemic would likely diminish the value of state-to-state mutual aid, an important tool in the response to localized incidents.[4]

The prolonged effects of a pandemic, coupled with potentially high absenteeism, could pose exceptional challenges in maintaining continuity of operations (COOP) for essential services, including, potentially, continuity of government.[5]

Since 2001, all states have received annual federal funding to plan for emergencies, including public health threats. Certain planning activities were required as a condition of the federal funds. These planning requirements have evolved from one year to the next. (See the **Appendix** for information regarding federal preparedness grants to states, and associated requirements.) But efforts to evaluate states' compliance with planning requirements, or the effectiveness of states' preparedness efforts in general, have not evolved concurrently.[6] This CRS report describes information that exists to date regarding evaluations of pandemic preparedness. It also presents an approach to the analysis of state pandemic plans, and the findings of that analysis.

CRS analyzed pandemic plans available as of July 2006. At that point, all states had been required to submit (to the U.S. Department of Health and Human Services) pandemic plans one year earlier, and all had done so. However, the states were not given specific direction regarding the content of the plans that were required in July 2005, and they were not required to update their plans during the subsequent grant funding cycle.[7] Since July 2006, states have received dedicated funding for pandemic preparedness through the federal public health and hospital preparedness grants, and additional guidance, emphasizing training and exercises, has been provided. Pandemic planning benchmarks have also been incorporated in a municipal homeland security grant program.

For additional background on the variety of pandemic planning activities discussed in this chapter, see the following CRS Reports:

- RL33145, *Pandemic Influenza: Domestic Preparedness Efforts;*
- RS22576, *Pandemic Influenza: Appropriations for Public Health Preparedness and Response;*
- RS22219, *The Americans with Disabilities Act (ADA) Coverage of Contagious Diseases;*
- RL3 3381, *The Americans with Disabilities Act (ADA): Allocation of Scarce Medical Resources During a Pandemic;*
- RL33201, *Federal and State Quarantine and Isolation Authority;*
- RL33609, *Quarantine and Isolation: Selected Legal Issues Relating to Employment;* and
- RS22453, *Avian Flu Pandemic: Potential Impact of Trade Disruptions.*

This analysis is not intended to grade or rank individual state pandemic plans or capabilities. Rather, its findings indicate that a number of challenges remain in assuring pandemic preparedness, and suggest areas that may merit added emphasis in future planning efforts.

CRS ANALYSIS: METHODS AND LIMITATIONS

In 2005, CRS retained a contractor, the National Opinion Research Center (NORC) at the University of Chicago,[8] to create a database that could be used to analyze state pandemic preparedness and response plans. NORC delivered the database to CRS, containing information abstracted from *one publicly available pandemic planning document* from each of the 50 states and the District of Columbia (DC), in August 2006.[9]

The most comprehensive publicly available document was used for analysis. Available documents varied, and included (1) comprehensive pandemic preparedness and response plans; (2) annexes to broader public health or emergency management plans; or (3) brief summaries of pandemic preparedness plans. Comprehensive pandemic plans were analyzed when available. When not, annexes were analyzed when available. Brief summaries were analyzed only when the other two options were not available. Broader public health or emergency management plans were not analyzed in any case. Often, they were not publicly available.

Of the 51 plans analyzed, 14 were referred to by the authoring state as draft pandemic plans, 14 as annexes to the state's all-hazards plan, and 13 as formally adopted influenza plans. Ten states did not specify.

The database was populated in July 2006. At that time, publication dates for the 51 plans ranged from 2002 through 2006, as follows:

- 2006: 29 plans;
- 2005: 16 plans, most pre-dating a key federal plan issued in November 2005;[10]
- 2004: 2 plans;
- 2003 and 2002: 1 plan each year; and
- Two plans were not dated.

A total of 66 variables were developed for analysis, to assess pandemic planning activities in the following eight topical areas:

(1) Leadership and Coordination;
(2) Surveillance and Laboratory Activities;
(3) Vaccine Management;
(4) Antiviral Drug Management;
(5) Other Disease Control Activities (e.g., isolation and quarantine);
(6) Communications Activities;
(7) Healthcare Services; and
(8) Other Essential Services (e.g., public utilities).

The 66 variables are *dichotomous*, that is, for each variable, plans were determined to contain substantive mention of a particular activity ("yes") or not ("no").[11] Variables were developed by CRS and the contractor to span a spectrum of pandemic planning activities. They were intended to reflect a variety of public health preparedness activities that were presented in federal pandemic planning guidance documents available at the time,[12] as well as a number of planning challenges and potential planning gaps that were the subject of ongoing policy discussions. While each individual variable was intended to reflect an essential element of pandemic preparedness, CRS did not attempt to weigh the relative importance of each variable with respect to the others.

The findings of this analysis are subject to a number of limitations. *First,* variables were developed intentionally to reveal planning gaps, rather than to document the universe of activities that may be described in the plans, or that may have been discussed in grant guidance. (See the Appendix.) *Second,* certain planning elements (e.g., reporting relationships between the health department and the governor, or plans for mass fatality management) may not be fleshed out in the pandemic plan, but may be laid out in a state's public health preparedness or general emergency management plan. These broader plans were not analyzed, and in many cases were (and are) not publicly available.

Third, some states have published only brief summaries of extant pandemic plans that are not publicly available. By their nature, these summaries did not typically make substantive mention of planning activities. *Fourth,* certain preparedness and response tasks may be delegated to local officials, and may not, therefore, be described in the state pandemic plan.[13] *Fifth,* states may have developed detailed operational plans for certain aspects of pandemic planning (such as ventilator triage), but may not have included them in the pandemic plan, or may not have updated the pandemic plan to reflect these narrowly tailored documents.

Sixth, while analyses began with keyword searches, "yes" findings were applied only to substantive discussions of relevant topics in the plan, not merely the finding of a keyword in a list, or another entry that lacked meaningful context for planning. While efforts were made to standardize analysis, these determinations were inherently subjective. *Finally,* this analysis reflects a snapshot in time, in what appears to be a dynamic national planning effort. The database contains state pandemic plans available as of July 2006. Since then, FY2006 supplemental funds for state pandemic preparedness were released, pandemic planning benchmarks were included in homeland security grant guidance, and at least 16 states have updated their pandemic plans.

Most of these limitations would have the likely effect of underestimating a state's planning efforts. Therefore, finding that a planning element is absent from a state's pandemic plan does not necessarily mean that the state has not addressed that element.

This analysis is not intended to grade or rank individual state pandemic plans or capabilities. There are not, at this time, the processes or standards to support such an evaluation. Rather, this analysis is premised on the idea that national preparedness for pandemic flu is, in part, dependent upon the preparedness of individual states. Variables in this analysis that yielded fewer "yes" responses overall may indicate areas that merit added emphasis in future planning efforts.

OTHER ANALYSES OF STATE PANDEMIC PLANNING

Analyses by Federal Agencies

Though the federal government has provided considerable funding and guidance for state pandemic preparedness, it has not published a comprehensive assessment of state pandemic planning efforts. Since FY2002, all states have received grants from two agencies in the

Department of Health and Human Services (HHS): the Centers for Disease Control and Prevention (CDC), to improve state and local public health capacity; and the Health Resources and Services Administration (HRSA), for hospital and healthcare system preparedness. The Department of Homeland Security (DHS) also provides preparedness grants to states and cities. A discussion of these grants, and associated federal requirements for pandemic planning, is provided in the **Appendix**. While each agency evaluates state compliance with those requirements, none has published assessments of states' performance.[14] The HHS Office of Inspector General has reported on the compliance of some individual states with certain requirements of the CDC and HRSA grants, but has not addressed pandemic planning specifically.[15] The White House Homeland Security Council has reported on federal progress to assist states in a variety of specific pandemic planning tasks laid out in the *National Strategy for Pandemic Influenza Implementation Plan* (Implementation Plan),[16] but has not evaluated state pandemic planning efforts.[17]

The Government Accountability Office (GAO) has published analyses of some aspects of federal pandemic preparedness,[18] but has not published a systematic analysis of state pandemic plans. GAO has also published analyses of the CDC public health and HRSA hospital preparedness grant programs, but these analyses have not included assessments of state pandemic preparedness.[19] GAO has not published information about the performance of individual states.

In 2006, DHS published the *Nationwide Plan Review*, the results of a comprehensive assessment of state preparedness for catastrophic events, regardless of cause.[20] While the review did not focus on pandemic preparedness, some of the methods used, and the findings, may nonetheless be of interest. DHS conducted its review in two phases: state self-assessments and validation site visits, conducted by teams of peer reviewers.[21] States were evaluated for a variety of benchmarks, and their planning status was graded as *fully, partially,* or *not sufficient*. Review teams focused on three health and medical benchmarks: (1) processes to maintain a patient tracking system; (2) procedures to license out-of-state medical volunteers; and (3) processes for mass fatality management. They found fewer than half of the states to be fully sufficient for each benchmark.[22] Results were published in aggregate (i.e., DHS did not publish the results for specific states).

Analyses by Nongovernmental Authors

Researchers from Research Triangle Institute International (RTI) published the findings of their analysis of 49 state pandemic plans, available as of early 2006, for planning elements including vaccination, surveillance and detection, and disease containment.[23] The authors found considerable variation among states, and posited two explanations: first, federalism, which places states in the lead in matters of public health; and second, limited scientific information about how flu is spread, and, therefore, which disease control practices are likely to be effective. The authors recommended that HHS publish more detailed planning guidance for states, and that there be more research on influenza, including the effect of interventions — such as use of masks and closure of schools — on disease transmission. Authors presented their findings for specific states for ten specific preparedness benchmarks, and published the findings for additional benchmarks in aggregate.

Trust for America's Health (TFAH), a not-for-profit public health advocacy group, has published annual "report cards" in which states were graded according to a set of preparedness criteria developed by the group.[24] As with prior reports, the 2006 report included primarily general — not pandemic-specific — public health criteria, but included a finding that four states do not test year-round for the flu, which is necessary to monitor for a pandemic outbreak. TFAH also created a model to assess potential economic losses caused by a severe pandemic, including state-bystate effects, and effects on 20 different industries, and on trade and worker productivity.[25] The model predicted that states with high levels of tourism and entertainment would be the hardest hit by the economic effects. Both reports included findings for specific states.

In December 2006, the Associated Press (AP) reported on the findings of interviews it conducted with health officials in every state regarding aspects of pandemic planning.[26] AP found that many states had not yet made investments of state funds for pandemic planning, but were reliant solely on federal funds. Health officials stressed that during a pandemic, shortages of healthcare workers would likely be the worst bottleneck in ramping up health system capacity. AP also found a lack of consensus on some planning elements, such as whether to close schools, or to stockpile antiviral drugs.

CRS ANALYSIS: RESULTS

The following sections tabulate and discuss findings for the 66 dichotomous variables. Findings of "yes" mean that a state pandemic plan makes substantive mention of the relevant subject matter. For each of the variables, 51 plans were analyzed. Tables are presented for each of eight topical areas studied. For most of the topical areas, plans were searched for *planning assumptions.* These are statements of generally accepted facts or circumstances that are used to achieve consistency and relevance in planning efforts, such as the assumption that a severe pandemic could result in absenteeism rates as high as 40%. Overarching planning assumptions for pandemic flu are provided in the HHS Pandemic Plan, and include the universal and near-simultaneous nature of a pandemic, and the expectation of shortages of vaccine and antiviral drugs.[27] In this analysis, state plans were searched for the presence of planning assumptions that were specific to the topical area being analyzed.

Leadership and Coordination

Often when emergency managers have reviewed the response to disasters, they have found the most serious shortcomings to involve unclear lines of authority, confusion about leadership, lack of mechanisms to coordinate multiple responding agencies, and other problems involving "command and control." In the 1970s, firefighters developed the *Incident Command System* (ICS) to address these problems in the management of rapidly moving wildfires. Since then, the nation's structures for coordinated incident response have evolved, incorporating lessons learned from a number of disasters and terrorist attacks. In 2002, Congress established DHS to serve as the focal point for the federal government's disaster preparedness and response activities, and tasked the Secretary of DHS to develop the

National Incident Management System (NIMS), to assure that responders from different jurisdictions and disciplines can work together effectively in disaster response. In addition, Congress has continued to refine the delegations of authority among key federal response agencies.[28] State response agencies have evolved similarly, and are in some cases required to adopt uniform emergency management practices as a condition of federal homeland security grant funding.

Table 1 presents the findings of this analysis for state designations of authority and coordinating mechanisms in the response to a flu pandemic. Generally, fewer than half of the plans made substantive mention of each of the leadership and coordination variables, such as the designation of specific responsible individuals or liaisons. About two-thirds of the plans mentioned the state's Emergency Operations Center and how it would be activated to coordinate response efforts during a pandemic.[29]

Only 16 of the plans mentioned the National Incident Management System (NIMS), though states were to address NIMS compliance as a requirement for FY2005 federal preparedness funds, made available in the spring of 2005.[30] Also, only 16 plans mentioned a possible role for the National Guard in pandemic response. Unless it is federalized, the National Guard is a state response asset under the control of the Governor.[31] There has been considerable discussion of the maintenance of civil order during a pandemic. While matters of incident management or deployment of the National Guard may be described in the state's general preparedness plan, a flu pandemic could have certain effects that are unlike other disasters. Hence, it could be helpful to describe specifically how the National Guard might be used, or how incident command could be established, during a pandemic. Only four state plans mentioned *both* NIMS and the National Guard.

Table 1. Leadership and Coordination

Leadership and Coordination Variable	No. of plans that address variable (N=51)
Provides general planning assumptions regarding pandemic flu	34
Designates a liaison between Health Department (HD) and Governor	10
Designates a liaison between HD and State Emergency Management Office	13
Designates an individual with authority to declare a public health emergency[a]	23
Mentions the National Incident Management System (NIMS)	16
Mentions role of the National Guard	16
Mentions NIMS *and* the National Guard	4
Mentions the State Emergency Operations Center (SEOC)	33
HD is represented in the SEOC	11
Healthcare system liaison is represented in the SEOC	6
Mentions pandemic flu exercises or drills	37

a. The designated individual is usually either the Governor or the State Health Official.

About three-fourths of the plans mentioned pandemic flu exercises or drills. States were required to conduct public health emergency response exercises, and to develop pandemic plans, as conditions of their FY2005 CDC public health grants, but they were not required, at that time, to conduct exercises specifically for a flu pandemic. As a requirement of FY2006 supplemental appropriations for pandemic flu, Congress called on the states to conduct pandemic flu exercises that would "enable public health and law enforcement officials to establish procedures and locations for quarantine, surge capacity, diagnostics, and communication."[32] CDC guidance accompanying the grants required states to test three aspects of pandemic response: control of community gatherings (e.g., school closings); medical surge capacity; and mass vaccination / mass prophylaxis.[33] The funds were made available to states in July 2006, the same time that the CRS pandemic plan database was constructed. While the requirement for multi-sector exercises by states is important, these exercises may be carried out individually by states. The only national multi-sector pandemic exercise reported to date has been a table-top simulation conducted by members of the Cabinet.[34]

Surveillance and Laboratory Activities

The CDC coordinates domestic surveillance for seasonal flu in people. State and local health departments and designated healthcare providers voluntarily report relevant information, such as laboratory results or hospital admissions, to several flu surveillance systems run by CDC. Information is gathered and analyzed weekly during the winter flu season. Monitoring for pandemic flu would be integrated into these existing systems. Key challenges in the rapid detection of novel flu viruses (i.e., those with "pandemic potential") are the vagueness of flu symptoms, which occur with many other diseases, and the difficulty in distinguishing specific flu strains of interest from the background of other strains commonly in circulation.[35]

Table 2 presents the findings of this analysis for state surveillance and laboratory activities in pandemic planning. Twenty-seven plans mentioned laboratory-based surveillance for flu-like illness. However, many of the plans predate 2006, when CDC reported that public health labs in all 50 states and the District of Columbia have the capability to test for H5N1 influenza.[36] Most state plans incorporated planning assumptions to guide flu surveillance. However, most state plans did not mention integration of human and animal flu surveillance data, or the use of "syndromic surveillance" to track flu.[37]

Table 2. Surveillance and Laboratory Activities

Surveillance and Laboratory Activities Variable	No. of plans that address variable (N=51)
Provides planning assumptions regarding surveillance	40
Mentions capacity to perform lab-based surveillance for flu-like illness	27
Mentions linkage of human and animal flu surveillance data	19
Mentions (existing or planned) use of syndromic surveillance to track flu	23

A previously published analysis of 49 state pandemic plans found that there was considerable variation among states in planning for surveillance and detection; all states planned to utilize some or all of the existing flu surveillance mechanisms during a pandemic; and few state plans mentioned procedures to screen arriving international travelers for influenza.[38]

Vaccine Management

Vaccination is considered the best preventive measure for influenza. But, because of continuous changes in the genes of flu viruses, vaccines must be "matched" to specific strains to provide good protection. Flu vaccine is currently produced using a time-consuming process with a six-month lead time. In the early months of a pandemic, vaccine would be in short supply. Policymakers have struggled to develop the best approaches for vaccine rationing when there are competing goals: maximizing lives saved, assuring the continuity of essential services, and maintaining perceptions of fairness, for example.[39]

Table 3 presents the findings of this analysis for variables regarding vaccine management before and during a pandemic.

While about two-thirds of the state plans discussed the matter of priority groups, only six attempted to enumerate the individuals in each group. Enumerating those in priority groups (i.e., knowing how many of a state's residents fall within each of the priority groups) is essential in executing a state's priority plan. Without that information, it would not be possible to match the magnitude of need to the actual number of doses of vaccine available, and to properly advise officials and the public regarding who should report for, request, or be given vaccination at specific points in time.

Table 3. Vaccine Management

Vaccine Management Variable	No. of plans that address variable (N=51)
Provides planning assumptions regarding vaccine management	28
Identifies priority groups	33
Identifies and enumerates priority groups	6
Describes plan for vaccine distribution	36
Describes multiple contingency plans for vaccine distribution	12
Describes plan for vaccine storage	20
Describes plan for vaccine security	17
Describes plan to implement Investigational New Drug (IND) protocol	15
Describes plan to track dose parity (first or second dose for an individual)	13
Describes plan to track vaccine-associated adverse events (VAEs)	34
Describes plan for IND protocol *and* tracking vaccine parity *and* VAEs	6
Delegates aspects of vaccine management and logistics to local HD	8

This analysis did not attempt to describe vaccine priority schemes for those states that proposed them. A previously published analysis of state pandemic plans found that most states planned to comport with vaccine priority guidelines laid out in the HHS Pandemic Plan[40] (if the state plan was published after the HHS plan), or with earlier federal recommendations.[41] In general, these federal recommendations call for healthcare workers, and sometimes other first responders, to be vaccinated first, in order that they can remain at work and not make others ill. Next in order of priority are those most vulnerable to serious complications from flu, based on annual experience with seasonal flu. Some have criticized this approach, saying that it fails to address other legitimate planning goals, such as the continuity of essential services, vaccination of populations that are most likely to spread flu, or the apparent poor immune response to the vaccine among some individuals in vulnerable priority groups.[42] A 2006 analysis of pandemic plans from 45 countries found marked variability in proposed vaccine priority schemes, in particular with respect to the priority ranking assigned to children, further demonstrating the lack of scientific and cultural consensus on this matter.[43]

While about three-fourths of state plans discussed vaccine procurement and distribution, 12 states appear to have kept their options open, and have planned to distribute vaccine, or coordinate its distribution, according to several different possible procurement scenarios. Fewer than half of the state plans discussed vaccine storage or security.

States' efforts to plan for vaccine procurement and distribution during a pandemic may have been complicated by uncertainty about the ways in which vaccine may be made available to states. To date, efforts to develop and stockpile candidate *pre-pandemic* (unmatched prototype) vaccines have been federally funded, and the vaccines are not commercially available. But it is not clear that the federal government would purchase matched vaccine during a pandemic. While having centralized control could simplify planning efforts, it could also carry significant cost for the federal government unless it were possible to use collateral financing sources — such as Medicare and private health insurance — when available to pay for the vaccine. The HHS Pandemic Plan states that during a pandemic, vaccine would be made available through existing commercial channels and distribution mechanisms.[44] This is the same system that has come under fire during recent shortages of seasonal flu vaccine, because of the difficulties faced by public health officials in trying to locate and redirect available vaccine to priority groups. In 2006, Congress passed the Pandemic and All-Hazards Preparedness Act (P.L. 109-4 17), which authorizes the Secretary of HHS, with the voluntary cooperation of manufacturers, wholesalers, and distributors, to track the initial distribution of federally purchased flu vaccine during a pandemic.[45]

If a pandemic were to spread swiftly, vaccine may be pressed into service before standard safety and efficacy tests could be completed. Such unlicensed vaccine could be used under the Food and Drug Administration's (FDA's) Investigational New Drug (IND) provisions.[46] These include requirements for strict inventory control, record keeping, informed consent, and adverse event tracking, all of which would pose an additional challenge for public health officials during a vaccination campaign. In addition, two doses of a pandemic flu vaccine may be needed to provide optimal protection. Consequently, an individual's "vaccine parity" — whether he or she has received no vaccine, one dose, or two doses — is vital information to assure the effective use of this finite resource within a population. As shown in **Table 3**, while two-thirds of state plans discussed vaccine adverse event tracking, most did not address the conduct of IND protocols or tracking of vaccine parity, and only six plans discussed all three planning elements.

Eight state plans made explicit mention that planning for vaccine management was delegated to local health departments. As with emergency response in general, local authorities would be responsible for carrying out most of the actual operations in a vaccination campaign, so coordination between state pandemic plans and local efforts is critical.

Antiviral Drug Management

Since "matched" pandemic flu vaccine would be unavailable in the early stages of a pandemic, governments and private parties have been interested in drugs that could treat or prevent serious illness from flu. The federal government has set a goal to stockpile antiviral medications adequate to treat 75 million persons (one-fourth of the population), divided between federal and state stockpiles.[47] States were expected to procure 31 million of the 75 million treatment courses, for which HHS would reimburse 25% of the cost. A May 2007 survey of state health officials found that 24 of them did not yet have sufficient funding from other sources to purchase the planned amounts of antiviral drugs.[48]

Table 4 presents the findings of this analysis for states' management of antiviral drugs before and during a pandemic. Many of the variables — such as the designation and enumeration of priority groups, and plans for distribution and security — are similar to those developed to analyze vaccine management.

Table 4. Antiviral Drug Management

Antiviral Drug Management Variable	No. of plans that address variable (N=51)
Provides planning assumptions regarding antiviral drug management	28
Priority groups identified	29
Priority groups specific for antiviral drugs	14
Priority groups same as for vaccine	15
Priority groups identified and enumerated	7
Describes plan for antiviral drug distribution	37
Distribution plan is specific for antiviral drugs	26
Distribution plan is same as for vaccine	11
Describes plan for drug storage	8
Describes plan for drug security	12
Creates a database or other antiviral drug tracking mechanism	17
Describes plan to implement Investigational New Drug (IND) protocol	8
Describes plan to track drug-associated adverse events	25
Describes plan for IND protocol *and* VAEs	6

In designating priority groups for antiviral drugs, HHS has proposed a slightly different scheme than that for vaccines, beginning with treatment for those who are admitted to hospitals with severe illness from flu.[49] Priority categories are otherwise fairly similar to those for vaccine. While 29 state plans addressed priorities for antiviral drugs, only seven enumerated the priority groups.

Almost three-fourths of the state plans discussed plans for antiviral drug distribution, though fewer than half of them discussed plans for storage, security, or tracking.

If unlicensed antiviral drugs were used under emergency authorities during a pandemic, their use would require Investigational New Drug (IND) protocols, including adverse event tracking, as discussed earlier with respect to vaccines. Most state plans did not address the implementation of IND protocols for unlicensed antiviral drugs, but about half of the plans did mention adverse event tracking, which could be useful whether the drugs used are licensed or unlicensed.

Other Disease Control Activities

In the United States, isolation and quarantine authority is generally based in state rather than federal law.[50] While isolation and quarantine were crucial in the worldwide response to SARS, these methods are less likely to be successful in controlling influenza. Influenza has a shorter incubation period than SARS, and is often contagious in the absence of symptoms or before symptoms appear, making it difficult to identify persons who should be quarantined. **Table 5** presents the findings of this analysis regarding the use of isolation, quarantine, and other so-called *non-pharmaceutical interventions* (NPI, i.e., interventions not involving drugs or vaccines) during a pandemic.

More than half of the plans discussed isolation and quarantine procedures whether voluntary or compulsory. Twenty one plans identified the state official who has authority to compel isolation and quarantine, though only two discussed the use of judicial review to assure the protection of civil liberties if such orders were made. Whether this signals a gap in state legal preparedness for public health threats, skepticism about the utility of constraining individual movement to limit the spread of pandemic flu, or other factors, cannot be determined from this analysis. Since the 2001 terrorist attacks, states have been active in revising their public health authorities, though the scope of authorities regarding disease control still varies from state to state.[51]

Table 5. Other Disease Control Activities

Other Disease Control Activities Variable	No. of plans that address variable (N=51)
Describes procedures for isolation and quarantine	29
Identifies locations for isolation and quarantine	9
Identifies individual(s) with authority to compel isolation and quarantine	21
Describes procedures for judicial review of due process protections	2
Describes plans for "snow days" or other social distancing measures	16

Only nine plans discussed designated locations in which isolation and quarantine could be carried out, and for several of them, "home" was the designated location. This comports with the planning assumption that the healthcare workforce could be overwhelmed during a pandemic of even modest severity. Those who were sufficiently ill could receive care, under feasible isolation protocols, within healthcare facilities. (These may include *alternate* facilities, which are discussed later in the section on healthcare services.) Those who were exposed but not ill, or who were mildly ill, would remain at home, receiving care from family and friends. Few plans discussed the use of large, congregate isolation or quarantine facilities for pandemic flu.

Fewer than one-third of the plans provided substantive descriptions of large- scale social distancing measures. Such measures include so-called "snow days," in which communities would close schools, cease non-essential operations, and enact other protocols that would have the effect of keeping people at home. In February 2007, after the creation of the CRS database, CDC published a planning guide for the phased use of interventions not involving drugs or vaccines, including isolation and quarantine, school closures, liberal work leave policies, and teleworking strategies.[52]

Communications Activities

Since FY2002, states have been required to develop plans for public health emergency risk communication (i.e., communication to the public). A flu pandemic would likely affect jurisdictions throughout the United States, though timing, severity, and other aspects of the outbreak could vary considerably. That complicates the delivery of a unified message. Public confidence could erode if neighboring jurisdictions recommended different approaches to school and business closures, though each jurisdiction's decision may be sound. Successful management of a pandemic would require public cooperation, especially if resources of various kinds were to become scarce. The HHS Pandemic Plan notes that effective risk communication during a pandemic could, among other things, help set realistic public expectations of the healthcare system, and promptly address rumors, inaccuracies and misperceptions.[53] States can offer considerable assistance to localities in managing public communication, such as maintaining a common website, and making experts and spokespersons available. **Table 6** presents the findings of this analysis regarding public communications during a pandemic.

About two-thirds of the plans designated the individual who would serve as the lead public information official. In most cases in which it could be determined, the designated individual was an employee of the state health department. Some plans mentioned the creation of a joint communications function (consistent with the National Incident Management System), in which the health department communications official would report to another public information officer, who would lead the state's multi-sector response.[54] Plans did not always explicitly address other aspects of public communication during a pandemic, namely: training and outreach to other responders; monitoring of information from official sources; maintenance of websites and other public information resources; or individual and family preparedness.

Table 6. Communications Activities

Communications Variable	No. of plans that address variable (N=51)
Provides planning assumptions regarding public communication	26
Designates a lead public information officer	34
Describes training or outreach to emergency response groups	17
Describes plan to monitor information from WHO, CDC, other official sources	30
Mentions websites, hotlines or other public information resources	30
Mentions individual / family preparedness	20

Healthcare Services

There is a growing concern that medical surge capacity could be the Achilles' heel of pandemic preparedness.[55] To contain costs, much of the nation's healthcare system functions at full capacity under normal conditions, and relies on a "just-intime" supply chain. The healthcare sector is also largely under private ownership, generally beyond the purview, and often beyond the expertise, of the public health officials who lead pandemic preparedness efforts. Though there are federal and state efforts to stockpile vaccines, drugs, ventilators, and other supplies, the healthcare workforce is likely to be the key limiting factor in ramping up healthcare service delivery during a pandemic.

An influenza pandemic of even limited magnitude has the potential to disrupt the normal workings of the healthcare system in a variety of ways. These may include deferral of elective medical procedures; diversion of patients away from overwhelmed hospital emergency departments and tertiary care facilities; protective quarantines of susceptible populations such as residents of long-term care facilities; and hoarding, theft or black-marketeering of scarce resources such as vaccines or antiviral drugs. The system's usual approaches to mass casualty management involve bringing in additional workers from other states, and diverting or evacuating patients to unaffected facilities. Because flu is a communicable disease, and because a pandemic could affect large areas of the United States simultaneously, these approaches may be ineffective, or even harmful, during a pandemic.

Options to expand healthcare capacity during a pandemic include stockpiling supplies beforehand (with considerable up-front cost), and *altering standards of care*, that is, implementing policies that change the way medicine is practiced. Approaches to altered standards of care include providing healthcare at alternate sites, such as gymnasiums; changing required staffing ratios; altering scopes of practice (e.g., permitting a nurse to perform certain procedures that normally could only be performed by a physician); withholding of certain services, such as diagnostic tests; and rationing of services. **Table 7** presents the findings of this analysis for variables regarding the provision of healthcare services during a pandemic.

Table 7. Healthcare Services

Healthcare Services Variable	No. of plans that address variable (N=51)
Mentions planning assumptions regarding healthcare services	26
Mentions deployment of the Strategic National Stockpile	35
Mentions stockpiling of routine drugs and supplies	22
Mentions stockpiling of antiviral drugs	20
Mentions procurement of medical supplies during a pandemic	19
Mentions plan for medical surge capacity	22
Mentions plan for health workforce surge capacity	10
Mentions alternate care sites	20
Mentions plan for altered standards of care	8
Mentions plan to monitor utilization and capacity (e.g., hospital beds)	7
Mentions plan for psycho-social support / mental health services for citizens	29
Mentions psycho-social support / mental health services for responders	18
Mentions mass fatality management	17

Most state plans discussed deployment of the Strategic National Stockpile (SNS), a civilian stockpile of drugs and supplies maintained by CDC for distribution to state officials during emergencies.[56] States were required to plan and exercise for receipt and distribution of SNS contents as a condition of their public health preparedness grants. This mechanism may be used to distribute vaccines and/or antiviral drugs during a pandemic. But the federal stockpile could not contain the amounts and variety of drugs and medical supplies needed to sustain general healthcare services across the nation during a pandemic. Fewer than half of state plans discussed state or local stockpiling of drugs and supplies, or their procurement during a pandemic in the event that supply chains were disrupted.

Fewer than half of state plans discussed each of several other approaches to expand healthcare capacity during a pandemic, including plans for: medical surge capacity in general; health workforce surge capacity; the use of alternate healthcare sites; altering standards of care; and tracking of capacity and utilization.[57]

While slightly more than half of the plans discussed providing for the mental health and psycho-social support needs of citizens, only about one-third of plans addressed this planning element specifically for responders.

Also, only one-third of the plans mentioned the management of mass fatalities. According to the HHS Pandemic Plan, a moderate pandemic could result in an estimated 209,000 deaths nationwide, and a severe pandemic, like that in 1918, could result in an estimated 1.9 million deaths.[58]

Other Essential Services

A severe pandemic could cause high absenteeism, with disruption of essential services, supply chains, and other consequences beyond the public health and healthcare sectors. The Secretary of HHS, Michael Leavitt, has said, "If a pandemic hits our shores, it will affect almost every sector of our society, not just health care, but transportation systems, workplaces, schools, public safety and more. It will require a coordinated government-wide response, including federal, state and local governments, and it will require the private sector and all of us as individuals to be ready."[59]

Following release of the National Strategy and the HHS Pandemic Plan in November 2005, HHS Secretary Michael Leavitt and other federal officials hosted pandemic planning summits in all 50 states, to support states' multi-sector planning activities. In July 2006, the National Governors Association, Center for Best Practices, developed a pandemic planning guide for governors and senior state officials,[60] and, in April 2007, launched a series of regional workshops to examine state pandemic planning in a number of non-health areas.[61] The workshops were designed to help governors' staff and state agencies examine issues such as governance; maintenance of essential services; and the coordination of response strategies among levels of government and across borders during a pandemic.

Table 8 presents the findings of this analysis regarding the continuity of services other than public health and healthcare services, during and after a pandemic. Findings show that few state plans mentioned other essential services during a pandemic, including planning assumptions for the continuity of essential services; emergency food distribution; the continuity of essential services, including public utilities; and the re-establishment of routine functions, such as schools and businesses, as a pandemic recedes.

CONCLUSIONS AND REMAINING ISSUES

The variables reported in this analysis were developed to reflect common concerns in pandemic flu planning, and to highlight gaps. Findings of "no" (not mentioned) were frequent. There are many possible explanations for this, other than "poor planning." As described in the section on methodology, the approach used for this analysis would have the likely effect of underestimating the robustness of state plans. Nonetheless, a plan is merely an essential first step in a competent response, and true weaknesses in planning could be magnified as responses unfold.

Table 8. Other Essential Services

Other Essential Services Variable	No. of plans that address variable (N=51)
Provides planning assumptions regarding continuity of essential services	11
Mentions plan for emergency food distribution	9
Mentions plan for continuity of essential services (including public utilities)	7
Mentions plan to re-establish schools and businesses as pandemic recedes	4

The state pandemic flu plans analyzed here reflected their authorship by public health officials. Many of them addressed core public health functions such as surveillance or vaccine management, though specific aspects of these functions were addressed in varying degrees of depth. This suggests that challenges remain even in areas that are familiar to public health planners, such as: developing schemes to prioritize or ration limited medical assets; coordinating surveillance to optimize early detection and ongoing disease monitoring; and legal liability and civil rights issues associated with disease control measures. Fewer plans addressed leadership and coordination, or the continuity of non-health services, subjects which may be unfamiliar to public health planners, or which may exceed their authority. These elements may require stronger engagement by emergency management officials and others in planning.

This analysis studied pandemic planning at the state level. As with any emergency response, most of the responsibility rests with local authorities. This analysis did not attempt to assess the status of local pandemic planning efforts, though such efforts are also likely to pose significant challenges. Just as public health authority is decentralized to state rather than federal authorities, it is also decentralized in some states, with local health departments having varying degrees of autonomy, further complicating planning efforts.[62]

Variability among states in pandemic planning has been noted in another analysis.[63] The decentralized nature of public health is often cited as an explanation. The federal government cannot directly dictate to states what they must do to prepare, though it can establish certain requirements as a condition of federal preparedness funding. Some flexibility in those requirements is helpful in allowing states to prepare differently for those threats — such as hurricanes, earthquakes and wildfires — that are likely to affect states differently. A pandemic, on the other hand, is more likely to affect states in similar ways that are, to some extent, predictable. This threat may be more amenable to standardized planning approaches, and to more directive federal requirements tied to funding. But the matter of what the states should do to be prepared for a pandemic is not always clear. For example, uncertainties about the ways in which flu spreads, the lack of national consensus in matters of equity in rationing, and a long tradition of federal deference to states in matters of public health, all complicate efforts to set uniform planning requirements for states.

The CRS database analyzed here contains state pandemic plans available as of July 2006. At that point, all states had been required to submit pandemic plans to HHS one year earlier, and all had done so. However, the states were not given specific direction regarding the content of the plans that were required in July 2005, and they were not required to update their plans during the subsequent FY2005 funding cycle.

The guidance that accompanied targeted pandemic funding for FY2006, in accordance with congressional report language, emphasized exercises, assessments, assistance to local jurisdictions in their planning efforts, and other specific tasks, but did not explicitly require that states update their plans, if needed, to keep them current to a certain date.[64] This may reflect a broader trend in disaster preparedness, in which planning is seen as the first step toward a competent response, but the assurance of actual response capability is focused instead on the development and evaluation of exercises, rather than on evaluation of plans.[65]

Exercises and drills test the ability of jurisdictions to execute their plans, and they detect planning gaps. Consequently, assessments of response capability rest not only on assessments of planning, but also on assessments of exercise programs, and integration of findings into subsequent rounds of planning.[66] DHS has developed the all-hazards Homeland Security

Exercise and Evaluation Program (HSEEP) to provide standardized policy, methodology, and language for designing, developing, conducting, and evaluating exercises.[67] But it has not published information about the specific application of this approach to pandemic flu preparedness. The RAND Corporation, under contract from HHS, developed the Public Health Preparedness Database, which incorporates evaluation criteria to be applied to exercises, and a searchable database of exercises (including orientations, table-top exercises, and drills) used to evaluate public health preparedness.[68] The database contains two local exercises specifically for pandemic flu, but none at the state level. Also, while pandemic influenza scenarios have been used to exercise specific elements of a public health response, such as distribution of stockpiled medications, there has been no national exercise to test a multi-sector, multi-jurisdictional response to a flu pandemic.

APPENDIX: FUNDING AND BENCHMARKS FOR PANDEMIC PLANNING

Federal Pandemic Planning

The United States has engaged in pandemic flu planning activities, with an emphasis on the public health sector, for several decades. The threat posed by H5N1 avian flu has heightened *multi-sector* preparedness activities in recent years. The federal government has been engaged in a coordinated, multi-sector, government- wide planning effort since 2005.[69] Prior to that, in 2004, the Department of Homeland Security (DHS) developed planning scenarios for 15 types of incidents, to assist emergency managers, public health officials, and others in planning across sectors and jurisdictions. A pandemic flu scenario was provided, along with scenarios for biological attacks, a major hurricane, a nuclear detonation, and other threats.[70]

Federal Funding for State Pandemic Preparedness

Since the terrorist attacks in 2001, Congress has provided almost $8 billion in grants to states to strengthen public health and hospital preparedness for public health threats. Beginning in FY2002, and each fiscal year subsequently, all states have received annual funding for these activities through two grant programs: one administered by the Centers for Disease Control and Prevention (CDC) to improve state and local public health capacity; the other administered by the Health Resources and Services Administration (HRSA) to prepare hospitals, clinics and other healthcare facilities for bioterrorism and other mass-casualty events.[71] Both agencies are in the Department of Health and Human Services (HHS). Grants for both programs are administered at the state level by the State Health Official, the senior official in charge of the state's department of public health. The grants include requirements for local consultation, and for some pass-through of funding to local authorities. HHS does not have any grant programs that directly fund local or municipal authorities for preparedness activities.

As a common requirement of the CDC and HRSA grant programs, all states and the District of Columbia (DC)[72] were required to develop pandemic flu plans, beginning with their FY2004 awards, and to submit the plans to CDC by July 2005.[73] The FY2004 guidance did not, however, stipulate any requirements for the content of the plans. While earlier guidance had been developed by CDC and state health officials to guide state planning efforts, pandemic planning was voluntary at that time, and the FY2004 requirement did not refer to the earlier voluntary guidance.[74]

All states and DC submitted plans by the July 2005 deadline. Many of the plans, some of which have been updated since the deadline, are publicly available on a pandemic flu information website created by HHS.[75]

The July 2005 deadline corresponded with the deadline for state applications for FY2005 cooperative agreement funds. The FY2005 cooperative agreement guidance reiterated that all states must have a pandemic flu plan, and cited the earlier voluntary pandemic guidance. The FY2005 guidance did not, however, require that states that had already submitted a plan for the July 2005 deadline (all of them had) revise the plan during the FY2005 funding cycle.

In November 2005, after the July 2005 deadline, HHS published the *HHS Pandemic Influenza Plan* (the HHS Pandemic Plan).[76] Part 2 of the plan, "Public Health Guidance for State and Local Partners," lays out, in a series of supplements, detailed activities to help state and local jurisdictions and healthcare facilities mount an effective response to a pandemic. Activities were provided in the following topical areas:

- Surveillance;
- Laboratory testing;
- Healthcare planning;
- Infection control;
- Clinical guidelines;
- Vaccine distribution and use;
- Antiviral drug distribution and use;
- Community disease control and prevention;
- Managing travel-related risk of disease transmission;
- Public health communications; and
- Workforce support: psychosocial considerations and information needs.

Subsequently, in May 2006, the White House Homeland Security Council published the *National Strategy for Pandemic Influenza, Implementation Plan* (the Pandemic Implementation Plan), which assigned more than 300 preparedness and response tasks to departments and agencies across the federal government, and provided planning guidance for state, local, and tribal entities, businesses, schools and universities, communities, and non-governmental organizations.[77]

In FY2006, Congress provided $6.1 billion in emergency supplemental funding exclusively for pandemic preparedness. These funds built upon earlier efforts to plan for public health emergencies in general, and pandemic flu in particular. The supplemental funding included $600 million for state and local pandemic preparedness, to be administered by the CDC through the public health preparedness grant program.[78] All states and territories received portions of the pandemic funding according to a formula, and were required by CDC to conduct a variety of activities involving community-wide (versus health-sector specific) planning, exercises and drills, preparedness of sub-state jurisdictions, and others.[79]

Supplemental funding was made available to states in phases, from the spring through the fall of 2006. An additional $175 million in FY2007 funds was made available in July 2007.[80]

Targeted state funding for pandemic preparedness was provided to states after the July 2005 deadline for them to submit their pandemic plans. Prior to the availability of this funding, states were expected to use unspecified amounts of their public health and hospital preparedness funds to carry out pandemic planning. As with emergency preparedness in general, pandemic planning efforts are expected to be ongoing, and supporting documents are to be continually updated ("evergreen") to reflect current developments.

The CRS database contains state pandemic plans available as of July 2006. At that point, all states had been required to submit pandemic plans to HHS one year earlier, and all had done so. However, the states were not given specific direction regarding the required content of the plans that were required in July 2005, and they were not required to update their plans during the FY2005 funding cycle. The guidance that accompanied targeted pandemic funding for FY2006, in accordance with congressional report language, emphasized exercises, assessments, assistance to local jurisdictions in their planning efforts, and other specific tasks, but did not explicitly require that states update their plans, if needed, to keep them current to a certain date. This is consistent with a broader trend in disaster preparedness, in which planning is seen as merely the first step toward a competent response, while the assurance of actual response capability may be better achieved through the development and evaluation of exercises, rather than through evaluation of plans.[81]

Mass Casualty Planning Grants to Municipalities

The Department of Homeland Security (DHS) administers a number of state, local and municipal grant programs intended to enhance homeland security.[82] One of them, the Metropolitan Medical Response System (MMRS) program, first incorporated pandemic planning in guidance to accompany FY2006 funds, and expanded the requirements in guidance for FY2007. Other homeland security grant programs may mention pandemic preparedness, but do not require specific activities or include specific benchmarks for this purpose.

The MMRS program began by awarding contracts to municipalities, requiring the submission of disaster response plans as the contract deliverable. The program's scope now includes planning as well as exercising, training, and equipment purchasing. Currently, MMRS awards are provided annually to 124 of the nation's most populous cities to develop plans and conduct related activities for mass casualty incidents by coordinating efforts among first responders, healthcare providers, public health officials, emergency managers, volunteer organizations, and other local entities.[83] In FY2007, each MMRS jurisdiction received $258,145 to establish or sustain local mass casualty preparedness capabilities. Each fiscal year, MMRS guidance explicitly requires grantees to update or revise their plans as needed to address new benchmarks.

MMRS guidance for FY2006 funds included an "overarching requirement" that MMRS jurisdictions address a number of pandemic preparedness matters in their planning and operations documents.[84] These matters included reviewing mutual aid agreements to clarify protocols for facility sharing or closure; planning for priority dispensing of flu vaccines and antiviral drugs to first responders; providing enhanced public safety services at mass casualty response facilities; and establishing the legal authorities necessary to allow alterations in standards of medical practice.

MMRS guidance for FY2007 reiterated the FY2006 requirements, and added the additional requirement that funded jurisdictions update their Continuity of Operations (COOP) and Continuity of Government (COG) plans to: define clear lines of succession for key positions; assure the protection of key records, facilities, equipment and personnel; address the operation of alternate facilities; and assure the functioning of emergency communications.[85] The FY2007 guidance also said that jurisdictions should attempt to use CDC funds for the purchase of antiviral drugs and ventilators, before using MMRS funds for that purpose.

Grantees' MMRS plans are not generally publicly available, and were not analyzed by CRS.

End Notes

[1] In this chapter, the term "pandemic" refers to pandemic influenza.

[2] For more information about the nation's public health system and public health preparedness, see CRS Report RL3 1719, *An Overview of the U.S. Public Health System in the Context of Emergency Preparedness*, by Sarah A. Lister.

[3] For a discussion of these approaches in the response to public health threats in general, see CRS Report RL33 579, *The Public Health and Medical Response to Disasters: Federal Authority and Funding*, by Sarah A. Lister.

[4] For more information about state-to-state mutual aid, see CRS Report RS2 1227, *The Emergency Management Assistance Compact (EMAC): An Overview*, by Keith Bea.

[5] See, for example, CRS Report RL32752, *Continuity of Operations (COOP) in the Executive Branch: Issues in the 109th Congress*, by R. Eric Petersen, and White House Homeland Security Council, "National Strategy for Pandemic Influenza: Implementation Plan," Chapter 9, "Institutions: Protecting Personnel and Ensuring Continuity of Operations," May 2006, at [http://www.pandemicflu.gov/plan/federal/index.html].

[6] See, for example, Nicole Lurie, Jeffrey Wasserman and Christopher D. Nelson, "Public Health Preparedness: Evolution or Revolution?" *Health Affairs*, vol. 25, no. 4, pp. 935-945, July/August 2006.

[7] States have generally received funding for the public health and hospital preparedness grants in the summer of each year.

[8] See [http://www.norc.org/homepage.htm].

[9] Reference in this chapter to "state plans" includes DC, and the total number of plans analyzed is 51. Plans analyzed were the most current publicly available plan available for each state, as of July 2006, on either the state's website, or on a federal pandemic flu website [http://www.pandemicflu.gov/plan/states/index.html]. The database was created and analyzed using Microsoft Office Access 2003 software.

[10] States were required to submit pandemic flu plans to the Department of Health and Human Services (HHS) by July 2005. The HHS pandemic plan for public health and medical preparedness, which included guidance for state planning, was published in November 2005, superceding a more cursory draft pandemic plan. Many states subsequently updated their plans to better coordinate with the HHS plan. See HHS, "HHS Pandemic Influenza Plan," November 2005, at [http://www.pandemicflu.gov].

[11] Additional categorical and free-text variables were also created, and were used to inform analysis of the dichotomous variables. In addition to the 66 dichotomous variables presented, selected cross-tabulations are also presented to show the interaction of certain variables.

[12] The set of variables was finalized in May 2006. See the Appendix for a discussion of federal guidance for state pandemic planning.

[13] Some local jurisdictions have published detailed pandemic plans. See, for example, Santa Clara County, California, "Pandemic Influenza Preparedness and Response Plan for Santa Clara County," at [http://www.sccphd.org/panflu].

[14] In December 2006, the Associated Press reported that HHS planned an evaluation of state pandemic preparedness, to be completed in spring 2007, based on a questionnaire that would "go beyond health care to ask how communities would keep the economy and society in general running." Lauran Neergaard, "State Preparations for Pandemic Vary Widely," *Associated Press*, December 16, 2006.

[15] See HHS, Office of Inspector General, reports on the HRSA Bioterrorism Hospital Preparedness Program, and the CDC Public Health Preparedness and Response for Bioterrorism Program, at [http://oig.hhs.gov/reports.html].

[16] White House Homeland Security Council, "National Strategy for Pandemic Influenza: Implementation Plan," May 2006, at [http://www.pandemicflu.gov/plan/federal/index.html].

[17] See White House Homeland Security Council, summary of progress on actions to be completed within 12 months of the release of the "National Strategy for Pandemic Influenza Implementation Plan," July 2007, at [http://www.pandemicflu.gov/plan/federal/ summaryprogress2007.html].

[18] See, for example, GAO: "Influenza Pandemic: Further Efforts Are Needed to Ensure Clearer Federal Leadership Roles and Effective National Strategy," GAO-07-781, August 14, 2007; "Influenza Pandemic: Efforts to Forestall Onset Are Under Way; Identifying Countries at Greatest Risk Entails Challenges," GAO-07-604, June 20, 2007; and "Avian Influenza: USDA Has Taken Important Steps to Prepare for Outbreaks, but Better Planning Could Improve Response," GAO-07-652, June 11, 2007.

[19] See, for example, GAO, "Public Health and Hospital Emergency Preparedness Programs: Evolution of Performance Measurement Systems to Measure Progress," GAO-07-485R, March 23, 2007.

[20] See DHS, "Nationwide Plan Review, Phase 2 Report," June 16, 2006, at [http://www.dhs.gov/xprepresp/programs/], hereinafter DHS Nationwide Plan Review.

[21] States were to assess their preparedness according to FEMA's "State and Local Guide (SLG) 101: Guide for All-Hazard Emergency Operations Planning," September 1996, at [http://www.fema.gov/pdf/plan/slg101 .pdf].

[22] DHS Nationwide Plan Review, pp. 27-28.

[23] Holmberg, S.D., Layton, C.M., Ghneim, G.S., and Wagener, D.K., "State Plans for Containment of Pandemic Influenza," *Emerging Infectious Diseases,* September 2006, at [http://www.cdc.gov/ncidod/EID/vol 1 2no09/06-0369.htm], hereinafter referred to as Holmberg et al.

[24] Trust for America's Health, "Ready or Not? Protecting the Public's Health from Disease, Disasters, and Bioterrorism, 2006," December 2006, available, along with comparable reports for 2003, 2004 and 2005, at [http://healthyamericans.org/reports/bioterror06/].

[25] Trust for America's Health, "Pandemic Flu and Potential for U.S. Economic Recession," March 2007, at [http://healthyamericans.org/reports/flurecession/].

[26] Lauran Neergaard, "State Preparations for Pandemic Vary Widely," *Associated Press,* December 16, 2006.

[27] HHS Pandemic Plan, Executive Summary, p. 5.

[28] See CRS Report RL33729, *Federal Emergency Management Policy Changes After Hurricane Katrina: A Summary of Statutory Provisions,* by Keith Bea, Coordinator, and CRS Report RL33579, *The Public Health and Medical Response to Disasters: Federal Authority and Funding,* by Sarah A. Lister. For more information about NIMS, see [http://www.fema.gov/emergency/nims/index.shtm].

[29] An Emergency Operations Center is the physical location where agency representatives assemble during an emergency to coordinate response and recovery actions and resources.

[30] See, for example, the announcement accompanying FY2005 guidance for the CDC public health grants to states, May 2005, pp 13-14, at [http://www.bt.cdc.gov/planning/ coopagreement/].

[31] For more information, see CRS Report RS22266, *The Use of Federal Troops for Disaster Assistance: Legal Issues,* by Jennifer K. Elsea.

[32] H.Rept. 109-359, to accompany H.R. 2863, Department of Defense, Emergency Supplemental Appropriations to Address Hurricanes in the Gulf of Mexico, and Pandemic Influenza Act, 2006, p. 523. See the Appendix for more information.

[33] CDC, "Pandemic Influenza Guidance Supplement: Phase 2," guidance for FY2006 funds, July 10, 2006, at [http://www.bt.cdc.gov/planning/coopagreement/].

[34] White House, "Press Gaggle after Avian Flu Tabletop Exercise with Homeland Security Advisor Fran Townsend, Secretary of Health and Human Services Michael Leavitt, and Secretary of Homeland Security Michael Chertoff," transcript, December 10, 2005, at [http://www.whitehouse.gov/news/releases/2005/1 2/2005121 0-2.html]. CDC has a comprehensive internal pandemic response plan, and has also conducted a series of internal pandemic preparedness exercises. See CDC podcast on pandemic preparedness, April 25, 2007, at [http://www2a.cdc.gov/podcasts/index.asp], and CDC, "Influenza Pandemic Operation Plan"(OPLAN), March 20, 2007, at [http://www.cdc.gov/flu/pandemic/ pdf/20MarchOPLAN.pdf].

[35] CDC, "Overview of Influenza Surveillance in the United States," June 26, 2006, at [http://www.cdc.gov/flu/weekly/pdf/flu-surveillance-overview.pdf].

[36] An H5N1 influenza diagnostic test, developed by CDC, was approved by the Food and Drug Administration (FDA) and delivered to laboratories in the national Laboratory Response Network, which includes public health labs in all 50 states, many federal labs, and others, in February 2006. See [http://www.bt.cdc.gov/lrn/factsheet.asp].

[37] "Syndromic surveillance" means tracking symptoms of illness, which could provide information faster than waiting for the results of laboratory testing. CDC's surveillance of sentinel healthcare providers gathers reports of "influenza-like illness" (ILI), which is a form of syndromic surveillance. Some have recommended that

during a pandemic, states should be able to expand surveillance of ILI to emergency departments and other healthcare facilities.

[38] Holmberg et al.

[39] See CRS Report RL3338 1, *The Americans with Disabilities Act (ADA): Allocation of Scarce Medical Resources During a Pandemic*, by Nancy Lee Jones.

[40] HHS Pandemic Plan, Part 1, Appendix D, "NVAC/ACIP Recommendations for Prioritization of Pandemic Influenza Vaccine and NVAC Recommendations on Pandemic Antiviral Drug Use," beginning on p. 59 of the pdf document.

[41] Holmberg et al.

[42] See, for example, Ezekiel J. Emanuel and Alan Wertheimer, " Who Should Get Influenza Vaccine When Not All Can?" *Science,* vol. 312, pp. 854-855, May 12, 2006.

[43] L. Uscher-Pines et al., "Priority Setting for Pandemic Influenza: An Analysis of National Preparedness Plans," *PLoS Medicine*, vol. 3, no. 10, October 17, 2006. The study also found variability among countries in their plans to prioritize the use of antiviral drugs.

[44] HHS Pandemic Plan, "Vaccine Production, Procurement and Distribution," p. S6-6 (p. 278 of the pdf document).

[45] See CRS Report RL33589, *The Pandemic and All-Hazards Preparedness Act (P.L. 109-41 7): Provisions and Changes to Preexisting Law*, by Sarah A. Lister and Frank Gottron.

[46] 21 C.F.R. 312.

[47] White House Homeland Security Council, "The National Strategy for Pandemic Influenza," p. 9. November 1, 2005, at [http://www.pandemicflu.gov/plan/federal/ index.html].

[48] Association of State and Territorial Health Officials, (ASTHO), "ASTHO Antiviral Survey Summary," May 2007, at [http://www.astho.org/pubs/ April07AntiviralSurveyResults05 1607.pdf]. Respondents included officials from all 50 states, the District of Columbia, and one territory. A baseline survey from October 2006 is at [http://www.astho.org/pubs/AntiviralSurvey121806.pdf].

[49] HHS Pandemic Plan, Part 1, Appendix D, "NVAC/ACIP Recommendations for Prioritization of Pandemic Influenza Vaccine and NVAC Recommendations on Pandemic Antiviral Drug Use," beginning on p. 59 of the pdf document.

[50] Both isolation and quarantine restrict the movement of those affected, but they differ depending on whether an individual has been exposed to a disease (quarantine), or is actually infected (isolation). Persons in isolation may be ill, and isolation sometimes occurs in healthcare settings. Those under quarantine are, by definition, not ill from the disease in question, though other health conditions may complicate the quarantine process. For more information, see CRS Report RL33201, *Federal and State Quarantine and Isolation Authority*, by Kathleen S. Swendiman and Jennifer K. Elsea.

[51] See status reports of two projects developed to assist states in revising their public health laws: the Model State Emergency Health Powers Act, developed by the Center for Law and the Public's Health; and the Turning Point Model State Public Health Act, funded by the Robert Wood Johnson Foundation, both at [http://www.publichealthlaw.net/ Resources/Modellaws.htm]. For more information about state emergency management and homeland security authorities, see CRS Report RL3 2287, *Emergency Management and Homeland Security Statutory Authorities in the States, District of Columbia, and Insular Areas: A Summary*, by Keith Bea, L. Cheryl Runyon, and Kae M. Warnock, in particular Table 1, listing individual state profiles and accompanying CRS report numbers.

[52] CDC, "Interim Pre-pandemic Planning Guidance: Community Strategy for Pandemic Influenza Mitigation in the United States — Early Targeted Layered Use of Non-Pharmaceutical Interventions," February 2007, at [http://www.pandemicflu.gov/].

[53] HHS Pandemic Plan, Part 2, "Public Health Communications," p. S 10-1 ff. (p. 359-396 of the pdf document).

[54] See, for example, the Virginia Department of Health's coordinated public information activities, including integration into the state's on-scene Joint Information Center (JIC), in response to the Virginia Tech shootings in April 2007, at [http://www.astho.org/ newsletter/newsletters/9/index.html].

[55] For more information on issues associated with medical surge capacity, see HHS, "Mass Medical Care with Scarce Resources: A Community Planning Guide," February 2007, at [http://www.ahrq.gov/research/mce/].

[56] See CDC, Strategic National Stockpile overview, at [http://www.bt.cdc.gov/stockpile/].

[57] Some states have created work groups to address specific aspects of surge capacity during a pandemic, such as rationing schemes for ventilators. See, for example, John L. Hick and Daniel T. O'Laughlin, "Concept of Operations for Triage of Mechanical Ventilation in an Epidemic," *Academic Emergency Medicine,* vol. 13, no. 2, pp. 223-229, published online January 6, 2006, at [http://www.aemj.org/cgi/content/abstract/1 3/2/223]; and New York State Department of Health, "New York State Health Department Releases Ventilator Allocation Guidelines for Comment," press release, March 16, 2007, at [http://www.health.state.ny.us/press/releases/2007/2007-03-1 6_ventilator_allocation.htm].

[58] HHS Pandemic Plan, p. 18.

[59] Remarks of HHS Secretary Michael Leavitt on "Avian Flu," National Press Club, October 27, 2005, CQ Transcriptions.

[60] National Governors Association, Center for Best Practices, "Preparing for a Pandemic Influenza: A Primer for Governors and Senior State Officials," July 2006, at [http://www.nga.org/Files/pdf/0607PANDEMICPRIMER.PDF].

[61] National Governors Association, "NGA Center Launches Pandemic Outbreak Workshops to Enhance State Readiness," press release, April 10, 2007, at [http://www.nga.org/portal/site/nga].

[62] For more information, see CRS Report RL31719, An Overview of the U.S. Public Health System in the Context of Emergency Preparedness, by Sarah A. Lister.

[63] Holmberg et al.

[64] The CRS database was created using plans available before the FY2006 guidance and funding were provided to states.

[65] See Nicole Lurie, Jeffrey Wasserman and Christopher D. Nelson, "Public Health Preparedness: Evolution or Revolution?" Health Affairs, vol. 25, no. 4, pp. 935-945, July/August 2006.

[66] Ibid.

[67] DHS, The Homeland Security Exercise and Evaluation Program (HSEEP), at [https://hseep.dhs.gov/].

[68] RAND, Public Health Preparedness Database, at [http://www.rand.org/health/projects/

[69] See White House Homeland Security Council, "National Strategy for Pandemic Influenza Implementation Plan, One Year Summary," July 2007, at [http://www.pandemicflu.gov/plan/federal/index.html]. See also CRS Report RL33 145, Pandemic Influenza: Domestic Preparedness Efforts, and CRS Report RS22576, Pandemic Influenza: Appropriations for Public Health Preparedness and Response, both by Sarah A. Lister.

[70] See DHS, Office of Inspector General, "A Review of the Top Officials 3 Exercise," p. 6, at [http://www.dhs.gov/xoig/assets/mgmtrpts/OIG_06-07_Nov05 .pdf].

[71] See CDC Cooperative Agreement Guidance for Public Health Emergency Preparedness, at [http://www.bt.cdc.gov/planning/#statelocal]; and HRSA emergency preparedness programs at [http://www.hrsa.gov/healthconcerns/default.htm]. See also Government Accountability Office (GAO), "Public Health and Hospital Emergency Preparedness Programs: Evolution of Performance Measurement Systems to Measure Progress," GAO-07-485R, March 23, 2007. Though commonly referred to as grants, these programs are actually cooperative agreements. Congress transferred the hospital preparedness program from HRSA to the HHS Assistant Secretary for Preparedness and Response, effective with FY2007 funds, in P.L. 109-417.

[72] According to the Public Health Service Act, the District of Columbia is considered a state for grant-making purposes.

[73] See CDC, "Continuation Guidance — Budget Year Five, Attachment H, Cross-cutting Benchmarks and Guidance," Cross-Cutting Critical Benchmark #6: Preparedness for Pandemic Influenza, June 14, 2004, at [http://www.bt.cdc.gov/planning/ continuationguidance/pdf/activities-attachh.pdf].

[74] CDC and the Council of State and Territorial Epidemiologists developed voluntary pandemic planning guidance for states in 1997, with sections on: command, control and management; surveillance; vaccine delivery; antiviral drugs; emergency response; and communications. CDC, National Vaccine Program Office, "Pandemic Influenza: A Planning Guide for State and Local Officials," version 1.1, January 1997, unpublished document. A subsequent version of the document (Draft 2.1, also unpublished) states: "The guide has not been formally approved or endorsed by any governmental or non-governmental organization, and should be considered only as an interim (draft) guidance document as national planning efforts are completed."

[75] See HHS, "State Pandemic Plans," at [http://www.pandemicflu.gov/plan/stateplans.html]. This site does not, however, consistently post the most current or complete plan for each jurisdiction.

[76] U.S. Department of Health and Human Services, "HHS Pandemic Influenza Plan," November 2005, at [http://www.pandemicflu.gov/plan/federal/index.html].

[77] White House Homeland Security Council, "National Strategy for Pandemic Influenza: Implementation Plan," May 2006, at [http://www.pandemicflu.gov/plan/federal/index.html].

[78] $350 million was provided in P.L. 109-148, and $250 million in P.L. 109-234. These funds are in addition to the approximately $8 billion provided through the public health and hospital preparedness grants from FY2002 through FY2007.

[79] See CDC, Cooperative Agreement Guidance for Public Health Emergency Preparedness, pandemic influenza guidance supplements, Phase 1 and 2, along with general program guidance for FY2005 and FY2006, at [http://www.bt.cdc.gov/planning/coopagreement/].

[80] See HHS, "HHS Announces $896.7 Million in Funding to States for Public Health Preparedness and Emergency Response," press release, July 17, 2007.

[81] See Nicole Lurie, Jeffrey Wasserman and Christopher D. Nelson, "Public Health Preparedness: Evolution or Revolution?" Health Affairs, vol. 25, no. 4, pp. 935-945, July/August 2006.

[82] See CRS Report RL33770, Department of Homeland Security Grants to State and Local Governments: FY2003 to FY2006, by Steven Maguire and Shawn Reese.

[83] For more information, see DHS, "FY 2007 Homeland Security Grant Program Allocation Overview," 2007, at [http://www.dhs.gov/xlibrary/assets/grants_st-local_fy07 .pdf].

[84] DHS, "FY2006 Homeland Security Grant Program, Program Guidance and Application Kit," pp. 99-100, December 2005, at [http://www.ojp.usdoj .gov/odp/docs/fy2006hsgp.pdf].

[85] DHS, "FY2007 Homeland Security Grant Program, Program Guidance and Application Kit," pp. 58-64, January 2007, at [http://www.ojp.usdoj .gov/odp/docs/fy07_hsgp_ guidance.pdf].

In: Influenza Pandemic - Preparedness and Response to ...   ISBN: 978-1-60692-953-7
Editor: Emma S. Brouwer pp.93-102   © 2010 Nova Science Publishers, Inc.

Chapter 4

WOULD AN INFLUENZA PANDEMIC QUALIFY AS A MAJOR DISASTER UNDER THE STAFFORD ACT?

Edward C. Liu

SUMMARY

This chapter provides a legal analysis of the eligibility of an influenza pandemic (flu pandemic) to be declared by the President as a major disaster under the Robert T. Stafford Disaster Relief and Emergency Assistance Act. In 1997, the discovery of a virulent H5N1 strain of avian influenza (bird flu) raised the possibility of a flu pandemic occurring in the United States. In such an event, the Stafford Act could provide authority for federal assistance. Although it is widely agreed that emergency assistance under the Stafford Act could be provided by the President in the event of a flu pandemic, questions remain as to whether major disaster assistance would be available. An analysis of the Stafford Act suggests that this issue was not addressed by Congress when it drafted the current definition of a major disaster, and that neither inclusion nor exclusion of flu pandemics from major disaster assistance is explicitly required by the current statutory language.

In the 109th Congress, § 210 of S. 3721 would have made any outbreak of infectious disease explicitly eligible for major disaster assistance, but it was not enacted.

THE THREAT OF AN INFLUENZA PANDEMIC

In 1997, a virulent strain of avian influenza (bird flu) was discovered in Asia. Hundreds of people in Europe and Asia have suffered from severe illness caused by the virus, but the virus has not, at this time, developed the ability to spread easily from person to person.[1] Were that to happen, a global pandemic could ensue. The Department of Health and Human Services (HHS) defines pandemic influenza as a "virulent human flu that causes a global outbreak, or pandemic, of serious illness. Because there is little natural immunity, the disease can spread easily from person to person."[2] According to HHS, an influenza pandemic (flu pandemic), "unlike natural disasters or terrorist events," could be widespread, affecting multiple areas of the United States and other countries at the same time. They postulate that a pandemic could be an extended event, with multiple waves of outbreaks in the same geographic area. HHS further maintains that each outbreak could last from six to eight weeks and waves of outbreaks may occur over a year or more.[3] In the event of a flu pandemic, the Robert T. Stafford Disaster Relief and Emergency Assistance Act could provide authority for federal assistance to individual victims and affected communities. The specific types of assistance that could be made available are discussed below.[4]

AN OVERVIEW OF THE STAFFORD ACT

The Robert T. Stafford Disaster Relief and Emergency Assistance Act (the Stafford Act)[5] authorizes the President to issue major disaster or emergency declarations in response to incidents that overwhelm state and local governments. Either type of declaration would authorize the distribution of a wide range of federal aid to individuals and families, certain nonprofit organizations, and public agencies, but major disaster and emergency classifications each trigger different kinds and amounts of assistance from the federal government.

Under the Stafford Act, a major disaster is defined as

> *any natural catastrophe* (including any hurricane, tornado, storm, high water, winddriven water, tidal wave, tsunami, earthquake, volcanic eruption, landslide, mudslide, snowstorm, or drought), *or, regardless of cause, any fire, flood, or explosion,* in any part of the United States, which in the determination of the President causes damage of sufficient severity and magnitude to warrant major disaster assistance under this chapter to supplement the efforts and available resources of States, local governments, and disaster relief organizations in alleviating the damage, loss, hardship, or suffering caused thereby.[6]

A major disaster declaration authorizes the President to offer a variety of federal assistance, although none is specifically required to be provided.[7] The types of general federal assistance available include directing federal agencies to support in assistance efforts, coordinating assistance efforts, providing technical and advisory assistance, and distributing supplies and emergency assistance. Under the major disaster classification, there are also more specific provisions, including repair and restoration of federal facilities, removal of debris, housing assistance, unemployment assistance, emergency grants to assist low-income migrant and seasonal farmworkers, food coupons and distribution, relocation assistance, crisis counseling assistance and training, community disaster loans, emergency communications, and emergency public transportation.[8]

In contrast the Stafford Act defines an emergency as

> *any occasion or instance* for which, in the determination of the President, Federal assistance is needed to supplement State and local efforts and capabilities to save lives and to protect property and public health and safety, or to lessen or avert the threat of a catastrophe in any part of the United States.[9]

An emergency declaration authorizes limited federal assistance when compared to a major disaster classification.[10] The emergency declaration would *not* authorize grants, unemployment assistance, food coupons, crisis counseling assistance and training, or community disaster loans as would be available through a major disaster declaration. An emergency declaration would authorize technical and advisory assistance to affected state and local governments for certain needs; emergency assistance through federal agencies; clearance of debris; housing assistance; and assistance in the distribution of medicine, food, and other consumable supplies. The total amount of assistance available is also limited in an emergency declaration to $5 million, "unless the President determines that there is a continuing need; Congress must be notified if the $5 million ceiling is breached."[11]

EXECUTIVE BRANCH RESPONSES TO POTENTIAL PANDEMICS

Although "neither disaster declarations nor congressional appropriations were issued for the 1957 Asian flu pandemic ... which resulted in almost 70,000 deaths in the United States [and] was one of the deadliest catastrophes of its time,"[12] emergency declarations under the Stafford Act in the event of an outbreak of infectious disease are not unprecedented. In 2000, the detection of West Nile virus in New York and New Jersey was used as the basis of an emergency declaration under the Stafford Act.[13] Despite the lack of a disaster declaration during the 1957 pandemic, a flu pandemic would likely qualify under the broad category of "any occasion or instance" in the statutory definition of an *emergency*.[14]

However, recent events have led to uncertainty over whether a flu pandemic is eligible for major disaster assistance under the Stafford Act.[15] In 2005, various federal agencies participated in TOPOFF 3, a national level exercise that simulated various security-related events, including a biological attack causing an outbreak of pneumonic plague in the United States.[16] The Federal Emergency Management Agency (FEMA), the agency responsible for administering the Stafford Act, was among the participants in that exercise. During TOPOFF 3, as well as during an earlier exercise, FEMA interpreted "biological disasters" as ineligible for major disaster assistance because such incidents were not explicitly mentioned in the Stafford Act.[17]

Subsequently, in May of 2006, the Homeland Security Council issued its *Implementation Plan for the National Strategy for Pandemic Influenza*,[18] which stated that "the President could declare either an emergency or a major disaster with respect to an influenza pandemic," potentially contradicting the earlier position adopted by FEMA during the TOPOFF exercises.[19] As discussed later in this chapter, it is debatable whether the Homeland Security Council's broad interpretation is supported by the text and legislative history of the Stafford Act.

Most recently, in March of 2007, FEMA issued a *Disaster Assistance Policy* (DAP) that "establishes the types of emergency protective measures that are eligible under the Public Assistance Program during a federal response to an outbreak of human influenza pandemic."[20] It is unclear whether this DAP is a departure from FEMA's prior assertions that biological disasters were ineligible for major disaster assistance. On one hand, the DAP states that it is "applicable to all major disasters and emergencies declared on or after the date of publication" and cites as authority the provisions of the Stafford Act authorizing major disaster assistance.[21] However, the only types of assistance offered by the DAP in the event of a flu pandemic are Emergency Protective Measures (Category B) provided by FEMA's Public Assistance Program.[22] Notably, Category B assistance may be offered during emergency declarations, and is not limited to major disaster incidents.[23] In fact, Category B assistance was precisely the type of assistance authorized during the emergency declarations for West Nile virus in 2000.[24] Therefore, this DAP is not necessarily inconsistent with the view that biological disasters are ineligible for major disaster assistance. Other guidance issued by FEMA does not mention flu pandemics, but may still be relevant. For example, the most recent working draft of the National Disaster Housing Strategy notes that quarantine and isolation facilities may be necessary "to meet the demands of major or catastrophic disasters."[25]

In summary, FEMA has historically excluded biological incidents from major disaster declarations under the Stafford Act, but the current presidential policy appears to consider biological incidents, or at least flu pandemics, to be eligible for major disaster assistance. The permissibility of both interpretations in light of the current statutory language is discussed below.

Recent Legislative Activity

A provision in S. 3721, introduced in the 109th Congress by Senator Collins of Maine, would have added the following to the definition of a major disaster:

> any act of domestic terrorism or international terrorism (as those terms are defined in section 2331 of title 18, United States Code) [and] *any outbreak of infectious disease*, or any chemical release, in any part of the United States.[26]

This provision would have made flu pandemics clearly eligible for major disaster assistance, but it was not enacted. A number of other modifications to the Stafford Act were ultimately added by the Post-Katrina Emergency Management Reform Act of 2006,[27] but no changes to the definition of a major disaster were made by that law.

Analysis

Under the standard procedure for a declaration under the Stafford Act, the governor of an affected state submits a request for either an emergency or major disaster declaration.[28] The Federal Emergency Management Agency then evaluates the incident and makes a recommendation to the President, with whom lies the ultimate discretion to make a declaration.[29] The Stafford Act precludes any judicial review of that decision.[30] Therefore, even though "it is emphatically the province and duty of the judicial department to say what the law is,"[31] a requesting governor or other affected party that disagrees with the executive's interpretation of what constitutes a major disaster is unlikely to be successful seeking a judicial remedy. Denials of declaration requests may be appealed and resubmitted to the President, but, again, there is no possibility of judicial review.[32]

Nevertheless, questions may arise among policymakers and other stakeholders as to which of the dueling interpretations of the Stafford Act are legally permissible: that is, whether the Stafford Act requires the conclusion that flu pandemics are either eligible or ineligible for major disaster assistance. The validity of an executive branch construction of a statute can be evaluated using the two-prong test laid out by the Supreme Court in *Chevron v. Natural Resources Defense Council*.[33] First, if the text and legislative history of the statute demonstrate that Congress has spoken directly on the issue, then that statutory language or history must control. However, under the second prong, "if ... Congress has not directly addressed the precise question at issue," the agency's interpretation will stand so long as it is a reasonable one.[34]

Both positions regarding the eligibility of flu pandemics for major disaster assistance are evaluated below using this two-prong test. But, regardless of what result the application of Supreme Court jurisprudence is likely to have in this case, it is important to note that Congress may come to its own conclusions as to whether a particular type of incident *should or should not* be considered a major disaster, and may amend the statutory definition if it deems it appropriate to do so.

Ambiguity of Congressional Intent

The first prong of the *Chevron* test asks whether Congress has directly spoken on the issue. If Congress has spoken, then the analysis ends, and the agency's interpretation must comport with that congressional intent. In this case, the inquiry is whether the statutory text and legislative history of the Stafford Act demonstrate that Congress addressed whether the definition of a major disaster includes a flu pandemic.

Statutory Text
The statutory definition of a major disaster confines its scope to "natural catastrophes ... or, regardless of cause, any fire, flood, or explosion." A flu pandemic is not a fire, flood, or explosion under the ordinary meaning of those three words. Therefore, a flu pandemic cannot qualify as a major disaster unless it can be considered a natural catastrophe, as that term is defined for purposes of the Stafford Act.

The text of the Stafford Act provides concrete examples of natural catastrophes,[35] but it does not appear to provide an exhaustive list of all qualifying events.[36] Based on a plain reading of the phrase, it is not clear whether a flu pandemic would be considered a natural catastrophe. Neither the Stafford Act nor any other provision of the U.S. Code provides a legal definition of a catastrophe. Dictionary definitions of a catastrophe range from "a momentous tragic, usually sudden, event marked by effects ranging from extreme misfortune to utter overthrow or ruin"[37] to a "sudden disaster, wide-spread, very fatal, or signal,"[38] either of which would seem to be applicable in the case of a flu pandemic. Additionally, many media reports colloquially refer to a pandemic as a catastrophe.[39] But, even though a pandemic likely has the potential to cause sufficient harm to meet the ordinary understanding of a *catastrophe*, the event would still need to be considered *natural* in order to be eligible for major disaster assistance.

The Stafford Act does not elaborate on the meaning of natural, but various dictionaries define it as "formed by nature; not subject to human intervention, not artificial,"[40] and "occurring in conformity with the ordinary course of nature."[41] As has been recently observed with the H5N1 strain of avian influenza, it is possible for virulent flu strains to develop without human intervention, and once infection occurs, the virus can continue to propagate and spread absent human intervention by virtue of the innate biological processes present in living persons. In response, one could argue that the widespread dispersal of a flu pandemic is likely dependent upon human vectors.

Recent attention garnered by actual and potential biological terrorism attacks raises the question whether an entirely man-made disease epidemic could be rightly described as a *natural* catastrophe. Initially, one should note that it is not necessary to conceptually view randomly occurring flu pandemics in the same category as intentional biological attacks. However, even if one were to treat all biological incidents as the same, other examples of known natural catastrophes are not necessarily disqualified because they may be partially caused by human actions. For example, landslides are statutorily identified as natural catastrophes,[42] even though human development may precipitate their occurrence.[43]

Textual arguments for excluding a flu pandemic from major disaster assistance may also be made. One could conclude from the statutory definition that a flu pandemic is not natural in the same way that a tornado or a hurricane is natural. *Ejusdem generis* is a canon of construction stating that "when a general word or phrase follows a list of specifics, the general word or phrase will be interpreted to include only items of the same type as those listed."[44] Applying this canon of construction, one interpretation is that the list following the phrase "natural catastrophe" limits its scope to geologic or climatic events that have the potential to cause extensive physical property damage. Furthermore, there is evidence that the threat of infectious outbreaks was not alien to Congress, specifically in light of its response to cholera and yellow fever during the latter half of the 19th century.[45] Consequently, the omission of infectious diseases from the list of explicit natural catastrophes bolsters the argument that outbreaks of infectious disease were seen by Congress as distinct from natural catastrophes.

Legislative History

Insofar as the text of the major disaster definition is susceptible to more than one interpretation, it may be helpful to examine the legislative history to further interpolate Congress's intent in drafting the provision. The current definitions of emergencies and major disasters were enacted in 1988 with passage of the Stafford Act. Prior to that, the definitions for both major disasters and emergencies declarations were contained in the Disaster Relief Act of 1974 (Disaster Relief Act), and had applied to

> any hurricane, tornado, storm, flood, high water, wind-driven water, tidal wave, tsunami, earthquake, volcanic eruption, landslide, mudslide, snowstorm, drought, fire, explosion, *or other catastrophe.*[46]

Conspicuously, the pre-Stafford definitions did not limit emergency or major disaster declarations to *natural* catastrophes. In 1980, a review of past emergency and major disaster declarations found that "Presidential authority to extend disaster assistance has been exercised almost exclusively in cases where damage was caused by or was closely related to some act of nature."[47] However, it appears likely that the amended definitions in the Stafford Act, which limited major disasters to natural catastrophes and created a new definition for emergencies, were partly enacted in response to the presidential use of the Disaster Relief Act authority to deal with certain man-made incidents.[48]

For example, in 1980, a large number of people fled Cuba and arrived in southern Florida. President Carter directed FEMA to provide temporary housing and shelter for these refugees, apparently under the authority of the Disaster Relief Act.[49] Also in 1980, FEMA assisted with the temporary relocation of families affected by the toxic waste deposits in the Love Canal neighborhood of Niagara Falls, New York.[50] Similarly, in 1983, FEMA assisted with the relocation of residents of Times Beach, Missouri, after the area had been contaminated with dioxin.[51] These incidents generated controversy in Congress, which expressed concern that

> in some instances aid has been extended by the President in *situations which resulted primarily, if not entirely, from human activity* rather than natural hazards.... Broadening the scope of the [Disaster Relief] Act to cover *both natural and non-natural* catastrophes has strained the capacity of programs designed to respond only to natural catastrophes.[52]

Following these declarations, an amendment to the definition of both emergencies and major disasters under the Disaster Relief Act was proposed, limiting such declarations to "physical or natural catastrophe[s]."[53] Although this amendment was not enacted, the debate regarding the amendment suggested that a chemical spill would have been considered a physical catastrophe, but not a natural one.[54] Further attempts to amend the definitions of major disasters and emergencies were introduced several times during the 1980s and permitted only "natural catastrophes." The definition was ultimately successfully amended by the 100th Congress as part of the passage of the Stafford Act in 1988.

An examination of this legislative history reaffirms the conclusion that the 100th Congress's principal intent in limiting major disaster assistance to "natural" incidents was to deny major disaster assistance to incidents that were caused by human activity. Furthermore, the legislative history provides at least two clear examples of Presidential declarations for which Congress likely found natural causes lacking: the mass arrival of political refugees and instances of chemical contamination. Nevertheless, it is likely inaccurate to say that by excluding these two types of incidents from major disaster assistance Congress clearly addressed the issue of flu pandemics or other biological incidents under the Stafford Act.

Reasonableness of Executive Branch Interpretations

The preceding analysis of the text and legislative history indicates that Congress did not directly address whether a flu pandemic is a natural catastrophe for purposes of the Stafford Act. Under the framework laid out by the Supreme Court in *Chevron*, the remaining question is whether a particular executive branch interpretation is "a reasonable choice within a gap left open by Congress."[55]

In this case, interpreting a flu pandemic as either a natural or non-natural catastrophe is arguably reasonable. On the one hand, the manner in which a flu pandemic is likely to propagate does not require human intervention. Making flu pandemics eligible for major disasters makes the maximum amount of resources available to avert the loss of life, human suffering, and loss of income that is likely to occur in the event of a flu pandemic. Some types of assistance that are only available in a major disaster declaration may be particularly useful in a flu pandemic. For instance, a flu pandemic is likely to result in a significantly reduced workforce as victims fall ill and others stay home to take care of them. The provision of unemployment assistance and emergency public transportation under the Stafford Act both may be an appropriate response, but are only available under a major disaster declaration.

On the other hand, a pandemic is substantially different than the climatic and geologic natural catastrophes listed by the Stafford Act, and many types of major disaster provisions, such as assistance to repair buildings or clear debris, are not likely to be necessary during a flu pandemic. Restricting flu pandemics to only emergency assistance arguably limits the burden on federal disaster relief funds. Additionally, other federal responses may be more appropriate to deal with a pandemic, such as the authority of the HHS Secretary to declare a public health emergency,[56] or impromptu legislation to provide assistance with respect to a particular incident.

Finally, it should be noted that the reasonableness of either interpretation is being evaluated under current law. Were Congress to conclude that flu pandemics categorically should or should not be eligible for major disaster assistance, it may amend the statute to explicitly say so. In that case, the clearly expressed intent of Congress would render any evaluation of an executive branch interpretation unnecessary, and Congress's intent would control.

End Notes

[1] Available at [http://www.pandemicflu.gov].

[2] *Id.*

[3] *Id.*

[4] Sadena Thevarajah contributed to portions of this chapter during her time as a law clerk in the American Law Division of the Congressional Research Service.

[5] *Codified at* 42 U.S.C. § 5121 *et seq.*

[6] 42 U.S.C. § 5 122(2) (emphasis added).

[7] Except in the case of food coupons and assistance to damaged federal facilities, the authority to determine what types of assistance to provide in the event of a major disaster declaration has been delegated to the Secretary of Homeland Security. Exec. Order No. 12148, § 4-203.

[8] 42 U.S.C. §§ 5172-5187.

[9] 42 U.S.C. § 5 122(1) (emphasis added).

[10] 42 U.S.C. § 5192.

[11] CRS Report RL33053, *Federal Stafford Act Disaster Assistance: Presidential Declarations, Eligible Activities, and Funding*, by Keith Bea, at 18, n.85.

[12] Keith Bea, *The Formative Years: 1950-1978*, in EMERGENCY MANAGEMENT: THE AMERICAN EXPERIENCE 81, 87 (Claire B. Rubin, ed., 2007).

[13] CRS Report RL33579, *The Public Health and Medical Response to Disasters: Federal Authority and Funding*, by Sarah A. Lister, at n.10 and accompanying text; and 65 Fed. Reg. 63589, 67747.

[14] Because declarations are ultimately subject to Presidential discretion, it is possible that some qualifying events may not be declared an emergency or a major disaster.

[15] *See* CRS Report RL33579, *The Public Health and Medical Response to Disasters: Federal Authority and Funding*, by Sarah A. Lister, at 9-11.

[16] DEP'T OF HOMELAND SECURITY, *A Review of the Top Officials 3 Exercise* (Nov. 2005), available at [http://www.dhs.gov/xoig/assets/mgmtrpts/OIG_06-07_Nov05 .pdf].

[17] *Id.* at 30.

[18] HOMELAND SECURITY COUNCIL, *Implementation Plan for the National Strategy for Pandemic Influenza*, at [http://www.whitehouse.gov/homeland/nspi_implementation.pdf]. This document "describes more than 300 critical actions, many of which have already been initiated, to address the threat of pandemic influenza."

[19] *Id.* at 212.

[20] FEDERAL EMERGENCY MANAGEMENT AGENCY, *Emergency Assistance for Human Influenza Pandemic*, Disaster Assistance Policy 9523.17, at 1 (Mar. 31, 2007).

[21] *Id.* However, this language and cited authority is not unique to this DAP and may simply be boilerplate used by the drafters.

[22] Category B assistance offers reimbursement to state or local entities for, among other things, the purchase and distribution of medicine and other consumables; management, control, and reduction of immediate threats to public health and safety; emergency medical care and temporary medical facilities; communicating health and safety information to the public; storage and internment of unidentified human remains; and recovery and disposal of animal carcasses. *Id.*

[23] *See* 42 U.S.C. § 5 170b(a)(3) (authorizing specific emergency protective measures to save lives and protect property) *and* 42 U.S.C. § 5192(b) (generally authorizing the President to provide assistance to save lives, protect property and public health and safety during an emergency declaration).

[24] 65 Fed. Reg. 63589, 67747.

[25] FEDERAL EMERGENCY MANAGEMENT AGENCY, *National Disaster Housing Strategy: Working Draft*, July 17, 2008, at 31.

[26] S. 3721, 109th Cong., § 210 (2006) (emphasis added).

[27] Enacted as part of the Department of Homeland Security Appropriations Act of 2007, P.L. 109-295, Title VI.

[28] 42 U.S.C. § 5170, 5191; 44 C.F.R. §§ 206.35-6.

[29] 44 C.F.R. § 206.37; Exec. Order No. 12148, § 4-203.

[30] 42 U.S.C. § 5148. *See, also, Kansas v. U.S.*, 748 F. Supp. 797, 799-800 (D. Kan. 1990) (holding that federal courts have no jurisdiction to review Stafford Act declaration decisions made by the President).

[31] *Marbury v. Madison*, 5 U.S. (1 Cranch) 137, 178 (1803).

[32] 44 C.F.R. § 206.46.

[33] *Chevron v. Nat'l Resources Def. Council*, 467 U.S. 837, 842-845 (1984). *See, also, Hawaii v. FEMA*, 294 F.3d 1152, 1159 (9th Cir. 2002) (applying *Chevron's* two-prong test to FEMA's interpretation of provisions of the Stafford Act).

[34] *Id.* Although this analysis uses a judicially created framework for evaluating an interpretation of a statute by the executive branch, this should not be taken to mean that FEMA or the President could be sued in state or federal court for failing to designate a flu pandemic as a major disaster. This analysis is solely included to provide a context with which policymakers and other stakeholders may view this issue.

[35] *Id.* ("any hurricane, tornado, storm, high water, winddriven water, tidal wave, tsunami, earthquake, volcanic eruption, landslide, mudslide, snowstorm, or drought" qualifies as a natural catastrophe).

[36] Note that the phrase natural catastrophe *includes* the enumerated incidents, but is arguably not limited to those events. *Id.*

[37] WEBSTER'S THIRD NEW INTERNATIONAL DICTIONARY 351 (1976).

[38] OXFORD ENGLISH DICTIONARY (Sept. 2008), available at [http://www.oed.com].

[39] *E.g.*, Diane Stafford, *Preparing for Catastrophe; Most U.S. Businesss are not ready for avian flu outbreak*, KANSAS CITY STAR, Dec. 13, 2005, at 1; Sabin Russell, *Statewide flu plan ready for public input*, SAN FRANCISCO CHRONICLE, Jan. 19, 2006, at B1; Lawrence K. Altman, M.D., *With Every Epidemic, Health Officials Face Tough Choices*, NEW YORK TIMES, Mar. 28, 2006, at 5.

[40] OXFORD ENGLISH DICTIONARY (Sept. 2008) available at [http://www.oed.com].

[41] WEBSTER'S THIRD NEW INTERNATIONAL DICTIONARY 1506-7 (1976).

[42] *See supra* note 35.

[43] *See* FEMA, *Landslide and Debris Flow (Mudslide)*, available at [http://www.fema.govhazard/landslide/] (noting that landslides may be activated by "steepening of slopes caused by erosion or human modification").

[44] *See* CRS Report 97-589, *Statutory Interpretation: General Principles and Recent Trends*, by Yule Kim, at n.49 and accompanying text. In this case, the general phrase "any natural catastrophe" actually precedes the list of specific examples, but the same interpretive principle applies.

[45] *See, e.g.*, An Act granting additional quarantine powers and imposing additional duties upon the Marine-Hospital Service, ch. 114, 27 Stat. 449 (1893).

[46] P.L. 93-288, 88 Stat. 143, at § 102 (emphasis added). Under the Disaster Relief Act, emergencies and major disasters were primarily distinguished by the severity of the incident.

[47] *See*, 126 CONG. REC. 27 664-6 (1980) (statement of Sen. Edward Zorinsky) (citing CRS Report LTR80-1 646, *"Other Catastrophe" Statutory Authority for Major Disaster Declarations*, by Clark Norton).

[48] U.S. GENERAL ACCOUNTING OFFICE, *Requests for Federal Disaster Assistance Need Better Evaluation*, CED-82-4, Dec. 7, 1981, at 39-40, available at [http://www.gao.gov/cgi-bin/getrpt?CED-82-4].

[49] Margot Hornblower, *Cuban Refugees Hold Emotional Mass, First Ever for Many*, WASHINGTON POST, May 5, 1980, at A2. *See, also*, Sen. Quentin Burdick, "Disaster Relief Acts of 1980," Senate debate, Congressional Record, vol. 126, part 21 (Sept. 26, 1980), at 27662.

[50] ENVIRONMENTAL PROTECTION AGENCY, *Press Release: EPA, New York State Announce Temporary Relocation of Love Canal Residents*, May 21, 1980, available at [http://www.epa.gov/history/topics/lovecanal/03.htm] (noting that "the temporary relocation will be assisted by the Federal Emergency Management Agency").

[51] ENVIRONMENTAL PROTECTION AGENCY, *Press Release: Joint Federal/State Action Taken to Relocate Times Beach Resident*, Feb. 22, 1983, available at [http://www.epa.gov/history/topics/times/02.htm].

[52] S.Rept. 100-524 at 2 (1988) (emphasis added).

[53] S. 3027, 96th Cong., § 2 (as reported in Senate).

[54] S.Rept. 96-891 at 3 (1980).

[55] *Chevron*, 467 U.S. at 866.

[56] For a more detailed discussion of authority and funding for public health emergencies, *see* CRS Report RL33 579, *The Public Health and Medical Response to Disasters: Federal Authority and Funding*, by Sarah A. Lister, at 4-7, 16-18.

In: Influenza Pandemic - Preparedness and Response to...
Editor: Emma S. Brouwer pp.103-157

ISBN: 978-1-60692-953-7
© 2010 Nova Science Publishers, Inc.

Chapter 5

INFLUENZA PANDEMIC: HHS NEEDS TO CONTINUE ITS ACTIONS AND FINALIZE GUIDANCE FOR PHARMACEUTICAL INTERVENTIONS

Government Accountability Office

WHY GAO DID THIS STUDY

The emergence of the H5N1 avian influenza virus (also known as "bird flu") has raised concerns that it or another virus might mutate into a virulent strain that could lead to an influenza pandemic. Experts predict that a severe pandemic could overwhelm the nation's health care system, requiring the rationing of limited resources. GAO was asked to provide information on the progress of the Department of Health and Human Services's (HHS) plans for responding to a pandemic, including analyzing how HHS plans to (1) use pharmaceutical interventions to treat infected individuals and protect the critical workforce and (2) use nonpharmaceutical interventions to slow the spread of disease. To conduct this work, GAO reviewed government documents and scientific literature, and interviewed HHS officials, state and local public health officials, and subject-matter experts on pandemic response.

WHAT GAO RECOMMENDS

GAO recommends that HHS expeditiously finalize guidance to assist state and local jurisdictions to determine how to effectively use limited supplies of antivirals and pre-pandemic vaccine in a pandemic, including prioritizing target groups for pre-pandemic vaccine. In comments on a draft of this chapter, HHS described additional actions it has taken and plans to take relating to GAO's recommendation, including releasing for public comment in the near future proposed guidance on pre-pandemic vaccine allocation.

WHAT GAO FOUND

HHS plans to make existing federal stockpiles of pharmaceutical interventions available for distribution once a pandemic begins. These interventions would include antivirals, which are drugs to prevent or reduce the severity of infection, and pre-pandemic vaccines, which are vaccines produced prior to a pandemic and developed from influenza strains that have the potential to cause a pandemic. HHS has established a national goal of stockpiling 75 million treatment courses of antivirals in the Strategic National Stockpile and in jurisdictional stockpiles. According to HHS, these public sector stockpiles are intended to be used primarily for the treatment of individuals sick with influenza. HHS intends to oversee the distribution and administration of pre-pandemic vaccine to individuals identified as members of the critical workforce. Members of the critical workforce—estimated to be about 20 million—include workers in sectors that are considered necessary to keep society functioning, such as health care and law enforcement personnel. HHS's strategy for using pre-pandemic vaccine is to keep society functioning until a pandemic vaccine—a vaccine specific to the pandemic-causing strain—becomes widely available. HHS anticipates that initial batches of a pandemic vaccine may not be available until 20 to 23 weeks after the start of the pandemic. As batches of the pandemic vaccine become available, HHS plans for state and local jurisdictions to provide it to members of targeted groups based on factors such as occupation and age, instead of making it available to the general public. HHS faces challenges implementing its strategy for using pharmaceutical interventions during a pandemic, including the lack of vaccine manufacturing capacity in the United States. HHS is currently making large investments to expand domestic vaccine manufacturing capacity. In 2008, HHS released guidance on prioritizing target groups for pandemic vaccine and draft guidance on antiviral use during a pandemic. HHS has not yet released draft guidance for public comment on prioritizing target groups for pre-pandemic vaccine.

HHS will rely on state and local jurisdictions to utilize nonpharmaceutical interventions, such as isolation of sick individuals and voluntary home quarantine of those exposed to the pandemic strain. To assist state and local jurisdictions with implementing nonpharmaceutical interventions, HHS has developed guidance that describes the department's "community mitigation framework." The framework involves the early initiation of multiple nonpharmaceutical interventions, each of which is expected to be partially effective and to be maintained consistently throughout a pandemic. HHS faces difficulties, including helping jurisdictions develop ways to ensure community compliance. HHS is investing in several initiatives to increase the nation's knowledge about the general use and effectiveness of nonpharmaceutical interventions. The findings from this research will be used to update existing guidance.

ABBREVIATIONS

CDC	Centers for Disease Control and Prevention
DHS	Department of Homeland Security
EMAC	Emergency Management Assistance Compact
FDA	Food and Drug Administration

FEMA	Federal Emergency Management Agency
HHS	Department of Health and Human Services
ICU	intensive care unit
mcg.	Microgram
PAHPA	Pandemic and All-Hazards Preparedness Act
SARS	severe acute respiratory syndrome
Stafford Act	Robert T. Stafford Disaster Relief and Emergency Assistance Act
SNS	Strategic National Stockpile

September 30, 2008

The Honorable Edward M. Kennedy
Chairman
The Honorable Michael B. Enzi
Ranking Member
Committee on Health, Education, Labor, and Pensions
United States Senate

The Honorable Bennie G. Thompson
Chairman
Committee on Homeland Security
House of Representatives

The emergence of the H5N1 avian influenza virus (also known as "bird flu") has raised concerns that it or another influenza virus might mutate into a novel and virulent strain that could lead to a human influenza pandemic[1] that would pose a grave threat to global public health. Pandemics occur when an influenza strain to which humans have little or no immunity begins to cause serious illness and spreads easily from person to person. In the United States alone, at least 675,000 people died during the 1918-19 pandemic, the deadliest pandemic in the twentieth century. The Department of Health and Human Services (HHS) has estimated that a pandemic similar to the severe 1918-19 pandemic would sicken 90 million people in the United States (30 percent of the population), of whom nearly 10 million would require hospitalization and almost 2 million would die.[2] Given that as of 2005 there were approximately 950,000 staffed hospital beds[3] in the United States, HHS's estimates indicate that the effects of a severe pandemic would far exceed the capacity of U.S. hospitals.[4]

HHS has made substantial progress in its preparedness for pandemic influenza. For example, since 2000, we had been urging HHS to complete its pandemic plan.[5] HHS released the *HHS Pandemic Influenza Plan* in November 2005. (See app. I for summaries of select federal pandemic documents.) We recently reported that HHS has improved its influenza surveillance and diagnostic testing capabilities.[6] Prompted by concerns regarding H5N1, HHS and its international partner organizations have increased efforts to enhance animal and human surveillance systems overseas. Additionally, in February 2006, the Food and Drug Administration (FDA)—an agency within HHS—approved a diagnostic test developed by the Centers for Disease Control and Prevention (CDC)— another agency within HHS—that recognizes H5 influenza viruses within 4 hours of testing; it previously would have taken 2 to 3 days.

Despite this progress, a severe pandemic would pose formidable challenges to the federal government's efforts to minimize damage to the public's health and the nation's economy. The single most important pharmaceutical intervention during a pandemic—a pandemic vaccine that is well-matched to the pandemic-causing strain—will not be available in large quantities in the initial stages of a pandemic. Other pharmaceutical interventions,[7] such as antivirals[8] and pre-pandemic vaccines (possibly less effective vaccines produced prior to the pandemic and based on strains experts believe may cause a pandemic) are also expected to be in limited supply and unavailable to the population at large.[9] In addition, although the ability to quickly increase the number of health care providers, called surge capacity, will be vital for treating the potentially large numbers of infected individuals, efforts to do so must overcome existing shortages of health care workers in the United States.[10] Similarly, because they are rarely used on a large scale, the effectiveness of large-scale implementation of nonpharmaceutical interventions, including closing schools and voluntary home quarantine, is uncertain. In addition, throughout the initial stages of a pandemic, crucial information—such as when and where to access medical care, and how to reduce the chances of infection—will need to be communicated to the public in a way that does not incite panic.

Given these obstacles and the possible risk that the best-made plans may still be ineffective in a severe pandemic, the federal government is taking steps to prepare the nation for a potential pandemic in hopes of lessening its overall impact. The *National Response Framework* charges the Secretary of the Department of Homeland Security (DHS) with responsibility for overall management and federal coordination of domestic incidents when needed,[11] the Federal Emergency Management Agency (FEMA) Administrator with responsibility as principal advisor to the President regarding emergency management, and the Secretary of HHS with responsibility for public health and medical response.[12] On November 2, 2005, the Secretary of HHS released the *HHS Pandemic Influenza Plan*, which provides HHS's plans for responding to a pandemic.[13] The document also provides pandemic response guidance to officials in state and local jurisdictions[14] and to health care facility officials. Since then, HHS has released five updates regarding the department's preparedness efforts and has released its *Pandemic Influenza Implementation Plan*. Despite these efforts, influenza and public health preparedness experts have raised concerns about the adequacy of HHS's plans and guidance to state and local officials and to health care facility officials.

Because of your interest in pandemic preparedness, we are providing information on the progress of HHS's plans and its guidance to state and local officials, and to health care facility officials, for responding to a pandemic outbreak. The focus of our work is on 4 key components taken from 5 of the 11 response elements critical for preparedness as described in the *HHS Pandemic Influenza Plan* (see table 5 in app. I for a list of all the response elements). Three components that we examined— pharmaceutical interventions (vaccines and antivirals), surge capacity of health care providers, and public communications—have repeatedly been found to need improvement by GAO and outside experts. In prior work, we reported on potential problems with pharmaceutical interventions during a pandemic, including vaccine shortages and the need for identifying target groups in advance.[15] Health care provider shortages, including nurses and physicians, have been reported for many years by GAO.[16] We reported that during the anthrax incidents of 2001, the media and the general public looked to CDC as the source for health-related information. However, CDC was not always able to successfully convey the information that it had.[17] We also reported on the significance of communicating clearly on response efforts during a pandemic.[18] The fourth component we focus on in our work—guidance for nonpharmaceutical interventions—is based on limited scientific evidence.

Specifically, for this chapter we analyzed how HHS plans to (1) use pharmaceutical interventions for treatment of infected individuals and to protect the critical workforce, (2) improve surge capacity of health care providers, (3) prepare state and local authorities to use nonpharmaceutical interventions for slowing the spread of disease, and (4) prepare to communicate with the public during a pandemic.

To determine how HHS plans to implement the four key components, we reviewed government documents related to a pandemic response. (See app. I for a description of each document.) In addition, to learn more about the elements needed for an effective public health emergency response, we reviewed related reports issued by GAO and HHS agencies, independent studies (including those from the Institute of Medicine, Congressional Research Service, and World Health Organization), and peer-reviewed journals. We interviewed officials from HHS offices, including the Office of the Assistant Secretary for Preparedness and Response, Office of the Assistant Secretary for Public Affairs, CDC, National Vaccine Program Office, National Institutes of Health, Agency for Healthcare Research and Quality, Health Resources and Services Administration, and FDA to learn more about their planning efforts. In addition, we interviewed state and local public health officials and members of the National Association of County and City Health Officials and the Association of State and Territorial Health Officials. We also interviewed officials from the American Hospital Association, American Medical Association, American Society For Microbiology, Council of State and Territorial Epidemiologists, Infectious Diseases Society of America, and Association of Public Health Laboratories. We also interviewed subject-matter experts to get their perspectives on HHS's planning efforts. We participated in relevant public meetings on pandemic preparedness, such as those sponsored by the Institute of Medicine, to gain knowledge of new scientific evidence on the effectiveness of planning efforts.

U.S. pandemic preparedness work is an ongoing process. The data in this chapter were last updated on August 2008. However, changes have continued to occur since completion of our data collection, and this chapter may not reflect all these changes. We conducted our work from April 2006 through September 2008 in accordance with generally accepted government auditing standards.

RESULTS IN BRIEF

Once a pandemic begins, HHS plans to make accessible to state and local jurisdictions federal stockpiles of antivirals and pre-pandemic vaccine until a pandemic vaccine becomes widely available. HHS has established a national goal of stockpiling 75 million treatment courses of antivirals in public-sector stockpiles—meaning those in the Strategic National Stockpile (SNS) and in jurisdictional stockpiles. HHS expects state and local jurisdictions to distribute antivirals received from the SNS as well as from stockpiles maintained by the jurisdictions. According to HHS, these public-sector stockpiles are intended to be used primarily for the treatment of sick individuals. HHS intends to oversee the distribution and administration of federally owned pre-pandemic vaccine to individuals identified as members of the critical workforce. Members of the critical workforce—estimated to be about 20 million—include workers in sectors that are considered necessary to keep society functioning, such as health care and law enforcement personnel. HHS's strategy for using pre- pandemic vaccine is to keep society functioning until a pandemic vaccine becomes widely available. However, HHS anticipates that initial batches of a pandemic vaccine may not be available for as long as 20 to 23 weeks after the start of the pandemic. HHS recommends that as batches of pandemic vaccine become available, state and local jurisdictions provide it to members of targeted groups based on factors such as occupation and age, instead of making the vaccine available to the general public. HHS faces challenges implementing its strategy for using pharmaceutical interventions during a pandemic, including the lack of vaccine-manufacturing capacity in the United States. HHS is currently making large investments in domestic vaccine manufacturing capacity. Additionally, we and others have reported since 2000 how problems can arise if potential target groups are not established in advance. In 2008, HHS released guidance on prioritizing target groups for pandemic vaccine and draft guidance on antiviral use during a pandemic. HHS has not yet released draft guidance for public comment on prioritizing target groups for pre-pandemic vaccine.

HHS has initiated efforts to improve the surge capacity of health care providers, but these efforts will be challenged during a severe pandemic because of the widespread nature of such an event, the existing shortages of health care providers, and the potential high absentee rate of providers. HHS is encouraging health care facilities to be capable of increasing the number of health care providers in the event of a pandemic through efforts such as using medical and nursing students to treat patients directly and cross training health care personnel. In addition, HHS's plans include using a national database to enable state and local officials to quickly identify licensed volunteers. However, there are concerns about the use of untrained health care personnel. Given the uncertain effectiveness of efforts to increase surge capacity, HHS has developed guidance to assist health care facilities in planning for altered standards of care; that is, for providing care while allocating scarce equipment, supplies, and personnel in a way that saves the largest number of lives in mass casualty events. For example, the HHS guidance recommends that, rather than treat all patients equally, health care facilities determine how to identify and treat the subset of patients who have a critical need for treatment and are likely to survive.

HHS will rely on state and local jurisdictions to utilize nonpharmaceutical interventions, such as isolation of sick individuals and voluntary home quarantine of those exposed to the pandemic-causing strain. To assist state and local jurisdictions with implementing nonpharmaceutical interventions, HHS has developed guidance that describes the department's "community mitigation framework." This framework is based upon a targeted, layered strategy involving the direct application of multiple nonpharmaceutical interventions, each of which is partially effective, initiated early and maintained consistently throughout a pandemic. However, HHS faces difficulties in helping state and local jurisdictions overcome implementation challenges, such as developing ways to help jurisdictions ensure community compliance. HHS is also investing in several initiatives to increase the nation's knowledge about the general use and effectiveness of nonpharmaceutical interventions. The findings from this research will be used to update existing guidance.

HHS has made progress in establishing roles, responsibilities, and procedures for communicating with the general public during a pandemic. For example, HHS's Office of the

Assistant Secretary for Public Affairs has responsibility for coordinating the public health and medical communications effort aimed at the general public. In addition, HHS has undertaken activities to better understand public perceptions and knowledge of pandemics, developed pandemic educational materials to communicate messages to the general public before and during a pandemic, and identified ways to disseminate these materials. Nevertheless, communications during a pandemic will be challenging, as a pandemic will create an immediate, intense, and sustained demand for information from the general public. HHS plans to communicate with the general public about sensitive and technical issues, which may include why a vaccine is not readily available to the population at large and why a pandemic may require allocating scarce health care resources in a way that saves the largest number of lives. The public may become confused if they receive inconsistent information from other sources, as HHS will not be able to ensure that messages delivered to the general public by nonHHS entities are consistent with HHS messages.

Although HHS has made progress in identifying issues that need to be addressed, significant challenges remain, many of which are beyond HHS's control or cannot be quickly addressed, such as the length of time it will take to develop a pandemic vaccine. However, among the important activities within HHS's control that HHS could address before a pandemic is finalizing the guidance on how limited pharmaceutical interventions should be used during a pandemic. Therefore, we are recommending that the Secretary of HHS expeditiously finalize guidance to assist state and local jurisdictions to determine how to effectively use limited supplies of antivirals and pre-pandemic vaccine in a pandemic, including prioritizing target groups for pre-pandemic vaccine.

In comments on a draft of this chapter, HHS described actions it has taken and plans to take relating to our recommendation. HHS also provided clarifications and additional details about its pandemic preparedness activities, which we incorporated where appropriate.

BACKGROUND

Pandemics occur when an influenza virus mutates into a novel strain that is highly transmissible among humans, leading to outbreaks worldwide. Because there is little or no pre-existing immunity in the population, the strain is highly pathogenic, thus causing disease among those who become infected. Infected individuals may be capable of transmitting the virus strain for 1 to 2 days before developing symptoms. Pandemics arise periodically but unpredictably and can cause successive waves of disease lasting for up to 3 years.

In recent years, the H5N1 strain and other strains of the influenza virus have emerged or re-emerged. Experts are concerned because of similarities between the H5N1 strain and the H1N1 strain, which caused the 1918-19 pandemic. For example, research suggests that both the H5N1 and H1N1 strains prompt an over-reaction of the inflammatory response in humans, causing rapid and severe damage to the lungs. Although the H5N1 strain has not been easily transmitted among humans, influenza experts believe that H5N1 or another new influenza strain may eventually mutate to become highly transmissible.

Pharmaceutical Interventions during a Pandemic

Pharmaceutical interventions available during a pandemic include vaccines and antivirals. Pharmaceutical interventions are the primary methods used to prevent the spread of disease as well as to reduce morbidity and mortality caused by the influenza virus. See table 1.

Vaccination is the primary method for preventing infection with the influenza virus. Vaccines reduce the severity of disease or provide immunity by causing the body to produce protective antibodies to fight off a particular virus strain.[19] In order for a vaccine to be most effective, it needs to be well-matched to a particular strain of the influenza virus so that the antibodies formed in response to the vaccine protect against that strain. However, existing strains of the influenza virus can mutate into new strains; in part, this is why a new vaccine is created each year for the upcoming influenza season. Much of what is known about the anticipated effectiveness of a pandemic vaccine is based on evidence from the annual seasonal vaccine.

During a pandemic, it may be necessary to use a vaccine that was developed prior to a pandemic and therefore may not be well-matched to the pandemic-causing strain. This vaccine, called a pre-pandemic vaccine, is developed using an influenza strain that experts believe is likely to cause the next pandemic.[20] Research exploring the use of a pre-pandemic vaccine based on strains of the H5N1 virus suggests that it may provide some protection against serious illness and death.[21] In contrast, a pandemic vaccine would be developed against an identified pandemic- causing strain and would likely provide better protection against the pandemic strain.

It is likely that seasonal influenza vaccine manufacturers will produce the vaccine used during a pandemic.[22] However, for the 2007-08 influenza season, only five vaccine manufacturers were licensed to produce seasonal influenza vaccine for the United States[23] and only one manufacturer produced its vaccine from start to finish in facilities within U.S. borders.[24] We also recently reported that experts are concerned that countries without domestic manufacturing capacity will not have access to vaccine in the event of a pandemic if the countries with manufacturing capacity prohibit the export of pandemic vaccine until their own needs are met.[25]

Antivirals can reduce symptoms and help prevent the spread of influenza by suppressing the growth of the influenza virus.[26] Unlike the immune response triggered by a vaccine, antivirals target the virus itself. For example, some antivirals interfere with the virus's ability to attach to cells, thereby preventing infection of human cells. Antivirals also differ from vaccines in that they do not need to be reformulated to match a specific influenza strain in order to be effective. In addition, antivirals can be manufactured and stockpiled in advance, making them potentially available at the beginning of a pandemic. HHS currently maintains a stockpile of antivirals in the SNS.[27]

However, as we have previously reported, there are limitations associated with relying on antivirals during a pandemic.[28] For example, the effectiveness of antivirals during seasonal influenza has been limited if they are used more than 48 hours after the onset of symptoms in an infected individual

Table 1. Comparison of Pharmaceutical Interventions for a Pandemic

Pharmaceutical interventions	How it works	Time frame for development	When it is expected to be available	Dosage	Known potential benefits	Known potential weaknesses
Antivirals	Disrupts viral infection of cells, such as the ability to bind to human cells or be released from an infected cell	Before a pandemic	Before and during a pandemic	Varies, depending on the type of antiviral used and age of patient	• May be used as a form of prophylaxis or treatment • May be made and stockpiled in advance of a pandemic	• Virus can develop resistance • Must be taken within 48 hours of developing symptoms for maximum effectiveness[a]
Pre-pandemic vaccine	Stimulates a human immune response	Before a pandemic	Early in a pandemic	Research on one type of vaccine suggests 2 doses of 90 micrograms (mcg.)[b]	• May prevent severe illness and death • May be made and stockpiled in advance	• May or may not be well-matched to the pandemic-causing strain
Pandemic vaccine	Stimulates a human immune response	During a pandemic	HHS estimates that initial doses will not be available until 20 to 23 weeks after the start of the pandemic	Unknown until actual pandemic-causing strain emerges	• Will help prevent infection or serious illness because the vaccine will be well-matched to the pandemic-causing strain	• Cannot be developed in advance • Will take months to develop

Source: GAO analysis of HHS documents and journal articles.

[a] Effectiveness estimate is based on antiviral use during seasonal influenza outbreaks.

[b] This dosing is based on the vaccine developed from an H5N1 strain and was approved by FDA for use in humans in the United States in April 2007.

For prophylactic use against seasonal influenza in healthy individuals, antivirals may not be as effective if they are not taken throughout the entire time an outbreak is present in a community. Some influenza strains have become resistant to the antivirals currently approved for prevention and treatment, and thus, the antivirals may not always be effective in preventing disease.[29] In addition, antivirals, like vaccines, take several months to produce, and the lead time needed to scale up production capacity may make it difficult to meet any large-scale, unanticipated demand immediately. As we recently reported, current antiviral production capacity is inadequate to meet expected demand during a pandemic.[30] Further, antivirals can be expensive to stockpile and difficult to administer, depending on the form in which they are given. For example, Tamiflu is given as a capsule or liquid and is relatively easy to administer, whereas, Relenza, is more difficult to administer because it is a powder that must be inhaled using a special device.

Since 2000, we and others have reported that federal, state, and local officials need to have information on target groups that have priority for receiving pharmaceutical interventions to know how, where, and to whom to distribute the interventions. We reported that having established target groups is particularly crucial in times of limited supply, such as during a pandemic, when a lack of specific guidance makes it difficult for federal, state, and local officials to plan. For example, in a prior report, we noted that health officials in one state did not know exactly how many individuals were considered a priority for receiving a vaccine.[31] In that case we found that it took state officials nearly a month to compile data on high-risk individuals, to decide how many doses of vaccine were needed in local areas, and to receive and ship vaccine to counties. State and local officials rely on federal guidance when making decisions on which groups should be targeted first for vaccination. For example, in a prior report on the 2004-05 influenza season, when the United States lost approximately half of its seasonal vaccine supply because of manufacturing difficulties, we found that CDC quickly revised its recommendations on who should be prioritized for vaccine.[32] CDC's changes decreased the targeted population from approximately 188 million to 98 million. State and local officials we spoke with for this chapter told us that they quickly adopted CDC's revised recommendations.

Surge Capacity of Health Care Providers

Since the terrorist attacks on September 11, 2001, public health departments and hospitals have been considered vital elements of emergency preparedness and response efforts. Surge capacity in public health departments and hospitals will be critical to pandemic response given the large number of people expected to require medical care. During a pandemic, hospitals will need to provide care for influenza patients as well as continue providing care for other patients.

A pandemic will put a severe strain on the health care system, which already is easily overwhelmed by seasonal influenza outbreaks. Seasonal influenza results in more than 200,000 hospital admissions and 36,000 deaths in the United States every year, and hospitals were stretched to capacity in some past seasonal influenza outbreaks. A severe pandemic would overwhelm hospitals in the United States. For example, using HHS's planning assumptions, authors of one study estimated that influenza patients would need the equivalent of 191 percent of available staffed non- ICU beds and 461 percent of available staffed ICU beds.[33]

A pandemic would occur in the context of existing health care provider shortages. Shortages of health care providers, including physicians and nurses, have been reported for many years by GAO and others.[34] For example, the Association of American Medical Colleges recently released a report summarizing studies issued by 15 states between 2000 and 2007 regarding physician shortages in the United States.[35] That report found that many of these states reported shortages of physicians in specialties such as primary care, cardiology, and endocrinology. Similarly, a recent survey of chief executive officers by the American Hospital Association found that as of December 2006, hospitals across the country reported having an estimated 116,000 registered nurse vacancies.[36] That survey also found that nearly half of emergency departments are operating at or above capacity.[37]

Partly in response to these workforce shortages, Congress passed the Pandemic and All-Hazards Preparedness Act (PAHPA) in December 2006.[38] Among other things, the law requires the Secretary of HHS by 2009 to identify strategies to recruit, retain, and protect the public health workforce from workplace exposures during public health emergencies, which would include pandemics.[39] In addition, PAHPA established the Office of the Assistant Secretary for Preparedness and Response to coordinate activities between HHS and other federal departments, agencies, and offices and state and local officials responsible for emergency preparedness.[40]

Nonpharmaceutical Interventions

Nonpharmaceutical interventions are measures used to reduce the impact of a communitywide infectious disease outbreak without the use of pharmaceuticals. Examples of nonpharmaceutical interventions include isolation, quarantine, social distancing, and infection control (see table 2).

Slowing the spread of disease during a pandemic will be particularly important given anticipated shortages of pharmaceutical interventions and the expectation that a severe pandemic will overwhelm the health care system. Experts have suggested that nonpharmaceutical interventions can help the health care system by reducing the anticipated influx of patients by limiting the rate of disease transmission (see figure 1).

In the past, nonpharmaceutical interventions have been used in some cases to successfully slow the spread of infectious disease outbreaks. For example, during the 1918-19 pandemic, local public health officials relied on nonpharmaceutical interventions—including rules forbidding overcrowding in streetcars and bans on public gatherings—to slow the spread of disease. More recently, during the global outbreak of severe acute respiratory syndrome (SARS) in 2003, nonpharmaceutical interventions were also implemented to slow the spread of disease. For example, we reported that nonpharmaceutical interventions, such as closing two hospitals to new admissions, appeared to be useful in Canada's management of the SARS outbreak.[41]

Table 2. Some Types of Nonpharmaceutical Interventions and Their Definitions

Type of Nonpharmaceutical Intervention	Definition
Isolation	The separation or restriction of movement of individuals ill with an infectious disease to prevent transmission to others.
Quarantine	The separation or restriction of movement of individuals exposed to an infectious disease, but not yet ill, who may become infectious to others.
Social distancing	Measures taken to decrease the frequency of contact among people, such as school closures.
Infection control	Hygiene measures to reduce the risk of transmission from infected individuals to uninfected individuals, including hand washing, cough etiquette, and disinfection.

Source: CDC.

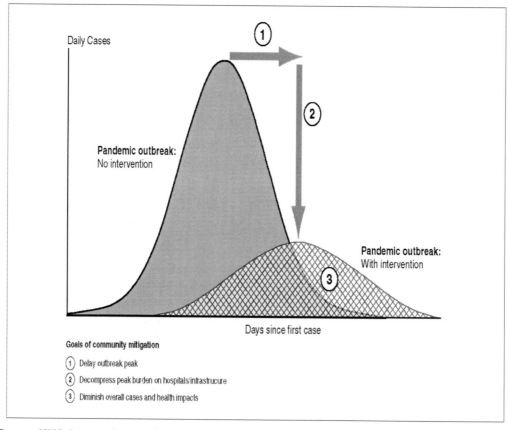

Source: HHS, *Interim Pre-Pandemic Planning Guidance: Community Strategy for Pandemic Influenza Mitigation in the United States - Early, Targeted Layered Use of Nonpharmaceutical Interventions*, Atlanta, Ga., 2007.

Figure 1. Potential Effect of Nonpharmaceutical Interventions on a Pandemic Outbreak

Communication with the Public

Public health emergencies such as the SARS outbreak in 2003 and the anthrax incidents in 2001 have demonstrated that communication with the public about a public health emergency by federal officials is a critical component of national preparedness. In July 2003, we reported that effective communication between health care providers and the public reinforced the need to adhere to infectious disease control measures and that rapid and frequent communications regarding SARS helped slow its spread.[42] In addition, in October 2003, we reported that the media and the public looked to CDC as the source for health-related information during the anthrax incidents, but that CDC was not always able to successfully convey the information that it had.[43]

As with the SARS outbreak and anthrax incidents, a pandemic will generate immediate, intense, and sustained demand for information. The public will want information quickly about the risks and status of the pandemic, what they can do to stay healthy, what is being done by the government to protect them, and where to go for medical services. Very technical points and sensitive political issues will need to be explained to the general public. If accurate and consistent information is not available and disseminated in a timely and efficient manner, rumors, myths, and misinformation may lead to unnecessary public anxiety and could result in mistrust of, and noncompliance with, the public health and medical measures that are recommended to save lives.

HHS PLANS TO MAKE FEDERAL STOCKPILES OF PHARMACEUTICALS ACCESSIBLE TO STATE AND LOCAL JURISDICTIONS, BUT FACES CHALLENGES WITH IMPLEMENTATION

Once a pandemic begins, HHS plans to make accessible to state and local jurisdictions[44] federal stockpiles of antivirals and pre-pandemic vaccine until a pandemic vaccine becomes widely available. According to HHS, public-sector stockpiles of antivirals are intended to be used primarily for the treatment of sick individuals. HHS intends to oversee the distribution and administration of federally owned pre-pandemic vaccine to individuals identified as members of the critical workforce; that is, workers in sectors that are necessary for society to continue functioning. HHS also plans to provide jurisdictions with doses of the pandemic vaccine as they become available. HHS recommends that state and local jurisdictions follow its list of targeted groups in administering the pandemic vaccine. However, HHS faces challenges with implementing its strategy for using pharmaceutical interventions, such as the lack of vaccine manufacturing capacity within U.S. borders and the length of time experts anticipate will be needed to manufacture a pandemic vaccine. Additionally, we and others have reported since 2000 how problems can arise if potential target groups are not established in advance. In 2008, HHS released guidance on prioritizing target groups for pandemic vaccine and draft guidance on antiviral use during a pandemic. HHS has not yet released draft guidance for public comment on prioritizing target groups for pre-pandemic vaccine.

HHS Plans to Distribute Antivirals from the SNS to Jurisdictions and Is Relying on Additional Stockpiles to Supplement These Drugs

Until a pandemic vaccine becomes widely available, one part of HHS's strategy for using pharmaceutical interventions involves distributing antivirals in the SNS to state and local jurisdictions. HHS has established a national goal of stockpiling 75 million treatment courses of antivirals in public-sector stockpiles—meaning those in the SNS and in jurisdictional stockpiles.[45] As of May 2008, HHS had stockpiled 44 million courses of antivirals for treatment in the SNS and is subsidizing the purchase of 31 million treatment courses by state and local jurisdictions for storage in their own stockpiles.[46] As of May 2008, state and local jurisdictions had collectively stockpiled nearly 22 million treatment courses of antivirals.[47]

Of the federally stockpiled antivirals, HHS has reserved 6 million courses for containment of an initial outbreak.[48] For example, these 6 million courses may be used to respond to initial outbreaks abroad and parts of the United States experiencing the earliest cases. Officials told us that after the department distributes these initial 6 million courses of antivirals, it plans to deliver the remaining antivirals in the SNS to all jurisdictions simultaneously for treatment of individuals sick with influenza. According to HHS's guidance, state and local jurisdictions will receive their allotments of antivirals on a per-capita basis and should prepare to receive their share of antivirals when a pandemic begins, either in the United States or overseas. According to HHS officials, the decision to release antivirals from the SNS will be made by the Secretary of HHS in conjunction with the Director of CDC. HHS officials estimate that it will take between 7 days and 1 month for all antivirals to be distributed to jurisdictions. HHS officials also told us that they have conducted several exercises to test HHS's plan to distribute antivirals to these jurisdictions during a pandemic. Antivirals from the SNS will be delivered to one location within each jurisdiction. According to HHS officials, state and local jurisdictions will distribute both the SNS antivirals and antivirals stored in their own stockpiles throughout their respective areas using pandemic-specific distribution plans.

HHS officials told us that the stockpiles of antivirals owned by state and local jurisdictions will provide the jurisdictions with more immediate access to the drugs during the initial stages of a pandemic. Because these stockpiles will be entirely under each jurisdiction's control, officials there may choose to use some of these antivirals as prophylaxis—as proposed in HHS's draft guidance on antiviral use during a pandemic—in an attempt to slow the spread of the pandemic by providing them to healthy individuals who have been exposed to the pandemic-causing strain. However, to ensure that stockpiles are not rapidly depleted, HHS currently recommends that jurisdictions use antivirals only for treatment. HHS also advises jurisdictions to begin deploying their respective antiviral stockpiles immediately when a pandemic has been confirmed.

In June 2008, HHS released draft guidance for the use of antivirals during a pandemic in the *Federal Register* for public comment. The draft guidance is consistent with HHS's previous recommendation that public-sector stockpiles be used primarily for treatment of individuals sick with influenza. In its draft guidance, HHS also acknowledged that more antivirals will be needed than will be available in public-sector stockpiles particularly if antivirals are used for prophylaxis. HHS proposes in its draft guidance that the private sector stockpile 110 million additional courses. HHS also suggests that antivirals in the private-sector stockpile be targeted for prophylactic use for health care and emergency services personnel, and in some circumstances, for persons with compromised immune systems as well as those living in group settings.[49] The purchasing, allocation, and distribution of private-sector stockpiles would be the responsibility of the owner of those stockpiles.

HHS Intends to Make Available Federally Owned Pre-Pandemic Vaccine to Protect the Critical Workforce

HHS's strategy also involves releasing federally owned pre-pandemic vaccine to specific locations in state and local jurisdictions for administration when it has been determined that sustained transmission of the pandemic virus has occurred. HHS intends to oversee distribution and administration of pre-pandemic to members of the critical workforce identified by a federal interagency group—the National Infrastructure Advisory Council. Workers considered critical consist of those necessary to maintain national or homeland security, economic survival, and the public health and welfare. These employees include emergency service providers, such as law enforcement, banking and financing personnel, and health care providers. The National Infrastructure Advisory Council estimates that the critical workforce includes about 20 million people.[50] HHS has a goal of stockpiling enough pre-pandemic vaccine to cover this group.[51] As of May 2008, HHS had purchased and stockpiled enough pre- pandemic vaccine for about 13 million people.[52] HHS's strategy for using pre-pandemic vaccine is to keep society functioning until a pandemic vaccine becomes widely available.

Table 3. HHS Target Groups for Pandemic Vaccination for a Severe Pandemic

Tier	Homeland and national security	Health care and community support services	Critical infrastructure	General population
Tier 1	• Deployed and mission critical personnel	• Public health personnel • Inpatient health care providers • Outpatient and home health care providers • Health care providers in long-term care facilities	• Emergency services sector personnel (Emergency Medical Services, law enforcement, and fire services) • Manufacturers of pandemic vaccine and antivirals	• Pregnant women • Infants and toddlers, 6 to 35 months old

Table 3 (Continued)

Tier 2	• Essential support and sustainment personnel • Intelligence services • Border protection personnel • National Guard personnel • Other domestic national security personnel	• Community support services and emergency management • Pharmacists • Mortuary services personnel	• Communications/information technology, electricity, nuclear, oil and gas, and water sector personnel • Financial clearing and settlement personnel • Critical operational and regulatory government personnel	• Household contacts of infants under 6 months old • Children 3 to 18 years old with high-risk conditions
Tier 3	• Other active duty and essential support	• Other important health care personnel	• Banking and finance, chemical, food and agriculture, pharmaceutical, postal and shipping, and transportation sector personnel • Other critical government personnel	• Children 3 to 18 years old without high-risk
Tier 4	• Not Applicable	• Not Applicable	• Not Applicable	• Persons 19 to 64 years old with high-risk condition • Persons over 65 years old
Tier 5	• Not Applicable	• Not Applicable	• Not Applicable	• Healthy adults, 19 to 64 years old

Source: HHS and DHS.

Note: Table was developed from *Guidance on Allocating and Targeting Pandemic Influenza Vaccine*, Washington, D.C., 2008.

State and local jurisdictions will receive allotments of pre-pandemic vaccine on a per-capita basis. According to HHS officials, stockpiles of pre-pandemic vaccine will be released for simultaneous distribution to selected sites in each jurisdiction. Currently, each vaccine manufacturer stores the doses of pre-pandemic vaccine that it produces. According to HHS, each manufacturer is assigned to supply this vaccine to certain jurisdictions using its established distribution channels. HHS officials also told us that they have a longer-term plan to distribute vaccine using a single distributor, based on CDC's Vaccine Management Business Improvement Project.[53] According to HHS officials, this centralized distribution system would be incorporated with its existing Vaccine Ordering and Distribution System, which allows for federal tracking of vaccine distribution. HHS anticipates having a centralized distribution system in place around 2010. HHS officials told us that utilizing this type of system would be beneficial during the early stages of a pandemic, when it is expected that maintaining central control of and securing vaccine will be a high priority.

HHS Plans to Distribute Pandemic Vaccine as It Becomes Available for Vaccination of Target Groups

HHS plans to provide pandemic vaccine as it becomes available to state and local jurisdictions for use among target groups. HHS has developed guidance for the prioritization system for administration of the pandemic vaccine. HHS has divided the entire U.S. population into four broad categories—homeland and national security, health care and community support services, critical infrastructure, and the general population. Within each category, groups are clustered into five tiers that correspond to the vaccination priority—or target group—for that specific category. (See table 3 for target groups for a severe pandemic.) These targeted groups were derived through consideration of four vaccination program objectives: (1) protecting those who are essential to the pandemic response and provide care for persons who are ill; (2) protecting those who maintain essential community services; (3) protecting children; and (4) protecting workers who are at greater risk of infection because of their job. In its guidance, HHS also proposed that not all targeted groups be vaccinated in every pandemic, depending on the severity of the pandemic.[54] For a less severe pandemic, for example, individuals in tiers 2 and 3 in the category of critical infrastructure would not be targeted for vaccination.[55] HHS also noted that the guidance will need to be reassessed periodically before a pandemic occurs to consider factors such as changes in vaccine production capacity. During a pandemic, guidance will also be modified based on additional factors that will not be known until a pandemic occurs, including the characteristics of pandemic illness.

HHS officials told us that should a pandemic occur in the near future, pandemic vaccine will likely be distributed from vaccine manufacturers directly to state and local jurisdictions using the same distribution systems the manufacturers regularly use for seasonal influenza vaccine.[56] As with pre-pandemic vaccine, HHS anticipates that eventually multiple manufacturers will produce pandemic vaccine. However, it anticipates utilizing a single, centralized distributor. HHS expects to have a centralized distribution system in place around 2010.

HHS Faces Challenges with Implementing Its Strategy for Using Pharmaceutical Interventions

HHS faces three challenges with implementing its strategy for using pharmaceutical interventions during a pandemic. The first challenge is associated with uncertainties about the effectiveness and clinical outcomes of the pharmaceutical interventions. For example, the uncertainty concerning which influenza strain will cause the next pandemic raises the possibility that the pre-pandemic vaccine currently being developed will not offer protection against the pandemic strain. Also, because the actual pandemic-causing strain has not yet surfaced, researchers can only estimate what amount of vaccine will actually be needed to stimulate a sufficient human immune response. Similarly, the appropriate dosage of antivirals or the exact length of the treatment course needed to make them effective will not be known until the actual pandemic-causing strain emerges. Further, the ability of influenza viruses to develop resistance to antivirals also raises questions about their effectiveness. In 2005, a group of global experts on antivirals noted that studies have suggested that different strains of the H5N1 avian influenza virus have developed resistance to different antivirals.[57]

There is also the potential for adverse outcomes that may result from large-scale administration of a newly developed vaccine, such as what occurred during the "swine flu" outbreak of 1976. The government's success in vaccinating large numbers of the public with the swine flu vaccine was negated by the development of Guillain-Barré syndrome among hundreds of immunized individuals, leading to several deaths.[58] This adverse event only became apparent when the vaccine had been administered to large numbers of people.[59]

A second challenge concerns difficulties with the production of pharmaceutical interventions, particularly vaccines. The United States lacks vaccine manufacturing capacity; for example, we found that for the 2007-08 influenza season only one influenza vaccine manufacturer had its production processes entirely within U.S. borders. Additionally, in 2007 we found that the lack of U.S. vaccine manufacturing capacity is cause for concern among experts because it is possible that countries without domestic manufacturing capacity will not have access to vaccine in the event of a pandemic if the countries with domestic manufacturing capacity prohibit the export of the pandemic vaccine until their own needs are met.[60]

According to HHS, exacerbating the lack of manufacturing capacity is the length of time experts anticipate will be needed to manufacture a pandemic vaccine. HHS estimates that it may take as long as 20 to 23 weeks after the start of the pandemic for the first doses of pandemic vaccine to become available.[61] Figure 2 shows how pharmaceutical manufacturers would proceed to develop and produce pandemic vaccine as well as when initial batches of vaccine are likely to become available.

In response to this lack of manufacturing capacity, HHS has established the long-term goal of domestically producing enough pandemic vaccine for 300 million people within 6 months of having a reference strain of the pandemic virus. HHS expects to reach this level of manufacturing capacity around 2010.[62] The department is currently making large investments in domestic vaccine manufacturing capacity for this purpose. (See app. II for a description of these investments.) HHS is doing this in part by supporting vaccine research with contracts that require manufacturers to establish vaccine-producing facilities within U.S. borders.[63] Through these contracts, one U.S. facility has expanded its manufacturing capacity and is expected to double its existing capacity by 2009 and triple its capacity by 2011. A second facility was recently established in the United States and is expected to manufacture a licensed product in 2010. HHS officials told us there had also been progress in expanding domestic manufacturing capacity for antivirals.

The third challenge HHS faces involves difficulties in stockpiling and distributing pharmaceutical interventions. The high costs of purchasing and storing antivirals calls into question HHS's plan to rely on state and local jurisdictions to acquire and store their own stockpiles of antivirals. For example, officials from one state we spoke with told us that the state was facing financial difficulty in determining how it will purchase its share of antivirals and in identifying and paying for adequate storage space. HHS officials have acknowledged that the cost of purchasing antivirals is high, but have also noted that the contract price HHS has negotiated for state and local jurisdictions is better than the retail price. No federal funding has been made available to aid state and local jurisdictions in building and maintaining storage capacity. In addition, should a pandemic occur in the near future, HHS plans to utilize multiple distributors for pre-pandemic and pandemic vaccines, allowing manufacturers to use existing processes with which they are familiar. However, HHS acknowledged that this process also has multiple weaknesses. For example, the current distribution plan requires extensive coordination between HHS and multiple manufacturers and distributors. It also requires that states and local jurisdictions manage vaccine shipments from multiple sources, which may complicate receipt and storage activities. In response, HHS is planning to centralize its distribution system through a single distributor.

HHS Has Made Progress on Revising Guidance for Target Groups for Use of Pandemic Vaccine, but Has Not Finalized Guidance for Using Pre-Pandemic Vaccine and Antivirals

HHS has made progress on revising its 2005 guidance to state and local jurisdictions for identifying target groups for the use of pandemic vaccine, but has not finalized guidance for using antivirals and pre-pandemic vaccine. Since 2000, GAO and others have reported on the importance of having pre-established target groups for pharmaceutical interventions to avoid problems deciding who should receive these interventions. In addition, during times of shortage, state and local public health officials look to the federal government for guidance, including when making decisions on which groups should be targeted for prioritization. For example, during the seasonal influenza vaccine shortage of 2004-05, state and local officials immediately adopted the revised guidance on who should be targeted for vaccination as recommended by CDC.[64] State and local public health officials and others have stressed that federal guidance on target groups is needed to aid in their pandemic planning efforts.

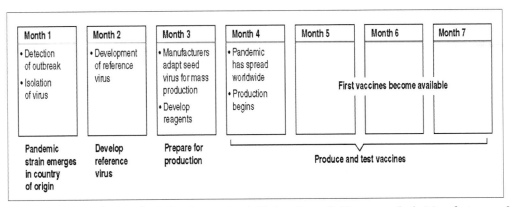

Source: GAO analysis of HHS, International Federation of Pharmaceutical Manufacturers & Associations, and World Health Organization data.

Figure 2. Pandemic Vaccine Production Timeline

HHS first published target groups for pandemic vaccine and antivirals in the *HHS Pandemic Influenza Plan* in November 2005.[65] These initial groups were identified to support a goal of reducing morbidity and mortality among those at greatest risk for developing complications from influenza, such as the elderly. Since the publication of the *HHS Pandemic Influenza Plan*, there has been wide recognition that other factors should be considered, such as protecting those critical workers needed to keep society functioning, including health care and law enforcement personnel. In addition, recent expansion in the production of antivirals has increased the amount available. Thus, HHS, in consultation with other federal agencies, was tasked by the *National Strategy for Pandemic Influenza Implementation Plan* and the *HHS Pandemic Influenza Implementation Plan* to revise the groups outlined in the *HHS Pandemic Influenza Plan*.[66] In July 2008, HHS released guidance on prioritizing target groups for pandemic vaccine. HHS released draft guidance for public comment in the *Federal Register* on how antivirals may be used during a pandemic in June 2008.

However, HHS has not yet released draft guidance identifying target groups for pre-pandemic vaccine. HHS officials told us they are working on draft guidance for pre-pandemic vaccine in collaboration with other federal agencies, such as DHS. According to officials, target groups for pre-pandemic vaccine are likely to resemble those for pandemic vaccine, but with more of a focus on the critical workforce rather than on the general population. HHS officials said a tiered structure, such as that used for the pandemic vaccine, would only be needed if a pandemic occurs before HHS has reached its goal of stockpiling enough doses for 20 million people.[67]

HHS EFFORTS TO IMPROVE SURGE CAPACITY OF HEALTH CARE PROVIDERS WILL BE CHALLENGED DURING A PANDEMIC

HHS has initiated efforts to improve the surge capacity of health care providers, but these efforts will be challenged during a severe pandemic. Surge capacity of health care providers will be hindered by existing shortages of health care providers and by the potentially high absentee rates of providers during a pandemic. Inadequate staffing of health care facilities will be likely, and the ability to deliver health care consistent with established standards of care may be compromised.[68] HHS's efforts include plans to supplement the number of health care providers with medical and nursing students. Given the uncertain effectiveness of efforts to increase surge capacity, HHS has developed guidance to assist health care facilities in planning for altered standards of care; that is, for providing care while allocating scarce equipment, supplies, and personnel in a way that saves the largest number of lives in mass casualty events, such as pandemics.

Surge Capacity during a Pandemic Will Be Hindered by the Potentially High Absentee Rate of Health Care Workers

In a severe pandemic, existing health-care provider shortages would worsen as health care providers become infected through exposure to infected patients or reach exhaustion because of longer working hours. The federal government assumes absenteeism among all workers, including health care providers, could be as high as 40 percent.[69] During the 2003 SARS outbreak (a disease that has a high mortality rate and poses a high risk for health care workers similar to a pandemic), health care workers accounted for more than 20 percent of the infected cases. During the epidemics in Toronto and Hong Kong, 51 percent and between

28 percent and 50 percent, respectively, of health care providers who treated SARS patients became infected with the SARS virus.[70]

Studies have shown that during extreme public health emergencies, such as a pandemic, some health care workers may be unable or unwilling to report to work.[71] For example, a survey of public health department workers, including communicable disease staff, nurses, and physicians, at three public health departments in Maryland found that approximately 46 percent would be likely not to report to work during a pandemic outbreak.[72] Similarly, in a survey of hospital personnel, including doctors and nurses, only half responded that they would be willing to report to work during a pandemic. Those who said they may be unlikely to report to work cited fear of contracting an illness as the reason.[73] These potential workforce shortages during a pandemic will affect care for all patients, not just those with influenza.

HHS's Efforts to Improve Surge Capacity during a Pandemic Will Face Challenges

HHS has initiated many efforts to increase the number of health care workers during a public health emergency by supplementing the workforce with federal response teams and by encouraging mutual aid between states. However, HHS faces challenges in improving surge capacity during a severe pandemic because of the widespread effects of a pandemic and the existing shortages of health care providers.

HHS's Plans for Surge Capacity of Health Care Providers during a Pandemic

HHS has planned four types of efforts to improve surge capacity during a pandemic. First, the *HHS Pandemic Influenza Plan* recommends that health care facilities use personnel available locally to increase the number of health care providers during emergencies. These recommendations include using trainees (such as medical and nursing students), patients' family members, and retired health care providers to provide support for essential patient care at times of severe staffing shortages. The plan recommends that hospital clinical administrators take on patient care responsibilities and that facilities recruit health care providers from other medical settings, such as medical offices and day surgery centers, to assist with patient care in the hospital setting. Additionally, the plan recommends that health care providers be cross- trained to provide support for essential patient care at times of severe staffing shortages. To assist with this effort, HHS's Agency for Healthcare Research and Quality has developed a video to help train health care workers who are not respiratory care specialists to provide basic respiratory care and ventilator management to adult patients during mass casualty events. In addition, the *HHS Pandemic Influenza Plan* recommends deployment of federal medical responders, such as members of the National Disaster Medical System, during the early stages of a pandemic to supplement the number of health care providers.

Second, the *HHS Pandemic Influenza Plan* encourages state and territory officials to use the Emergency System for Advance Registration of Volunteer Health Professionals program, which enables state and territory officials to quickly identify licensed volunteer professionals to work in areas with shortages. This program is state-based systems that provide advanced registration and the credentialing information of clinicians needed to augment health care facilities during a declared emergency. The program enables the sharing of pre-registered health care professionals across state lines. According to HHS, as of February 2008, 40 state and territorial jurisdictions had begun to implement the program; all states and territories are required to have this program fully operational by August 2008.

Third, HHS has advised state officials to incorporate the Emergency Management Assistance Compact (EMAC) in their plans as another vehicle for obtaining medical assistance during a pandemic. Once a governor declares a state of emergency, a state can request that EMAC address its need for resources, such as health care providers. EMAC personnel will find states that have health care providers who can be deployed across state lines. EMAC was established in 1996 and is administered by the National Emergency Management Association. All 50 states, the District of Columbia, Puerto Rico, and the U.S. Virgin Islands have enacted legislation providing authority to join EMAC.

Fourth, HHS encourages state and local officials to use other mechanisms to expand surge capacity of health care providers for providing care to less severely ill patients during a pandemic. These mechanisms would encourage home care of less severely ill patients and include "telehealth" (also known as "telemedicine"), which allows health care providers in hospitals to care for and monitor patients at home with the use of electronic information and telecommunications technologies; and call centers (similar to nurse advice lines), which will allow patients at home to contact health care providers in hospitals in order to obtain medical advice regarding home care.

Challenges to Efforts to Increase Surge Capacity during the Initial Outbreak of a Pandemic

HHS faces several challenges in its efforts to increase surge capacity of health care providers during a pandemic. There are concerns that the use of untrained personnel may reduce the capacity of trained health care providers to deliver needed care. For example, officials from one professional association told us that using such individuals would require training and supervision, which would actually increase the workload of the health care facilities' staff. They also told us that cross-training personnel to provide support for essential patient care during a mass casualty event may be infeasible because health care providers will be busy caring for patients in their own areas of expertise. Cross-training of health care providers needs to be done in advance, but this may be infeasible because it would take providers away from their daily patient- care responsibilities, and this may be difficult to do given current workforce shortages.

Furthermore, health care providers from other areas may not be available for deployment in a severe pandemic. Members of response teams, such as those of the National Disaster Medical System, already have full-time jobs in health care. Therefore, these teams would not necessarily add to the nation's overall number of health care providers who would be available to treat influenza patients. We were told by HHS and FEMA officials that the National Disaster Medical System response teams will not likely be deployed during a pandemic outbreak because of the widespread nature of a pandemic and the need for those responders in their own regions. Similarly, while the EMACs make it easier for health care providers to work in states other than those in which they are licensed, given the widespread nature of pandemics, health care providers likely will be needed in their own home regions.[74]

HHS Has Issued Guidance Regarding Implementation of Altered Standards of Care to Be Used If There Is Inadequate Staffing of Health Care Facilities

During a severe pandemic, inadequate staffing of health care facilities will be likely despite efforts to improve surge capacity. Thus, the ability to deliver health care consistent with established standards of care for all patients may be compromised.[75] HHS officials told us they believe that decisions on the allocation of scarce resources—such as equipment, supplies and personnel—are best made at the local level.[76] Therefore, the *HHS Pandemic Influenza Implementation Plan* recommends that health care facilities plan ahead for providing altered standards of care;[77] that is, for providing care while allocating scarce resources in a way that saves the largest number of lives in mass casualty events.[78] With altered standards of care, instead of treating the sickest or most injured patients first, health care providers would identify and treat patients who have a critical need for treatment and would be likely to survive. Complicating conditions, such as an underlying chronic disease that may impact an individual's ability to survive, would be considered in the decision-making process. Resources being used by current patients, such as those recovering from surgery, would also become part of the overall resource allocation decisions and might be re-allocated to patients with a more critical need for treatment and a higher likelihood to survive. Altered standards of care would be implemented on a temporary basis. Once the event wanes and more resources become available, provision of health care would return to established standards of care used in normal situations.

HHS has issued two guidance documents, *Altered Standards of Care in Mass Casualty Events and Mass Medical Care with Scarce Resources: A Community Planning Guide*, to assist health care facilities to plan for providing altered standards of care.[79] *Altered Standards of Care in Mass Casualty Events* provides health care facilities guiding principles for developing altered standards of care. Additionally, it includes a discussion of the authority to activate the use of altered standards of care and the associated legal and regulatory issues, including the possible need for liability protection for health care providers and facilities.[80] *Mass Medical Care with Scarce Resources* expands on the *Altered Standards of Care in Mass Casualty Events* report. It provides a discussion of the circumstances that communities would face as a result of a mass casualty event, approaches and strategies that could be used to provide the most appropriate standards of care possible under the circumstances, examples of tools and resources available to help state and local officials in their planning process, ethical considerations in planning for a mass casualty event, and a pandemic case study.

Long-Term Efforts to Increase the Number and Enhance the Preparedness Level of Health Care Providers

PAHPA calls for HHS's Assistant Secretary for Preparedness and Response to lead and coordinate HHS emergency preparedness and response activities.[81] Accordingly, the Assistant Secretary is engaged in efforts to increase the number and enhance the preparedness level of health care providers for public health emergencies. As part of this effort, HHS officials told us that they have begun to examine issues related to recruitment, retention, and protection of the public health workforce with the goal of identifying strategies to overcome workforce shortages. In addition, to encourage health professionals to enter employment in a state or local public health agency, PAHPA authorizes HHS to award grants to states to assist in operating public health workforce loan repayment programs for individuals who serve in health professional shortage areas or in areas at high risk of a public health emergency.[82]

PAHPA also authorized HHS to develop Centers of Public Health Preparedness at accredited schools of public health.[83] HHS intends that these centers will help to train and educate health professionals to prepare for and respond to public health emergencies, including a pandemic. As part of this effort, CDC will develop core emergency preparedness and response curriculums, identify performance goals, and develop health systems research projects. HHS has already incorporated standardized benchmarks and performance measures into existing grant programs.[84]

HHS HAS PROVIDED GUIDANCE TO HELP STATE AND LOCAL JURISDICTIONS OVERCOME DIFFICULTIES WITH IMPLEMENTING NONPHARMACEUTICAL INTERVENTIONS

HHS will rely on state and local jurisdictions to utilize nonpharmaceutical interventions to help slow the spread of disease and to lessen the burden on the nation's health care system until a pandemic vaccine is widely available. HHS has developed guidance and is investing in research on the general use and effectiveness of nonpharmaceutical interventions, thereby helping jurisdictions make more informed decisions. According to HHS, the findings from this research will be used to update existing guidance. However, HHS faces difficulties in helping state and local jurisdictions overcome implementation challenges, such as identifying steps for ensuring community compliance.

HHS Will Rely on State and Local Jurisdictions to Utilize Nonpharmaceutical Interventions to Help Slow the Spread of Disease

The authority to implement nonpharmaceutical interventions—such as decisions on school closures—to slow the spread of disease and lessen the burden on the nation's health care system until a pandemic vaccine is available rests with state and local jurisdictions. To assist state and local authorities with their current planning efforts for using nonpharmaceutical interventions, HHS published a guidance document in February 2007—the *Interim Pre-pandemic Planning Guidance: Community Strategy for Pandemic Influenza Mitigation in the United States – Early, Targeted, Layered Use of Nonpharmaceutical Interventions*.[85] HHS officials told us that the recommendations in the guidance are for pre-pandemic contingency planning and are intended to provide state and local jurisdictions with a conceptual framework to guide their planning. In this guidance, HHS introduces its "community mitigation framework" that is based upon a targeted, layered strategy involving the direct application of multiple, partially-effective nonpharmaceutical interventions, initiated early and maintained consistently throughout a pandemic. Specifically, HHS's guidance describes four interventions: (1) isolation (either at home or in a health care setting) and treatment (as appropriate) with antivirals of all individuals with confirmed or probable infections; (2) voluntary home quarantine of members of households exposed to the disease and consideration of combining this intervention with antivirals, provided sufficient amounts are available and can readily be distributed; (3) school closures (including public and private schools as well as colleges and universities) accompanied by closures of other public settings (e.g., shopping malls and movie theaters) to prevent out-of-school social contacts; and (4) adult social distancing to reduce contact among adults in the community and workplace.

HHS officials and other experts have acknowledged the significance of implementing certain nonpharmaceutical interventions in order to maximize the available public health benefit while minimizing adverse secondary effects of the interventions. Thus, HHS recommends that state and local jurisdictions consider the severity of the pandemic when making decisions about how to respond to the outbreak. For example, for a less severe pandemic, HHS recommends voluntary home isolation of sick individuals, but generally does not recommend measures that may be more burdensome, such as voluntary quarantine of exposed household members, school closures, and adult social distancing. HHS recommends that state and local jurisdictions implement those additional measures and others in a more severe pandemic.

Department officials and experts have also stressed the importance of balancing the need to intervene early enough for nonpharmaceutical measures to be effective, while at the same time not causing unnecessary hardship by implementing them too early. HHS and other federal agencies released guidance in March 2008—the *Federal Guidance to Assist States in Improving State-Level Pandemic Influenza Operating Plans*[86]—that included information to assist state and local jurisdictions in determining when to implement certain nonpharmaceutical interventions. For example, this guidance recommends implementing voluntary quarantine and administering antivirals to individuals exposed to the pandemic virus when a case of novel influenza is detected in an area, including before sustained human-to-human transmission has been established.

Once a pandemic is underway, HHS anticipates providing technical assistance to state and local jurisdictions on the implementation of nonpharmaceutical interventions. This technical assistance would include assessing the specific epidemiological characteristics of the pandemic, such as how the pandemic-causing strain is transmitted, and consulting with state and local jurisdictions on the effectiveness of the nonpharmaceutical interventions that had been implemented. Because it is not possible to accurately predict the severity of a pandemic, HHS officials told us the recommendations in the guidance may change significantly during an actual pandemic, based on data HHS gathered from providing technical assistance as well as from data from initial outbreak investigations or from routine surveillance systems.

HHS's Guidance on Nonpharmaceutical Interventions Is Based on Inconclusive Scientific Evidence

HHS officials acknowledge that the recommendations in its guidance are not specific because the scientific evidence on the use and effectiveness of nonpharmaceutical interventions is limited, and therefore inconclusive. The research to date using mathematical modeling and analysis of historical data of past pandemics suggests that utilizing multiple nonpharmaceutical interventions simultaneously and early in a pandemic may aid in slowing disease transmission.[87] For example, historical studies of the 1918-19 pandemic describe how some cities reduced death rates by successfully implementing multiple nonpharmaceutical interventions, including social distancing, mandated mask wearing, and case isolation.[88] However, because of incomplete historical records, researchers are not able to determine precisely, where, when, and for how long these interventions were implemented.

HHS has supported several research initiatives to establish a stronger evidence base concerning the implementation and effectiveness of nonpharmaceutical interventions, thereby helping jurisdictions to make more informed decisions. For example, in October 2006, HHS awarded $5.2 million to support eight research projects on topics ranging from the role hand hygiene can play in reducing disease transmission to examining upper respiratory infections in families. According to HHS, the findings from this research will be used to update existing guidance. HHS and other experts have stressed the need for additional research to, for example, better inform the assumptions used in mathematical models.[89] HHS listed other key areas for further research in its guidance, such as understanding fundamental questions regarding influenza transmission and the potential psychosocial effects of certain nonpharmaceutical interventions, such as prolonged voluntary home quarantine and social distancing.

HHS Faces Difficulties in Assisting State and Local Jurisdictions to Overcome Implementation Challenges

HHS faces difficulties in helping state and local jurisdictions implement nonpharmaceutical interventions. First, as HHS acknowledged in its guidance, there is the potential for state and local jurisdictions to implement these interventions in an uncoordinated, untimely, and inconsistent manner, thereby dramatically reducing their effectiveness. For example, if one jurisdiction implements a voluntary quarantine of sick individuals and a neighboring jurisdiction does not, the overall movement of sick individuals in the area may not be sufficiently reduced. HHS hopes that state and local jurisdictions will follow its guidance and act in concert, but HHS cannot compel jurisdictions to do so.

Second, HHS faces the challenge of helping state and local jurisdictions identify specific thresholds for implementing and ending nonpharmaceutical interventions, such as at what point to close schools. The Federal Guidance to Assist States in Improving State-Level Pandemic Influenza Operating Plans provides general guidance to state and local jurisdictions on when to consider beginning to implement nonpharmaceutical interventions. However, this guidance does not provide details on when to implement specific interventions. For example, the guidance recommends state and local officials begin to consider closing schools when transmission of a pandemic virus occurs, but does not identify a specific absentee rate at which officials should take action. Experts have noted that determining specific triggers is difficult, partly because the data currently available are imperfect and sparse, requiring decision-makers to make assumptions regarding the transmission rate of the pandemic-causing strain as well as the effects of other community behaviors during the pandemic. In addition, state and local officials generally do not have the capabilities to collect the data that federal authorities will need to develop specific triggers during an actual pandemic. For example, one local official noted that one method of determining specific community triggers would be to use prevalence rates, which measure the percentage of the population infected with disease. However, state and local areas do not have surveillance systems capable of providing this level of detail in real-time.

Third, HHS faces the challenge of helping state and local jurisdictions convince residents to comply with its requests regarding nonpharmaceutical interventions. This task is especially difficult because restrictions on public activities to combat a pandemic may need to be in place for several months. During the 1918-19 pandemic, nonpharmaceutical interventions were implemented for 2 to 8 weeks. However, researchers have suggested that such interventions would need to be implemented for a longer period for a future pandemic in order to prevent another increase in transmission after the interventions are discontinued.[90] In the 1918-19 pandemic, nonpharmaceutical interventions were lifted. In some cases, the public became fatigued with the interventions, leading to public opposition and noncompliance when authorities found it necessary to reimpose the restrictions.

A fourth challenge HHS faces is that these restrictions may have negative impacts on the nation's economy and on the financial well-being of individual households. For example, nonpharmaceutical interventions may exacerbate worker absenteeism as parents stay home to care for their children when schools are closed. This could eventually result in disruptions in the provision of essential services, such as law enforcement. Similarly, lengthy nonpharmaceutical interventions could financially strain individuals and families. For example, while an HHS-sponsored study on public perceptions regarding a pandemic found a generally high willingness to comply with public health recommendations, it also found a decrease in reported ability to comply with recommended measures when financial constraints were considered.[91] Thus, 57 percent of respondents said they would have problems complying with recommended measures because of financial difficulties if they had to be out of work for 1 month, with 76 percent reporting problems if they had to miss 3 months.

A fifth challenge for HHS is the lack of trust by U.S. citizens of federal government public health authorities. A recent study found that only 40 percent of the U.S. population would trust federal government public health authorities as a source for accurate information.[92] The authors of this study assert that this lack of trust may have been exacerbated by the public's negative perceptions of the government's response to Hurricane Katrina in 2005 and that the U.S. population may now be less willing to cooperate with some public health requirements in the future, including isolation of sick individuals.

HHS IS DEVELOPING MESSAGES AND PROCEDURES FOR COMMUNICATING TO THE PUBLIC DURING A PANDEMIC BUT CHALLENGES REMAIN

HHS has made progress by establishing roles, responsibilities, and procedures for communicating messages to the general public during a pandemic. HHS has also developed pandemic educational materials to communicate messages to the general public before and during a pandemic and has identified ways to disseminate these materials. In addition, HHS has engaged the general public on pandemic issues to better understand public perceptions and knowledge. Nonetheless, communicating sensitive and complex issues to the general public during a pandemic will be challenging.

Roles, Responsibilities, and Procedures Have Been Established for How HHS Plans to Communicate with the General Public about a Pandemic

HHS has assigned roles and responsibilities, and developed procedures, for how HHS plans to communicate with the general public about a pandemic. Under the *National Response Framework*, HHS is the lead federal agency for public health and medical services, and as such, HHS is the federal agency responsible for communicating with the general public about the public health and medical aspects of a pandemic before and during an outbreak. In addition, the *HHS Pandemic Influenza Plan* identified activities that should be undertaken to prepare HHS to communicate with the general public before and during a pandemic.

In November 2006, HHS completed the *U.S. Department of Health and Human Services Pandemic Influenza Communications Plan* which lays out detailed roles, responsibilities, and procedures to guide HHS communications with the general public.[93] For example, this plan assigned HHS's Office of the Assistant Secretary for Public Affairs responsibility for coordinating pandemic health messages across all HHS agencies and with state and local communications staff in order to ensure that all HHS agencies work closely together to make public statements that are timely, consistent, and accurate.

HHS has named spokespersons within HHS to deliver messages to the public before and during an outbreak.[94] HHS has trained federal, state, local, and private sector public affairs officials to communicate with the general public about a pandemic. The Crisis and Emergency Risk Communication training modules developed by HHS clarify the role of spokespersons, describe the psychology of communicating during a crisis, and provide best practices for working with the media during a crisis. HHS has held 10 Crisis and Emergency Risk Communication training sessions for nearly 500 senior federal officials and public affairs staff, and 11 regional training sessions for approximately 900 state and local leaders. Two additional trainings are scheduled in 2008. HHS also held Crisis and Emergency Risk Communication training sessions in June 2007 for Red Cross leaders and in January 2007 for stakeholders. Nearly 900 training sites participated in these sessions via the Internet.

During a pandemic, the HHS communications effort will operate out of its Emergency Communications Center. The center's capabilities include originating or accessing video feeds, news conferencing, posting mass electronic mailings, responding to media telephone inquiries, receiving, vetting, and clearing messages to be released by HHS. HHS will use a departmental public affairs conference line to provide telephone connections for public affairs staff throughout the department. These phone connections will allow HHS public affairs personnel to work from dispersed sites during the crisis, coordinate messages, receive guidance or direction, and provide information to those needing it. The DHS National Incident Communications Conference Line will also be used by HHS to exchange information with other federal agencies.

In addition, the Office of the Assistant Secretary for Public Affairs conducts media outreach to strengthen the relationship between the media and HHS and to support pandemic planning and education. Periodic briefings are scheduled between senior department officials, including the HHS Secretary, and members of the press. For example, in early 2007 HHS held a series of roundtable discussions on pandemics with the major broadcast and cable television networks, wire services, and bloggers to raise awareness of pandemics; the secretaries of HHS and Department of Agriculture participated. HHS press-office staff members also talk to the media regularly to answer questions and provide updates on pandemic planning and related issues. In January 2007, HHS began holding a series of tabletop exercises[95] with key media leaders and senior government officials in six major cities to facilitate effective communication to help insure the timely dissemination of accurate information to the general public through the use of media outlets during a pandemic.

HHS Has Developed Pandemic Educational Materials to Communicate Messages to the General Public before and during a Pandemic

HHS has developed and disseminated educational materials for communicating critical information to the general public and is in the process of developing additional materials. HHS has identified some of the critical information that the general public will require during a pandemic and has developed message maps—communications tools used to help organize complex information—to convey that information in a concise format before an outbreak. HHS has developed 82 message maps. HHS's message maps are each designed to distill three primary, easily understood messages on issues such as the differences between avian influenza, pandemic influenza, and seasonal influenza, as well as what HHS is doing to prepare for a pandemic. Each of these primary messages has three supporting messages that can be used as appropriate to provide context for the issue being mapped.[96] HHS message maps take the form of a series of questions and answers and are made public so that spokespersons from across the government or from private organizations can use the maps to convey accurate and consistent background information to their constituents before an outbreak. Table 4 shows an example of an HHS message map.

Table 4. Example of an HHS Message Map

How fast would pandemic influenza spread?
1 When a pandemic influenza begins, it is likely to spread very rapidly.
• Influenza is a contagious disease of the lungs.
• Influenza usually spreads by infected people coughing and sneezing.
• Most people will have little or no immunity to pandemic influenza.
2 Efforts to prepare for pandemic influenza are continuing.
• Public health officials are building on existing disease outbreak plans, including those developed for SARS.
• Researchers are working to produce additional vaccine more quickly.
• Countries are working together to improve detection and tracking of influenza viruses.
3 Public participation and cooperation will be important to the response effort.
• Severe pandemic influenza could produce changes in daily life, including limits on travel and public gatherings.
• Informed public participation and cooperation will help public health efforts.
• People should stay informed about pandemic influenza and be prepared as they would for any emergency.

Source: HHS.

Note: *HHS Pandemic Influenza Pre-Event Message Maps*, Washington, D.C., 2006.

HHS has several means of disseminating information regarding a pandemic. HHS manages www.pandemicflu.gov, the official U.S. government Web site for disseminating information on pandemics to the public before and during a pandemic. The Web site is updated with new information as it becomes available and provides the public, public health and emergency preparedness officials, government and business leaders, school systems, and local communities with comprehensive governmentwide information on a pandemic. In addition, HHS will use a variety of other information systems to distribute pandemic information including telephone hotlines, such as 1-800-CDC-INFO; educational sessions through teleconferencing, such as the Clinician Outreach and Communication Activity to which the public can call-in; satellite informational broadcasts; and radio and television public service announcements.

HHS has developed public service announcements for use on television and radio that urge the general public to learn about and prepare for a pandemic and has created an archive of materials—video footage, posters, and fact sheets—for conveying key pandemic messages to the general public. HHS also has developed planning checklists for specific audiences—such as medical providers, schools, and businesses—to raise awareness and to assist these audiences in preparing for a pandemic.[97] For example, the planning checklists identify issues that should be considered, such as storing additional infection control supplies (such as hand cleansing products and tissues); establishing pandemic-specific policies, procedures, and roles and responsibilities; planning to maintain continuity of operations; coordinating activities with local stakeholders; practicing infection control; and developing communications plans.

Despite HHS's Preparations, Communicating with the General Public during a Pandemic Will Be Challenging

HHS officials told us that communicating messages to the general public during a pandemic will be challenging despite the department's preparations. The first challenge is that a pandemic will create an immediate, intense, and sustained demand for information from both the general public and the groups to whom the public will be turning for information, such as the media and health care community. In addition, the general public will likely turn to numerous sources other than HHS for information, including other federal agencies, state and local authorities, the media, health care providers, the Internet, hotlines, employers, peers, family, and community leaders. HHS will not be able to ensure that messages delivered to the general public by non-HHS entities are coordinated and consistent with HHS messages, and the communications may cause confuse the general public.[98]

A second challenge concerns the public's reception to HHS's communications. HHS has found a low level of public understanding on pandemic issues, some unwillingness to comply under certain circumstances with the messages that HHS plans to deliver, and anxiety over particular messages (such as why pre-pandemic vaccines and some antivirals will not be made available to the general public). For example, a nationally representative survey on pandemic issues found that 58 percent of the general public in the United States did not know what a pandemic is.[99] The survey also found that the public is less willing or is unable to follow some of the recommendations that HHS plans to communicate during a pandemic. For example, HHS plans to recommend that sick individuals who do not require hospital care observe voluntary home isolation and treatment; however, 24 percent of the people surveyed said that they did not have someone to take care of them in their homes. The same study also found that 35 percent of respondents would go to work if requested by their employer even if public health officials recommended that people stay at home during a pandemic.

Furthermore, HHS tabletop exercises have identified several issues that will prove challenging when communicating with the public during a pandemic, particularly the sensitivity of certain messages, the use of specialized public health terms in the messages, and the inadequacy of HHS message maps to address the complexity of the issues being communicated. Discussions during these tabletop exercises will help HHS to develop plans to resolve these identified challenges. For example, HHS's messages will have to communicate clearly the difference between specialized terms such as isolation and quarantine, and the meaning of the phrase "altered standards of care." Because of the complexity of the issues in its message maps, HHS plans to develop additional educational materials to distribute to the public before a pandemic in order to make these complexities more comprehensible.

CONCLUSIONS

Although HHS has made progress in identifying issues that need to be addressed and in funding research and vaccine production, significant challenges remain, many of which are beyond HHS's control or which cannot be quickly addressed. Such challenges include coping with the potentially high absentee rate among health care providers during a pandemic and the length of time it will take to develop a pandemic vaccine once the virus is identified. One important activity, however, that is within HHS's control that HHS could address before a pandemic is finalizing the guidance on how limited pharmaceutical interventions should be used during a pandemic.

A severe pandemic, such as that of 1918-19, has the potential to result in widespread illness and death and is expected to overwhelm the nation's ability to respond. According to HHS, initial batches of the most effective protective measure—a pandemic vaccine—may take as long as 20 to 23 weeks after the start of the pandemic to become available. Although the federal government has provided some guidance, final decisionmaking will fall on state and local officials who will have to decide how to allocate pharmaceutical interventions and whom interventions should go to first, and when.

HHS, in consultation with other federal agencies, has been tasked with revising guidance to assist state and local jurisdictions in identifying groups that should be considered a priority for receiving limited pharmaceutical interventions. In 2008, HHS released guidance on prioritizing target groups for pandemic vaccine and draft guidance for public comment on how antivirals may be used during a pandemic. However, HHS has not yet released draft guidance for public comment on prioritizing target groups for pre-pandemic vaccine. We and others have reported since 2000 how problems related to pandemic planning—such as those problems with the distribution and administration of pharmaceutical interventions—can arise if target groups are not established in advance. This lack of essential information could slow the initial response at the state and local levels and complicate the general public's understanding of the necessity for rationing these interventions. Additionally, the general public should continue to be engaged in the process of priority setting, as public participation is an essential component for acceptance of tough decisions that will be required unless and until greater capacity or a universal vaccine can be developed.

RECOMMENDATION FOR EXECUTIVE ACTION

To improve the nation's preparedness for a pandemic, we are recommending that the Secretary of HHS expeditiously finalize guidance to assist state and local jurisdictions to determine how to effectively use limited supplies of antivirals and pre-pandemic vaccine in a pandemic, including prioritizing target groups for pre-pandemic vaccine.

AGENCY COMMENTS AND OUR EVALUATION

HHS provided written comments on a draft of this chapter which we have reproduced in appendix III. HHS also provided technical comments, which we have incorporated as appropriate.

In its comments, HHS noted that it has taken and plans to take additional actions related to our recommendation since we provided the draft report to the department for its review. HHS indicated that the final guidance for pandemic vaccine allocation was released on July 23, 2008, and that this guidance describes the groups who should be targeted and prioritized for receiving pandemic vaccine. HHS also indicated that the department released draft guidance on how antivirals may be used during a pandemic in June 2008, and that HHS will release for public comment proposed draft guidance on pre-pandemic vaccine allocation in the near future. We updated the text of the report to reflect these developments. We also revised the wording of our recommendation in light of HHS's comment that HHS recommends that antivirals in public-sector stockpiles should be used primarily for the treatment of individuals sick with influenza. We first identified the need for finalized guidance on how limited pharmaceutical interventions should be used during a pandemic, including target groups where appropriate, in 2000. We believe that finalizing guidance on the use of pharmaceutical interventions will be crucial for responding to a pandemic outbreak and that the necessary guidance documents should be finalized as soon as possible.

Throughout its comments, HHS described aspects of its pandemic preparedness activities that it believed could be presented more clearly in our report and presented additional details about its activities. We have revised the language in the report to reflect HHS's comments where it was necessary. In particular, we revised our discussion of pharmaceutical interventions to clarify our presentation of the three types of pharmaceuticals and how pre-pandemic vaccine will be distributed and administered during a pandemic. We also revised the report to reflect HHS's objection to our statement that the use of antivirals early in a pandemic could slow the spread of the pandemic. HHS commented that the magnitude of the impact of pharmaceuticals on pandemic spread is uncertain given "...limited countermeasure supplies, unclear effectivenesss, and operational challenges..."

Many of HHS's comments addressed the scope of the department's actions in relation to the responsibilities of states and local jurisdictions. For example, HHS noted that it will directly oversee the administration of pre- pandemic vaccine to members of the critical workforce, rather than fully delegate that task. For antivirals, HHS agreed that states are free to administer antivirals in their own stockpiles to anyone they like, but also noted that state plans have been reviewed by CDC to ensure that the plans reflect the national recommendation to use antivirals primarily for treatment of individuals sick with influenza. Thirdly, HHS emphasized that health care personnel surge capacity in a pandemic is a local responsibility. Although the 2005 *HHS Pandemic Influenza Plan* recommends deployment of federal medical responders to supplement the number of health care providers, HHS noted that the federal government does not have adequate health care personnel to provide surge capacity. On that topic, HHS also noted that its planning documents for allocating scarce health care resources were intended as "...planning documents for consideration by communities, not for the purposes of establishing definitive standards."

Finally, HHS proposed alternate terms for some of the concepts in our report (we have noted these instances in the report). For example, HHS disagreed with our use of the term "altered standards of care" and said that the more appropriate term is "standards of care appropriate to the situation." Because we believe that "altered standards of care" is an accurate description of what may happen as the result of the allocation of scarce health care resources in a pandemic emergency and because HHS used this phrase in its guidance to state and local jurisdictions, we did not make this change.

We are sending copies of this chapter to the Secretary of HHS and to interested congressional committees. We will also make copies available to others on request. In addition, the report will be available at no charge on GAO's Web site at http://www.gao.gov.

If you or your staff have any questions about this chapter, please contact me at (202) 512-7114 or CrosseM@gao.gov. Contact points for our Offices of Congressional Relations and Public Affairs may be found on the last page of this chapter. GAO staff who made major contributions to this chapter are listed in appendix IV.

Marcia Crosse
Director, Health Care

APPENDIX I. SUMMARIES OF SELECT FEDERAL DOCUMENTS RELEVANT FOR PREPARING FOR AND RESPONDING TO INFLUENZA PANDEMIC

National Response Framework

The *National Response Framework* lays out, in part, the manner in which the federal government responds to domestic incidents.[100] The plan is a guide for an all-hazards response, categorizing the types of federal assistance into specific emergency support functions. Primary and supporting agencies are listed for each emergency support function. "Emergency Support Function #8 – Public Health and Medical Services Annex" of the *National Response*

Framework directs the Department of Health and Human Services (HHS) to provide support as the primary agency, with 16 other agencies, including the Departments of Homeland Security and Agriculture.

The *National Response Framework* replaced the *National Response Plan* in March 2008, which, in turn, replaced the *Federal Response Plan* in April 2005. The *Federal Response Plan*, originally drafted in 1992 and revised in 1999, established the process and structure for the federal government's provision of assistance in response to any major disaster or emergency declared under the Robert T. Stafford Disaster Relief and Emergency Assistance Act (Stafford Act). The purpose of the Stafford Act is "to provide an orderly and continuing means of assistance by the federal government to state and local governments in carrying out their responsibilities to alleviate the suffering and damage which result" from disasters and emergencies.[101]

National Strategy for Pandemic Influenza

On November 1, 2005, the President of the United States released the *National Strategy for Pandemic Influenza*, which provides a framework for future planning efforts for how the country will prepare for, detect, and respond to an influenza pandemic.[102] The strategy reflects the federal government's approach to the pandemic threat and is based on three main types of activities: (1) preparedness and communication, (2) surveillance and detection, and (3) response and containment.

National Strategy for Pandemic Influenza Implementation Plan

On May 3, 2006, the President of the United States released the *National Strategy for Pandemic Influenza Implementation Plan*, which further clarifies the roles and responsibilities of governmental and nongovernmental entities—including federal, state, local, and tribal authorities and regional, national, and international stakeholders—and provides preparedness guidance for all segments of society.[103] This plan addresses the following topics: U.S. government planning and response; international efforts and transportation and borders; protecting human health; protecting animal health; law enforcement, public safety, and security; and institutional considerations. The federal government has identified approximately 300 action items to address the threat of a pandemic. These items include 199 action items led or co-led by HHS. As stated in the plan's preface, the plan will be reviewed on a continuous basis and revised as appropriate to reflect changes in the understanding of the threat and the development of new technologies.

Since the release of the implementation plan, the Homeland Security Council released the *National Strategy for Pandemic Influenza Implementation Plan One Year Summary* on July 17, 2007.[104] This document summarizes the federal government's efforts to prepare for an influenza pandemic.

HHS Pandemic Influenza Plan

Because HHS has primary responsibility for coordinating the nation's response to public health emergencies under "Emergency Support Function #8," the department has developed the *HHS Pandemic Influenza Plan*.[105] The first part of this plan provides HHS's strategic plan for dealing with an influenza pandemic. This includes information on recommendations on the use of vaccines and antivirals, legal authorities, key HHS activities, HHS research activities, and international partnerships on avian and pandemic influenza. Preparing for and responding to a pandemic will not be purely a federal responsibility; it will primarily be a local response. And because a pandemic is likely to occur in multiple areas simultaneously, resources cannot be geographically shifted as is often done with other emergencies; every community will need to rely on its own planning and resources to respond to the outbreak. Therefore, the second part of the *HHS Pandemic Influenza Plan* consists of 11 supplements that provide guidance to state and local officials on response elements necessary for preparation for a pandemic (see table 5).

The third part of the plan, which details the critical actions items for which HHS has the lead as described in the *National Strategy for Pandemic Influenza Implementation Plan*, was produced as a separate plan—the *Pandemic Influenza Implementation Plan*—and was released in November 2006.[106] The *Pandemic Influenza Implementation Plan* also includes a second part that contains the HHS agencies' operational plans.

The *HHS Pandemic Influenza Plan* will be reviewed on a continuous basis and revised as appropriate to reflect changes in the understanding of the threat and new technologies. HHS has released five updates regarding the progress of the department's preparedness efforts on March 13, 2006; June 29, 2006; November 13, 2006; July 18, 2007; and March 17, 2008, respectively.

Homeland Security Presidential Directive-21: Public Health and Medical Preparedness

On October 18, 2007, the President of the United States released the *Homeland Security Presidential Directive-21: Public Health and Medical Preparedness*,[107] which provides a strategy for protecting the health of the U.S. population against all disasters, including a pandemic. This directive describes four critical components of public health and medical preparedness: biosurveillance, countermeasure distribution (including pharmaceuticals), mass casualty care, and community resilience. All four critical components will include coordination of efforts at the federal, state, and local levels, as well as with private sector, public health, and medical disaster response resources.

Guidance on Allocating and Targeting Pandemic Influenza Vaccine

On July 23, 2008, HHS, in coordination with DHS, released the *Guidance on Allocating and Targeting Pandemic Influenza Vaccine*.[108] This guidance provides a framework to state and local jurisdictions on how to allocate limited supplies of pandemic vaccine to targeted groups, with the goal of providing this vaccine to all who choose to receive it. According to the guidance, groups targeted for vaccination varies depending on the severity of the pandemic.

Table 5. Response Elements Needed for Preparing for and Responding to an Influenza Pandemic and Examples of Priority Activities for Each Response Element

Response elements	Examples of priority activities
Pandemic influenza disease surveillance	• Health departments provide weekly reports on the overall level of influenza in their states and territories • State and local officials implement virologic, outpatient, hospital, and mortality surveillance
Laboratory diagnostics	• Clinical and hospital laboratories work with state and local health departments to train personnel in management of respiratory specimens during an influenza pandemic • Clinical and hospital laboratories will send selected specimens from possible pandemic influenza patients to state or local health departments
Healthcare planning	• Healthcare facilities' officials will develop planning and decision-making structures for responding to pandemic influenza • Healthcare facilities' officials will identify and isolate all potential patients with pandemic influenza
Infection control	• Patients with known or suspected pandemic influenza should be isolated for a minimum of 5 days from the onset of symptoms • Follow standard facility procedures for post-discharge cleaning of an isolation room
Clinical guidelines	• State and local public health agencies will help educate health care providers about pandemic influenza • Health care providers will report pandemic influenza cases or fatalities as requested by health departments
Vaccine distribution and use	• HHS agencies will work with manufacturers to expedite public-sector vaccine purchasing contracts during a pandemic • HHS agencies will revise recommendations on vaccination of priority groups, guided by epidemiologic information about the pandemic virus
Antiviral drug distribution and use	• HHS, in concert with the Congress and in collaboration with the states in advance of an influenza pandemic, will acquire sufficient quantities of antivirals to treat 25 percentof the U.S. population • HHS will revise recommendations for treatment and prophylaxis with antivirals for priority groups, if necessary, guided by accumulating data about the pandemic virus
Community disease control and prevention	• Community officials will help identify potential isolation and quarantine facilities • Community officials will help ensure that legal authorities and procedures exist for various levels of movement restrictions
Response elements	**Examples of priority activities**
Management of travel-related risk of disease	• State and local officials will work with the Centers for Disease Control and Prevention quarantine stations and federal partners to

transmission	evaluate and manage arriving ill passengers who might be infected with influenza strains with pandemic potential • State and local officials will evaluate the need to implement or terminate travel-related containment measures as the pandemic evolves
Public health communications	• State and local officials will assess and monitor readiness to meet communications needs in preparation for an influenza pandemic, including regular review and update of communications plans • State and local officials will tailor communications services and key messages to specific local audiences
Psychosocial workforce support services	• HHS agencies will create, collect, and provide educational and training materials on psychosocial issues related to pandemic influenza for use by hospital administrators, emergency department staff, safety and security professionals, behavioral health providers, social workers, psychologists, chaplains, and others • Health care institutions, state and local agencies, first responder organizations, and employers of essential service workers will provide psychological and social support services for employees and their families

Source: HHS.

Note: *HHS Pandemic Influenza Plan*, Washington, D.C., Nov. 2005.

APPENDIX II. HHS ACTIVITIES FOR ACQUIRING PHARMACEUTICAL INTERVENTIONS FOR AN INFLUENZA PANDEMIC WITHIN THE UNITED STATES

According to HHS officials, it is important to have a stockpile of pharmaceutical interventions, when possible, for use during the early stages of a pandemic. HHS allotted portions of its total fiscal year 2006 appropriation for pandemic-related purposes—$5.683 billion—to the acquisition and development of pharmaceutical interventions.[109] Specifically, approximately $1.1 billion was targeted for investment in antivirals and approximately $3.2 billion was dedicated for vaccines.[110] HHS has also established goals for amounts of pharmaceutical interventions to be stockpiled nationally (see table 6).

HHS has invested millions of dollars into the stockpiling of antivirals to achieve its two goals for antivirals. Table 7 summarizes the approximate number of courses stockpiled as of May 2008. In addition, in March 2006, HHS allotted $200 million dollars to the development of additional antivirals, and in January 2007, the department awarded a 4-year contract of about $103 million for further development of the new antiviral peramivir.

HHS has also awarded contracts to purchase pre-pandemic vaccines from manufacturers to add to the federal stockpile. See table 8 for HHS's efforts to stockpile pre-pandemic vaccines. HHS officials told us that the greatest challenge to preparing for an influenza pandemic and implementing its plans for using pharmaceutical interventions is the lack of vaccine manufacturing capacity within the United States. We found in prior work that the lack of U.S. vaccine manufacturing capacity is cause for concern among experts because it is possible that countries without domestic manufacturing capacity will not have access to vaccines in the event of a pandemic if the countries with domestic manufacturing capacity prohibit the export of the pandemic vaccine until their own needs are met.[111]

Table 6. HHS Goals for Amounts of Pharmaceutical Interventions to Be Stockpiled Nationally

Antiviral goal 1	To provide 75 million treatment courses of antivirals
Antiviral goal 2	To provide antivirals for strategic use for limited containment at the onset of a pandemic – 6 million treatment courses
Vaccine goal 1	To establish and maintain a pre-pandemic influenza vaccine stockpile sufficient for 20 million persons[a] (at 2 doses per person)
Vaccine goal 2	To provide pandemic vaccine to all U.S. citizens within 6 months of a pandemic declaration – 600 million doses of pandemic vaccine

Source: HHS.

Note: Statement by Gerald W. Parker, Principle Deputy Assistant Secretary, Office of the Assistant Secretary for Preparedness and Response on Pandemic Influenza Preparedness: Update on the Development and Acquisition of Medical Countermeasures before the Committee on Appropriations, Subcommittee on Labor, Health and Human Services, Education, and Related Agencies, U.S. Senate, Jan. 24, 2007.

[a] In May 2006, the Secretaries of HHS and DHS tasked the National Infrastructure Advisory Council with, among other things, providing recommendations regarding the prioritization and distribution of pharmaceutical countermeasures to the critical workforce. According to this Council's report, the number of the most essential critical infrastructure workers is approximately 12 million. See National Infrastructure Advisory Council, The Prioritization of Critical Infrastructure for a Pandemic Outbreak in the United States Working Group: Final Report and Recommendations by the Council. Washington, D.C.: Jan. 16, 2007. According to HHS, the 20 million people in the critical workforce include the approximately 12 million identified by the National Infrastructure Advisory Council as the most critical as well as other essential personnel such as military personnel, including the National Guard and critical government workers, such as border protection personnel.

Table 7. Approximate Number of Treatment Courses of Antivirals in the Strategic National Stockpile as of May 2008

Antivirals	Approximate number of treatment courses available
Neuraminidase inhibitors	
Oseltamivir (Tamiflu)	40 million
Zanamivir (Relenza)	10 million

Source: HHS.

Other HHS activities to enhance domestic vaccine manufacturing capacity include investing in vaccine development and research. For example, HHS has invested over $1 billion in development of a cell-based approach to influenza vaccine manufacturing, which it claims will modernize the current egg-based production process (see table 10). The current manufacturing process uses chicken eggs, and egg-based vaccines can easily become contaminated. Cell-based technology does not have these sterility issues and allows for faster development and greater production capacity. Although cell-based vaccine production has been used for other vaccines, it has not been approved for use in developing influenza vaccines. However, according to HHS, it anticipates that a licensed cell- based influenza vaccine will be manufactured in 2010. Also, in January 2007, HHS awarded contracts totaling approximately $133 million to vaccine manufacturers for development of pre-pandemic vaccines, containing adjuvants—substances that may be added to a vaccine to increase the body's immune response, thereby necessitating a lower dose of vaccine.

Table 8. HHS Efforts to Acquire Pre-Pandemic Vaccine as of August 2007

Viral strain for pre-pandemic vaccine	Number of awarded contracts	Value of awarded contracts	Duration of contracts	Goals	Progress
H5N1 Vaccine Clade 1[a](2004)[b]	1	$21 million	2004-08	Provide 0.47 million doses at 90 micrograms (mcg.) per dose	As of May 2008, HHS hassto-ckpiled enough of this pre-pand-emic vaccine for at least 13 mill-ion people or 26 million doses.
H5N1 Vaccine Clade 1 (2005)	2	$243 million	2005-08	Provide 8 million dos-es at 90 mcg. per dose	
H5N1 Vaccine Clade 2 (2006)	3	$241 million	2006-08	Provide 4.9 million dos-es at 90 mcg. per dose	As August 2007, HHS has stockpiled enough vaccine for 3 million people or approximately 6 million doses.
H5N1 Vaccine (2007)	To be determined	To be determined	Intended to cover 2007-09	Intended to provide doses for pre-pande-mic stock-pile using H5N1	Not applicable

Source: GAO analysis of HHS data.

[a] Clades refer to different circulating viral strains of a single virus. For example, researchers have divided the H5N1 avian influenza virus into 2 clades – clade 1 refers to the H5N1 virus strain circulating in Cambodia, Lao People's Democratic Republic, Malaysia, and Vietnam, while clade 2 refers to the H5N1 virus strain circulating in Africa, Europe, Indonesia, and the People's Republic of China.

[b] In April 2007, HHS announced that the Food and Drug Administration licensed the first vaccine based on the 2004 H5N1 strain for humans in the United States.

Table 9 describes other HHS initiatives to establish domestic manufacturing infrastructure for vaccine production.

Table 9. HHS Efforts in Establishing Domestic Infrastructure for Vaccine Manufacturing as of June 2007

Project	Number of awarded contracts	Value of awarded contracts	Duration of contracts	Goals	Progress
Retrofit existing manuf-acturing facilities	2	$132.5 million	2007-13	• Increase dom-estic influenza vaccine capacity to produce 125 million doses of egg-based pandemic vaccine	• In June 2007, HHS announced it had awarded contracts to prov-ide funding for renovation of domestic manufa-cturing facilities and for providing warm-base opera-tions for manuf-acturing pande-mic accines.[a] Once operational, thes-efacilities are expected to expa-nd domestic pandemic vaccine manufacturing capacity by 16 percent.
Build new cell-based vaccine facilities	Request for Proposal expected in fiscal year 2007	To be deter-mined	Intended to cover 2008-13	• Intended for the building of domestic cell-based influenza manufacturing capacity to sup-port pandemic needs	• Not applicable

Source: GAO analysis of HHS data.

[a] In warm-base operations, the contractor provides year-round vaccine production.

Table 10. HHS Progress on Vaccine Development Projects

Project	Number of awarded contracts	Value of awarded contracts	Duration of contracts	Goals	Progress
Egg-based supply	1	$43 million	2004-2008	• Provide year-round egg supply for influenza vaccine manufacturing • Provide vaccines for use in clinical studies • Stockpile other vaccine manufacturing supplies, such as vials, caps, and stoppers • Develop and manufacture pandemic vaccine candid-ates for clinical investingation	• In April 2005, a secureyear-round egg supplyfor domes-tic influenza vaccine manu-facturingwas established • Two pandemic vaccine candidates – H5N1 clade 2 and H7N7 – have been produced for clinical investigations
Cell-based vaccine	6	$1.1 billion	2005-2011	• Expand domestic influenza manufacturing capacity • Establish capacity to produce 475 million doses of pandemic vaccine by 2013 • Require commitments from manufacturers to establish U.S.-based manufacturing facilities with vaccine prod-ucing capacity of at least 150 million doses within 6 months of a pandemic	• As of January 2007, six manufacturers were in Phase 1 clinical trials[a]in the United States using cell-based production methods
Adjuvant-conta-ining[b] vaccine	3	$133 million	2007-2012	• Reduce amount of vaccine needed in order to increase the number of doses that can be produced • Support further development of adjuvant-containing vaccine for U.S. licensure	• Initial studies have shown that addition of adjuvants to H5N1 vaccines have reduced 10-to-20 fold the amount of antigen needed per dose in order to stimulate an immune response believed to be acceptable during a pandemic
Project	Number of awarded contracts	Value of awarded contracts	Duration of contracts	Goals	Progress

Table 10 (Continued)

				• Require each company to build capacity to produce within 6 months of the onset of a pandemic either (1) 150 million doses of a pandemic vaccine containing adjuvant or (2) enough adjuvant to be stockpiled for 150 million doses of a pandemic vaccine • Require each company to provide its proprietary adjuvant for U.S. government-sponsored, independent evaluation with influenza vaccines from other manufacturers	• Phase 1 and 2 clinical studies[c] are planned in 2007 with three new adjuvants
Next gene-ration[d]	Request for Proposal in fiscal year 2007	To be deter-mined	200 7- 201 2	• Diversify influenza vaccine manufacturing • Reduce manufacturing time	• Not Applicable

Source: GAO analysis of HHS data.

[a] Clinical trials test potential treatments in human volunteers to see if they should be approved for wider use in the general population. In Phase 1 trials, researchers attempt to determine dosing, document how a drug is metabolized and excreted, and identify acute side effects. Usually, a small number of healthy volunteers (between 20 and 80) are used in Phase 1 trials.

[b] Adjuvants are substances that may be added to a vaccine to increase the body's immune response to the vaccine's active ingredient, called an antigen.

[c] Phase 2 trials include more participants (about 100-300) who have the disease or condition that the product potentially could treat. In Phase 2 trials, researchers seek to gather further safety data and preliminary evidence of the drug's beneficial effects (efficacy), and they develop and refine research methods for future trials with this drug.

[d] Next generation vaccines refer to vaccines, such as DNA vaccines, developed using new technologies.

APPENDIX III. COMMENTS FROM THE DEPARTMENT OF HEALTH AND HUMAN SERVICES

THE SECRETARY OF HEALTH AND HUMAN SERVICES
WASHINGTON, DC 20201

AUG 0 7 2008

Marcia Crosse
Director, Health Care
U.S. Government Accountability Office
441 G Street, N.W.
Washington, D.C. 20548

Dear Ms. Crosse:

Enclosed are the comments of the U.S. Department of Health and Human Services (HHS) on the Government Accountability Office's (GAO) draft report entitled: "Influenza Pandemic: HHS Needs to Continue Its Actions and Finalize Guidance for Pharmaceutical Intervention" (GAO 08-671).

The Department appreciates the opportunity to comment on this draft before its publication.

Sincerely,

Vincent J. Ventimiglia, Jr.
Assistant Secretary for Legislation

Enclosure

GENERAL COMMENTS OF THE US DEPARTMENT OF HEALTH AND HUMAN SERVICES (HHS) ON THE GOVERNMENT ACCOUNTABILITY OFFICE'S (GAO) DRAFT REPORT ENTITLED: "INFLUENZA PANDEMIC: HHS NEEDS TO CONTINUE ITS ACTIONS AND FINALIZE GUIDANCE FOR PHARMACEUTICAL INTERVENTIONS" (GAO 08-671)

General Comments – Overview

The Department of Health and Human Services (HHS) appreciates the opportunity to comment on the above-referenced Government Accountability Office (GAO) draft report.

In the draft report HHS was given to review, GAO recommended that "...the Secretary of HHS expeditiously issue final guidance to assist state and local jurisdictions in identifying target groups for receiving supplies of pandemic vaccine, antivirals, and pre-pandemic vaccine." On July 23, 2008, HHS and DHS released final guidance on pandemic vaccine allocation. This *Guidance on Allocating and Targeting Pandemic Influenza Vaccine* provides a planning framework to help state, tribal, local and community leaders ensure that vaccine allocation and use will reduce the impact of a pandemic on public health and minimize disruption to society and the economy. The guidance's vaccination structure defines four broad target groups: people who 1) maintain homeland and national security, 2) provide health care and community support services, 3) maintain critical infrastructure and 4) are in the general population. Everyone in the United States is included in at least one vaccination target group. People who are not included in any occupational group would be vaccinated as part of the general population based on their age and health status.

In the near future HHS will release for public comment proposed guidance on pre-pandemic vaccine allocation.

In June 2008, HHS released for public comment three draft guidance documents related to antiviral drugs and respiratory protection devices: *Proposed Guidance on Antiviral Drug Use during an Influenza Pandemic, Proposed Considerations for Antiviral Drug Stockpiling by Employers In Preparation for an Influenza Pandemic* and *Interim guidance on the use and purchase of facemasks and respirators by individuals and families for pandemic influenza preparedness.* HHS is now updating these three guidance documents based on comments submitted by the public.

General Comments – Supplementary Information to Be Considered

Medical Countermeasures

The GAO draft report incorrectly asserts that the use of vaccines and antiviral drugs early in an influenza pandemic is to slow the spread of the pandemic. While there is some modeling work that suggests that the use of vaccines or antiviral prophylaxis might have such an effect, a 2006 Institute of Medicine report pointed out the uncertainties associated with the predictive ability of pandemic influenza modeling. HHS strategies for vaccination and antiviral treatment are predicated on their direct effects in reducing the health, societal and economic impacts of a pandemic. Uncertainties regarding the magnitude of impact on pandemic spread given limited countermeasure supplies, unclear effectiveness and operational challenges support the recommended approach.

GENERAL COMMENTS OF THE US DEPARTMENT OF HEALTH AND HUMAN SERVICES (HHS) ON THE GOVERNMENT ACCOUNTABILITY OFFICE'S (GAO) DRAFT REPORT ENTITLED: "INFLUENZA PANDEMIC: HHS NEEDS TO CONTINUE ITS ACTIONS AND FINALIZE GUIDANCE FOR PHARMACEUTICAL INTERVENTIONS" (GAO 08-671)

HHS vaccine prioritization guidance, in addition to being firmly rooted in the most up-to-date scientific information available, also directly reflects the values of our society and the ethical issues involved in planning a phased approach to pandemic vaccination. As a key part of developing the guidance, HHS held day-long public engagement and stakeholder meetings throughout the country and received more than 200 written public comments on the goals and objectives of pandemic vaccination. In all the meetings, stakeholders and the public identified the same four vaccination program objectives as the most important:

- Protect persons critical to the pandemic response and who provide care for persons with pandemic illness,
- Protect persons who provide essential community services,
- Protect persons who are at high risk of infection because of their occupation, and
- Protect children.

Using pandemic vaccine to slow the spread of a pandemic also was considered but was rated by the public and stakeholders as a less important objective.

It is important to distinguish HHS policies for the use of antiviral drugs in public stockpiles from what it has proposed for private sector stockpiles in *Proposed Guidance on Antiviral Drug Use during an Influenza Pandemic* and *Proposed Considerations for Antiviral Drug Stockpiling by Employers In Preparation for an Influenza Pandemic*. As published in the *HHS Pandemic Influenza Plan* and the *Implementation Plan for the National Strategy* public sector stockpiles are intended to be used primarily for the treatment of ill individuals. Stockpile targets were estimated based on the expected demand for treatment. Treatment should be based on medical need and is not intended to be allocated to target groups. In contrast, prophylactic antiviral drug use in the proposed guidance and the guidance to employers outlines occupational target groups that could be covered by private sector stockpiles of antiviral drugs. The national stockpiling goal in support of treatment is a combined (between Federal and Project Area stockpiles) total of 75 million treatment regimens. HHS has stockpiled an additional 6 million regimens of antiviral drugs to assist in containment activities; these antiviral drugs may be used for both treatment and prophylaxis and combined with the treatment stockpiles round out our national goal of 81 million stockpiled regimens.

The GAO draft report discusses that State and Territorial stockpiles of antiviral drugs, purchased in support of the HHS-established goal of 31 million state-owned treatment regimens, will not be in Federal hands, and therefore, jurisdictions may choose to use these public stockpiles of antiviral drugs for prophylaxis rather than for treatment. State pandemic plans, which have been reviewed by CDC for compliance with national guidance recommendations, focus on using antiviral drugs for treatment, not prophylaxis. Should States decide to use antiviral drugs for prophylaxis rather than for treatment, those States and/or Territories would exhaust their stockpiles quickly and would not have enough antiviral drugs to treat ill individuals as the pandemic evolved. The same situation applies to those States and Territories that do not stockpile their full proportion of the 31 million regimen goal.

The GAO draft report states that "Once a pandemic begins, HHS expects to make existing federal stockpiles of pharmaceutical interventions available to state and local jurisdictions to distribute to

**GENERAL COMMENTS OF THE US DEPARTMENT OF HEALTH AND
HUMAN SERVICES (HHS) ON THE GOVERNMENT ACCOUNTABILITY
OFFICE'S (GAO) DRAFT REPORT ENTITLED: "INFLUENZA PANDEMIC:
HHS NEEDS TO CONTINUE ITS ACTIONS AND FINALIZE GUIDANCE FOR
PHARMACEUTICAL INTERVENTIONS" (GAO 08-671)**

targeted groups. These interventions would include antivirals, . . . and pre-pandemic vaccines," As
outlined above, antiviral drugs from the HHS Strategic National Stockpile (SNS) and other public
stockpiles managed by Project Areas are not intended for target groups, rather, they are to be dispensed
for treatment of ill individuals based on medical need.

The GAO draft report suggests that pre-pandemic vaccine will be administered by State and local
officials to targeted individuals who have been identified to receive the vaccine based on HHS
recommendations. This process is not described correctly in the draft report. Federal and State points
of distribution (POD) will receive pre-pandemic influenza vaccine from vaccine manufacturers under
HHS oversight and administer vaccination to critical workforce members as described in the HHS pre-
pandemic vaccine prioritization schedule, which will be released soon for public comment. The GAO
report should be clear that the role of HHS, in coordination with DHS and other key Federal partners,
is to identify the categories of workers that should be considered for vaccination. Work is ongoing to
provide guidance to critical infrastructure businesses on identifying individuals for pre-pandemic and
pandemic vaccination and to develop a system that will identify them at sites where vaccine is
administered.

Surge Capacity

Although the GAO draft report makes no specific recommendation related to surge capacity, the draft
report fails to accurately capture a number of key surge capacity concepts including strategies, roles
and responsibilities, and terminology.

The GAO draft report correctly states that HHS has initiated efforts to improve surge capacity but
incorrectly suggests that HHS is responsible for healthcare personnel surge capacity. Providing for
healthcare personnel surge capacity for an influenza pandemic is a local responsibility and will need to
be built locally. The Federal government can assist, but does not have adequate personnel to provide
for healthcare personnel surge during an influenza pandemic. The role of HHS is to provide tools to
support localities in developing their healthcare personnel surge planning.

The GAO draft report states that two documents issued by HHS (1) *Altered Standards of Care in Mass
Casualty Events*; and (2) *Mass Medical Care with Scarce Resources: A Community Planning Guide*
provide a "framework" for the allocation of scarce resources and standards of care appropriate to the
situation. HHS provided these documents as planning guidance for consideration by communities, not
for the purposes of establishing definitive standards. States in conjunction with professional societies
will determine the appropriate standards of care for the situation – not HHS or the Federal
government. Also, throughout the draft report, GAO report uses the phrase "altered standards of care,"
rather than the more appropriate phrase, "standards of care appropriate to the situation."

The GAO draft report states that HHS will deploy U.S. Public Health Service (PHS) Commissioned
Corps officers and National Disaster Medical System (NDMS) personnel to support healthcare
personnel surge capacity. While HHS plans to utilize these personnel during the early stages of a

GENERAL COMMENTS OF THE US DEPARTMENT OF HEALTH AND HUMAN SERVICES (HHS) ON THE GOVERNMENT ACCOUNTABILITY OFFICE'S (GAO) DRAFT REPORT ENTITLED: "INFLUENZA PANDEMIC: HHS NEEDS TO CONTINUE ITS ACTIONS AND FINALIZE GUIDANCE FOR PHARMACEUTICAL INTERVENTIONS" (GAO 08-671)

severe influenza pandemic, these personnel will not be available for deployment once the pandemic is spreading within the United States. Furthermore, NDMS personnel are primarily local healthcare providers who will be needed by their local communities and healthcare systems during a widespread influenza pandemic, and therefore, will unlikely be deployed elsewhere. Likewise, PHS officers who provide healthcare to tribal communities will be needed in those communities. PHS officers also serve essential functions within HHS agencies, and considering that personnel at HHS and other Federal Departments will be impacted by the pandemic, many PHS personnel will not be available for deployment.

GAO may want to consider some of the other mechanisms HHS has been exploring to expand healthcare personnel surge capacity. For example:

a. A new report that emphasizes the role of home care during a pandemic was released by HHS in July 2008 and can be found at http://www.pandemicflu.gov/plan/healthcare/homehealth.html. Home care may keep the less-severely ill out of the hospitals. One of the major points in this report is that telehealth can be used to support personnel surge since the health care provider would not need to visit each household and could provide care to more people.

b. In September 2007, HHS released a report that suggests the use of call centers as intervention that can be used to keep the less severely ill out of the hospital and enhance the ability of providers to maximize the number of people who receive information that allows them to receive the highest possible standard of care under the austere conditions of the pandemic. The report can be found at http://www.ahrq.gov/prep/callcenters/callcenters.pdf.

c. Another approach to expanding personnel surge is just-in-time training to assure that individuals are able to provide the highest possible standard of care under the austere conditions of a pandemic. One such program is Project Xtreme http://www.ahrq.gov/prep/projxtreme/.

APPENDIX IV. GAO CONTACT AND STAFF ACKNOWLEDGMENTS

Related GAO Products

Influenza Pandemic: Federal Agencies Should Continue to Assist States to Address Gaps in Pandemic Planning. GAO-08-539. Washington, D.C.: June 19, 2008.

Emergency Preparedness: States Are Planning for Medical Surge, but Could Benefit from Shared Guidance for Allocating Scarce Medical Resources. GAO-08-668. Washington, D.C.: June 13, 2008.

Influenza Pandemic: Efforts Under Way to Address Constraints on Using Antivirals and Vaccines to Forestall a Pandemic. GAO-08-92. Washington, D.C.: December 21, 2007.

Influenza Pandemic: Opportunities Exist to Address Critical Infrastructure Protection Challenges That Require Federal and Private Sector Coordination. GAO-08-36. Washington, D.C.: October 31, 2007.

Influenza Vaccine: Issues Related to Production, Distribution, and Public Health Messages. GAO-08-27. Washington, D.C.: October 31, 2007.

Influenza Pandemic: Further Efforts Are Needed to Ensure Clearer Federal Leadership Roles and an Effective National Strategy. GAO-07-781. Washington, D.C.: August 14, 2007.

Emergency Management Assistance Compact: Enhancing EMAC's Collaborative and Administrative Capacity Should Improve National Disaster Response. GAO-07-854. Washington, D.C.: June 29, 2007.

Influenza Pandemic: DOD Combatant Commands' Preparedness Efforts Could Benefit from More Clearly Defined Roles, Resources, and Risk Mitigation. GAO-07-696. Washington, D.C.: June 20, 2007.

Influenza Pandemic: Efforts to Forestall Onset Are Under Way; Identifying Countries at Greatest Risk Entails Challenges. GAO-07-604. Washington, D.C.: June 20, 2007.

Emergency Management: Most School Districts Have Developed Emergency Management Plans, but Would Benefit from Additional Federal Guidance. GAO-07-609. Washington, D.C.: June 12, 2007.

Avian Influenza: USDA Has Taken Important Steps to Prepare for Outbreaks, but Better Planning Could Improve Response. GAO-07-652. Washington, D.C.: June 11, 2007.

The Federal Workforce: Additional Steps Needed to Take Advantage of Federal Executive Boards' Ability to Contribute to Emergency Operations. GAO-07-515. Washington, D.C.: May 4, 2007.

Influenza Pandemic: DOD Has Taken Important Actions to Prepare, but Accountability, Funding, and Communications Need to be Clearer and Focused Departmentwide. GAO-06-1042. Washington, D.C.: September 21, 2006.

Influenza Pandemic: Applying Lessons Learned from the 2004-05 Influenza Vaccine Shortage. GAO-06-221T. Washington, D.C.: November 4, 2005.

Influenza Vaccine: Shortages in 2004-05 Season Underscore Need for Better Preparation. GAO-05-984. Washington, D.C.: September 30, 2005.

Influenza Pandemic: Challenges in Preparedness and Response. GAO-05-863T. Washington, D.C.: June 30, 2005.

Influenza Pandemic: Challenges Remain in Preparedness. GAO-05-760T. Washington, D.C.: May 26, 2005.

Infectious Disease Preparedness: Federal Challenges in Responding to Influenza Outbreak. GAO-04-1100T. Washington, D.C.: September 28, 2004.

Bioterrorism: Public Health Response to Anthrax Incidents of 2001. GAO-04-152. Washington, D.C.: October 15, 2003.

Infectious Diseases: Gaps Remain in Surveillance Capabilities of State and Local Agencies. GAO-03-1176T. Washington, D.C.: September 24, 2003.

SARS Outbreak: Improvements to Public Health Capacity Are Needed for Responding to Bioterrorism and Emerging Infectious Diseases. GAO-03-769T. Washington, D.C.: May 7, 2003.

Bioterrorism: Preparedness Varied across State and Local Jurisdictions. GAO-03-373. Washington, D.C.: April 7, 2003.

Hospital Emergency Departments: Crowded Conditions Vary among Hospitals and Communities. GAO-03-460. Washington, D.C.: March 14, 2003.

Nursing Workforce: Emerging Nurse Shortages Due to Multiple Factors. GAO-01-944. Washington. D.C.: July 10, 2001.

Nursing Workforce: Recruitment and Retention of Nurses and Nurse Aides Is a Growing Concern. GAO-01-750T. Washington, D.C.: May 17, 2001.

Flu Vaccine: Supply Problems Heighten Need to Ensure Access for High- Risk People. GAO-01-624. Washington, D.C.: May 15, 2001.

GAO's Mission

The Government Accountability Office, the audit, evaluation, and investigative arm of Congress, exists to support Congress in meeting its constitutional responsibilities and to help improve the performance and accountability of the federal government for the American people. GAO examines the use of public funds; evaluates federal programs and policies; and provides analyses, recommendations, and other assistance to help Congress make informed oversight, policy, and funding decisions. GAO's commitment to good government is reflected in its core values of accountability, integrity, and reliability.

End Notes

[1] In this chapter, the term "pandemic" will refer to a human influenza pandemic.

[2] Department of Health and Human Services, *HHS Pandemic Influenza Plan* (Washington, D.C.: November 2005). HHS also estimated that 1,485,000 people would require care in an intensive care unit (ICU) and 742,500 people would require mechanical ventilation.

[3] The term "staffed bed" means that there are health care staffs available to attend to a patient occupying the bed.

[4] HHS estimates show that the effects of even a moderate pandemic would exceed the capacity of U.S. hospitals, with 865,000 people requiring hospitalization, 128,750 people requiring care in an ICU, 64,875 people requiring mechanical ventilation, and 209,000 deaths.

[5] GAO, *Influenza Pandemic: Plan Needed for Federal and State Response*, GAO-01-4 (Washington, D.C.: Oct. 27, 2000), 27 and GAO, *Influenza Pandemic: Challenges Remain in Preparedness*, GAO-05-760T (Washington, D.C.: May 26, 2005), 17.

[6] GAO, *Influenza Pandemic: Efforts Under Way to Address Constraints on Using Antivirals and Vaccines to Forestall a Pandemic*, GAO-08-92 (Washington, D.C.: Dec. 21, 2007), 30-32, 36.

[7] HHS refers to pharmaceutical interventions as medical countermeasures.

[8] Antivirals are drugs designed to prevent or reduce the severity of a viral infection, such as influenza. Vaccines are drugs used to stimulate the response of the human immune system to help protect the body from disease.

[9] For more detailed information on the use of antivirals and vaccines in a pandemic, see GAO-08-92, 4.

[10] Surge capacity may also include the ability to acquire other resources such as hospital beds, pharmaceuticals, and equipment, and to allocate scarce resources and provide care outside of the normal health care delivery system and infrastructure. For the purpose of this chapter, we refer to surge capacity in the context of the ability to increase the number of health care providers.

[11] Federal assistance can be provided to state, local, and tribal jurisdictions through mechanisms and authorities that do not require coordination of federal response activities and can be provided without a Presidential declaration of a major disaster or emergency. For example, federal assistance can be provided through the National Search and Rescue Plan and the Maritime Security Plan.

[12] Department of Homeland Security, *National Response Framework* (Washington, D.C.: 2008). The *National Response Framework* replaced the *National Response Plan* in March 2008. See app. I for details regarding the genesis of the plan.

[13] This is only part of the federal government's planning efforts for responding to a pandemic. The President of the United States released two documents for a broader response: (1) the *National Strategy for Pandemic Influenza*, which provides a framework for future planning efforts for how the country will prepare for, detect, and respond to a pandemic and (2) the *National Strategy for Pandemic Influenza Implementation Plan*, which further clarifies the roles and responsibilities of governmental and nongovernmental entities and provides preparedness guidance for all segments of society. See app. I for general descriptions of these documents.

[14] For this chapter, we use the term "state and local jurisdictions" to refer to state, local, territorial, and tribal areas. For the allocation of pharmaceutical interventions during a pandemic, "state and local jurisdictions" refers to state, local, and territorial areas. Tribal populations are included in states' populations. HHS uses the term "Project Areas" when discussing the allocation of antivirals and points of distribution when discussing pre-pandemic and pandemic vaccines.

[15] See GAO-08-92, 4; GAO, *Influenza Pandemic: Applying Lessons Learned from the 2004-05 Influenza Vaccine Shortage*, GAO-06-221T (Washington, D.C.: Nov. 4, 2005), 2, 10; GAO, *Influenza Pandemic: Challenges in Preparedness and Response*, GAO-05-863T (Washington, D.C.: June 30, 2005), 6-9, 11-12; and GAO, *Influenza Pandemic: Challenges Remain in Preparedness*, GAO-05-760T (Washington, D.C.: May 26, 2005), 12-15. For additional information, see *Related GAO Products* at the end of this chapter.

[16] See GAO-05-863T, 13; GAO-05-760T, 16-17; GAO, *Infectious Diseases: Gaps Remain in Surveillance Capabilities of State and Local Agencies*, GAO-03-1176T (Washington, D.C.: Sept. 24, 2003), 9-10; GAO, *Bioterrorism: Preparedness Varied across State and Local Jurisdictions*, GAO-03-373 (Washington, D.C.: Apr. 7, 2003), 17-18, 2 1-22; GAO, *Nursing Workforce: Emerging Nurse Shortages Due to Multiple Factors*, GAO-01-944 (Washington, D.C.: July 10, 2001), 6-12; and GAO, *Nursing Workforce: Recruitment and Retention of Nurses and Nurse Aides Is a Growing Concern*, GAO-01-750T (Washington, D.C.: May 17, 2001), 4-14.

[17] GAO, *Bioterrorism: Public Health Response to Anthrax Incidents of 2001*, GAO-04-152 (Washington, D.C.: Oct. 15, 2003), 24.

[18] GAO-05-863T, 9-11.

[19] An antibody is a molecule produced by the immune system that helps fight infections. The ability of influenza vaccine to protect a person depends on the age and health status of the person getting the vaccine and the similarity or "match" between the virus strain(s) in the vaccine and those in circulation. For example, when the seasonal influenza vaccine and circulating virus strains are well-matched, the vaccine will prevent illness in approximately 70 percent to 90 percent of healthy adults under the age of 65. The protection drops to about 30 percent to 40 percent for the elderly. Vaccine effectiveness can also be lower for individuals with medical conditions such as compromised immune systems.

[20] Experts believe that a strain of the H5N1 influenza virus is the most likely candidate to cause a pandemic; thus, pre-pandemic vaccines currently under development are based on this virus. However, experts remain concerned that other influenza viruses—such as the H2N2, H7N7, and H9N2—have the potential to cause a pandemic.

[21] See, for example, Robert G. Webster and Elena A. Govorkova, "H5N1 Influenza— Continuing Evolution and Spread," *New England Journal of Medicine*, vol. 355, no. 21 (2006) 2174-77 and Aleksandr S. Lipatov, Richard J. Webby, Elena A. Govorkova, Scott Krauss, and Robert G. Webster, "Efficacy of H5 Influenza Vaccines Produced by Reverse Genetics in a Lethal Mouse Model," *Journal of Infectious Diseases*, vol. 191 (2005), 1216- 20.

[22] We previously reported that seasonal vaccine manufacturers for the U.S. market have agreed in principle to switch to production of pandemic vaccine should the need arise and compensation and indemnification be provided. Our prior work noted, therefore, that it would probably be unnecessary for the federal government to nationalize vaccine production, although a senior HHS official indicated that the federal government has the authority to do so if circumstances warrant it. GAO-05-863T, 5.

[23] The five vaccine manufacturers were GlaxoSmithKline plc (which includes its subsidiary ID Biomedical Corporation of Quebec), MedImmune Vaccines, Inc., Novartis Vaccines and Diagnostics Limited, sanofi pasteur, Inc. (the policy of this company is to spell its name without capital letters), and CSL Limited.

[24] This manufacturer is sanofi pasteur, Inc. in Swiftwater, Pa., and it produces a vaccine that is injected into muscle. The injectable vaccine represents the large majority of influenza vaccine administered in this country. Throughout this chapter, vaccine refers to the injectable form.

[25] GAO-08-92, 26.

[26] The amount of antiviral administered is measured in treatment courses. One treatment course is the number of doses of the antiviral needed to treat one person.

[27] The SNS is a federal repository of pharmaceuticals and medical supplies that can be delivered to the site of a bioterrorist attack or other event.

[28] See *Related GAO Products* at the end of this chapter.

[29] Two classes of antivirals are currently approved by the FDA for prevention and treatment of influenza. The first, older class is called adamantanes, which includes two drugs called amantadine and rimantadine. This class of antivirals has been affected by the emergence of drug-resistant influenza viruses. Antiviral resistance is the result of viruses changing in ways that reduce or eliminate the effectiveness of antiviral agents to prevent or treat infections. The second class of antivirals is called neuraminidase inhibitors. This relatively newer class of antivirals includes two drugs—oseltamivir (Tamiflu) and zanamivir (Relenza)—and are associated with fewer side-effects than the older class of antivirals. However, concerns regarding Tamiflu and Relenza have recently increased. In 2006, FDA announced a change to the prescribing information for Tamiflu to include a precaution about neuropsychiatric events. The revision is based on postmarketing reports of self- injury and delirium with the use of Tamiflu primarily in pediatric patients with influenza. In 2007, FDA's Pediatric Advisory Committee recommended stronger warning labels for both Tamiflu and Relenza because of reports of neuropsychiatric problems in children and teens.

[30] GAO-08-92, 23.

[31] GAO-05-863T, 8.

[32] GAO-05-984, 11-12.

[33] See Eric Toner and Richard Waldhorn, "What hospitals should do to prepare for an influenza pandemic," *Biosecurity and Bioterrorism: Biodefense Strategy, Practice, and Science,* vol. 4, no. 4 (2006).

[34] See GAO-05-863T, 13; GAO-05-760T, 16-17; GAO-03-1176T, 9-10; GAO-03-373, 17-18, 21-22; GAO-01-944, 6-12; and GAO-01-750T, 4-14. Also, Trust for America's Health, *Ready or Not? Protecting the Public's Health From Diseases, Disasters, and Bioterrorism* (Washington, D.C.: 2006); and American Hospital Association, *Taking the Pulse: The State of America's Hospitals* (Washington, D.C.: 2005).

[35] Association of American Medical Colleges, *Recent Studies and Reports on Physician Shortages in the U.S.* (Washington, D.C.: 2007).

[36] To identify nursing shortages as of December 2006, the American Hospital Association sent a survey to approximately 5,000 community hospital chief executive officers in late February 2007 and collected data through March 2007. The association received 840 responses for a response rate of approximately 17 percent.

[37] Hospital capacity is the number of staffed beds.

[38] Pub. L. No. 109-417, 120 Stat. 2831 (2006).

[39] Pub. L. No. 109-417, § 103, 120 Stat. 2836.

[40] Pub. L. No. 109-417, § 101, 120 Stat. 2833.

[41] GAO, *SARS Outbreak: Improvements to Public Health Capacity Are Needed for Responding to Bioterrorism and Emerging Infectious Diseases,* GAO-03-769T (Washington, D.C.: May 7, 2003), 4.

[42] GAO-03-1058T, 15-16.

[43] GAO-04-152, 24.

[44] For the allocation of pharmaceutical interventions during a pandemic, "state and local jurisdictions" refers to state, local, and territorial areas. Tribal populations are included in states' populations.

[45] In the draft guidance released for public comment in June 2008, HHS proposed increasing the national goal to 79 million.

[46] HHS has allocated $170 million to subsidize state and local jurisdictions in purchasing up to 31 million treatment courses of antivirals at 25 percent off the federal contract price. According to HHS officials, there is no current need for additional federal funding to be allocated towards this subsidy program.

[47] Of this nearly 22 million, almost 21 million treatment courses were purchased by state and local jurisdictions using the federal government subsidy of 25 percent. Separately, jurisdictions have purchased about 879,000 additional treatment courses without the use of the federal subsidy but under the contracts governing the program. Approximately 121,000 treatment courses of antivirals have been purchased on the open market, that is, separately from the governing contracts.

[48] These 6 million courses are included in addition to the 44 million treatment courses already purchased by HHS for storage in the SNS, for a total of 50 million courses of antivirals. The containment strategy is based on studies suggesting that efforts centered on using antivirals to prevent infection as well as to treat cases might contain a pandemic at the site of the outbreak or at least slow its spread.

[49] HHS also released a second draft guidance that includes advice for employers, other than health care providers and emergency services personnel, to help employers determine if antivirals would be useful in their plans to protect critical operations and personnel. The guidance does not recommend that all employers use antivirals. Rather, it recommends that maintaining critical infrastructure and operations should be strongly considered in deciding how to allocate antivirals for prophylactic use. Additionally, the guidance does not recommend all employers use antivirals because other measures, such as nonpharmaceutical measures, may be implemented instead.

[50] In May 2006, the Secretaries of HHS and DHS tasked the National Infrastructure Advisory Council with, among other things, providing recommendations regarding the prioritization and distribution of pharmaceutical interventions to the critical workforce. According to this Council's report, the number of the most essential critical-infrastructure workers is approximately 12 million. See National Infrastructure Advisory Council, *The Prioritization of Critical Infrastructure for a Pandemic Outbreak in the United States Working Group: Final Report and Recommendations by the Council*, (Washington, D.C.: Jan. 16, 2007). According to HHS, the 20 million people in the critical workforce include the 12 million identified by the National Infrastructure Advisory Council as the most critical as well as other essential personnel such as military personnel, including the National Guard and critical government workers, such as border protection personnel.

[51] The Office of Biomedical Advanced Research and Development Authority within HHS manages contracts for the manufacturing and stockpiling of pre-pandemic vaccine. See app. II for more information on these contracts.

[52] Each individual would require two doses of vaccine, according to the dosing instructions for the pre-pandemic vaccine developed from an H5N1 strain and approved by FDA for use in humans in the United States. Thus, in order to vaccinate 13 million people, HHS has stockpiled 26 million doses of vaccine. HHS has also awarded contracts to vaccine manufacturers for the development of pre-pandemic vaccines containing adjuvants—substances that may be added to a vaccine to increase the body's immune response, thereby necessitating a lower dose of vaccine. According to HHS officials, if FDA approves the use of adjuvants in these vaccines and adjuvants were obtained, there would be enough pre-pandemic vaccine in the current stockpile for more than 75 million people.

[53] The Vaccine Management Business Improvement Project is a collaborative effort between HHS, state and local immunization program managers, and the private sector to improve vaccine management processes at the federal, state, and local levels. Goals of the project include simplifying processes for the ordering, distribution, and management of vaccines to enhance response to public health emergencies, such as vaccine shortages.

[54] HHS created the Pandemic Severity Index to aid in determining the severity of a pandemic. This index is primarily based on case-fatality ratios. CDC defines case-fatality ratio as the proportion of deaths among clinically-ill persons.

[55] However, these individuals would be targeted under the category of general population for this scenario.

[56] HHS has exercised this distribution plan for pandemic vaccine several times. Also, HHS officials told us that manufacturers will provide the syringes and needles needed for administration when the pandemic vaccine is distributed.

[57] For example, the H5N1 viral strains in circulation in Thailand, Vietnam, and Cambodia are resistant to the older class of antivirals, adamantanes, which includes amantadine and rimantadine. In contrast, the H5N1 virus strain that emerged in 2004 has shown in a few cases to have some resistance to oseltamivir (Tamiflu), one of the relatively newer classes of antivirals. However, all strains of H5N1 currently are susceptible to zanamivir (Relenza). Frederick Hayden, Alexander Klimov, Masato Tashiro, Alan Hay, Arnold Monto, Jennifer McKimm-Breschkin, Catherine Macken, Alan Hampson, Robert G. Webster, Michèle Amyard, and Maria Zambon, "Neuraminidase Inhibitor Susceptibility Network position statement: antiviral resistance in influenza A/H5N1 viruses," *Antiviral Therapy*, vol. 10 (2005), 873-77.

[58] Guillain-Barré syndrome is a disorder in which the body's immune system attacks part of the peripheral nervous system. Symptoms include varying degrees of weakness or tingling sensations in the legs, which in many cases spreads to the arms and upper body.

[59] Elissa A. Laitin and Elise M. Pelletier, *Drugs and Devices Information Line*, "The Influenza A/New Jersey (Swine Flu) Vaccine and Guillain-Barré Syndrome: The Arguments for a Causal Association," (1997): p. 1-11 and David J. Sencer and J. Donald Millar, *Emerging Infectious Diseases*, "Reflections on the 1976 Swine Flu Vaccination Program," vol. 12, no. 1 (2006), 29-33.

[60] GAO-08-92, 26.

[61] The time required to produce vaccine depends, in part, on the satisfactory growth and yield of the virus in chicken eggs, the number of doses required to build immunity, and access to raw materials. Other factors that affect timing of vaccine production include testing by FDA and manufacturers to determine vaccine strength and the development of a reagent for such testing. A reagent is a substance used in a chemical reaction to detect, measure, examine, or produce other substances. Reagents are used to determine the purity and strength of influenza vaccine and must be developed each year for the specific new annual influenza vaccine.

[62] In order to provide enough pandemic vaccine for 300 million people, HHS has established a goal of producing 600 million doses to provide two doses per person. The 2010-2011 time frame is based on vaccine production

without adjuvants. According to HHS officials, if adjuvants were to be used, lowering the amount of vaccine needed to promote an immune response, HHS could reach its production goal in 2008 or 2009.

[63] HHS's investments in research have also resulted in FDA-approved products. In April 2007, FDA approved the first influenza vaccine based on an H5N1 strain for human use in the United States.

[64] GAO-05-984, 11-12.

[65] Department of Health and Human Services, *HHS Pandemic Influenza Plan* (Washington, D.C.: Nov. 2005).

[66] Homeland Security Council, *National Strategy for Pandemic Influenza Implementation Plan* (Washington, D.C.: May 3, 2006) and Department of Health and Human Services, *Pandemic Influenza Implementation Plan* (Washington, D.C.: Nov. 2006).

[67] According to HHS, if adjuvants are approved for use in pre-pandemic vaccine, it could in turn alter the prioritization and increase the population groups included in receiving pre- pandemic vaccine.

[68] A standard of care is the diagnostic and treatment process that a clinician should follow for a certain type of patient, illness, or clinical circumstance. It is how similarly qualified health care providers would manage the patient's care under the same or similar circumstances.

[69] Homeland Security Council, *National Strategy for Pandemic Influenza Implementation Plan* (Washington, D.C., 2006), 13.

[70] Henry Masur, Ezekiel Emanuel, and H. Clifford Lane, "Severe Acute Respiratory Syndrome: Providing Care in the Face of Uncertainty," *Journal of the American Medical Association*, vol. 289, no. 21 (2003): 2861-2863.

[71] Charlene Irvin, Lauren Cindrich, William Patterson, Angela Ledbetter, and Anthony Southall, "Hospital Personnel Response during a Hypothetical Influenza Pandemic: Will They Come to Work?" *Academic Emergency Medicine*, vol. 14, no. 5, suppl.1 (2007): S13; K. Qureshi, R.R.M. Gershon, M.F. Sherman, T. Straub, E. Gebbie, M. McCollum, M.J. Erwin, and S.S. Morse, "Health Care Workers' Ability and Willingness to Report to Duty During Catastrophic Disasters," *Journal of Urban Health*, vol. 82, no. 3 (2005), 378-388; Kristine A. Qureshi, Jacqueline A. Merrill, Robyn R. M. Gershon, and Ayxa Calero-Breckheimer, "Emergency Preparedness Training for Public Health Nurses: a Pilot Study," *Journal of Urban Health*, vol. 79, no. 3 (2002), 413-416; and Yaron Shapira, Baruch Marganitt, Ilan Roziner, Tzippora Shochet, Yael Bar, and Joshua Shemer, "Willingness of Staff to Report to Their Hospital Duties Following an Unconventional Missile Attack: A State-Wide Survey," *Israel Journal of Medical Sciences*, vol. 27 (1991), 704-711.

[72] Ran D. Balicer, Saad B. Omer, Daniel J. Barnett, and George S. Everly, Jr., "Local Public Health Workers' Perceptions Toward Responding to an Influenza Pandemic," *BioMedCentral Public Health*, vol. 6, no. 99 (2006), 3.

[73] Irvin, Cindrich, Patterson, Ledbetter, and Southall, S13.

[74] GAO, *Emergency Management Assistance Compact: Enhancing EMAC's Collaborative and Administrative Capacity Should Improve National Disaster Response*, GAO-07-854 (Washington, D.C.: June 29, 2007), 32.

[75] Established standards of care are the allocation of appropriate health and medical resources to improve the health status or save the lives of all patients under normal conditions.

[76] GAO recently reviewed emergency preparedness planning documents for 20 states and found that only 7 of the 20 states had adopted or were drafting altered standards of care for specific medical issues. See GAO, *Emergency Preparedness: States Are Planning for Medical Surge, but Could Benefit from Shared Guidance for Allocating Scarce Medical Resources*, GAO-08-668 (Washington, D.C.: June 13, 2008), 2 1-22.

[77] Altered standards of care are also referred to as "standards of care appropriate to the situation."

[78] Altered standards of care can be thought of in terms of triage, which refers to the process of sorting victims according to their need for treatment and the resources available. Triage is often done in emergency rooms, disasters, and wars when limited medical resources must be allocated to maximize the number of survivors.

[79] Health Systems Research Inc., *Altered Standards of Care in Mass Casualty Events*, a special report prepared at the request of the Department of Health and Human Services, the Agency for Healthcare Research and Quality (Rockville, Md.: 2005) and Health Systems Research Inc., *Mass Medical Care with Scarce Resources: A Community Planning Guide*, a special report prepared at the request of the Department of Health and Human Services, the Agency for Healthcare Research and Quality (Rockville, Md.: 2007).

[80] The uncertainty of emergency situations, the need for altered standards of care, and the unpredictability of injuries during emergencies may raise liability fears and may deter health care providers and facilities from participating. Therefore, laws and regulations governing the delivery of health care under normal conditions may need to be modified or enhanced to address a mass casualty event.

[81] Pub. L. No. 109-417, § 102, 120 Stat. 2833.

[82] Pub. L. No. 109-417, § 203, 120 Stat. 2849.

[83] Pub. L. No. 109-417, § 304, 120 Stat. 2860.

[84] See Department of Health and Human Services, *Pandemic and All-Hazards Preparedness Act Progress Report* (Washington, D.C.: Nov. 2007), 11.

[85] Department of Health and Human Services, *Interim Pre-pandemic Planning Guidance: Community Strategy for Pandemic Influenza Mitigation in the United States – Early, Targeted, Layered Use of Nonpharmaceutical Interventions* (Washington, D.C.: February 2007).

[86] U.S. government, *Federal Guidance to Assist States in Improving State-Level Pandemic Influenza Operating Plans* (Washington, D.C.: Mar. 11, 2008).

[87] Martin C. J. Bootsma and Neil M. Ferguson, "The effect of public health measures on the 1918 influenza pandemic in U.S. cities," *Proceedings of the National Academy of Sciences of the United States of America*, vol. 104, no. 18 (2007), 7588-93; Richard J. Hatchett, Carter E. Mecher, and Marc Lipsitch, "Public health interventions and epidemic intensity during the 1918 influenza pandemic," *Proceedings of the National Academy of Sciences of the United States of America*, (2007), 1-6; Michael J. Haber, David K. Shay, Xiaohong M. Davis, Rajan Patel, Xiaoping Jin, Eric Weintraub, Evan Orenstein, and William W. Thompson, "Effectiveness of Interventions to Reduce Contact Rates during a Simulated Influenza Pandemic," *Emerging Infectious Diseases*, vol. 13, no. 4 (2007), 58 1-89; Howard Markel, Alexandra M. Stern, J. Alexander Navarro, Joseph R. Michalsen, Arnold S. Monto, and Cleto DiGiovanni, Jr, "Nonpharmaceutical Influenza Mitigation Strategies, US Communities 1918- 1920 Pandemic," *Emerging Infectious Diseases*, vol. 12, no. 12 (2006), 196 1-64; Robert J. Glass, Laura M. Glass, Walter E. Beyeler, and H. Jason Min, "Targeted Social Distancing Design for Pandemic Influenza," *Emerging Infectious Diseases*, vol. 12, no. 11 (2006): 1671- 81; and Joseph T. Wu, Steven Riley, Christophe Fraser, and Gabriel M. Leung, "Reducing the Impact of the Next Influenza Pandemic Using Household-Based Public Health Interventions," *Public Library of Science*, vol. 3, no. 9 (2006), 1-9.

[88] Bootsma and Ferguson, 7588 and Hatchett, Mecher, and Lipsitch, 1.

[89] A report by the Institute of Medicine identified major limitations with the current use of mathematical models, particularly with the uncertainty associated with many of the assumptions made by researchers regarding key parameters, such as the transmissibility of the virus, the effectiveness of social distancing interventions, and compliance with these interventions. For example, results from a model with the assumption that most viral transmission occurs among children in schools will differ from a similar model with the assumption that most transmission occurs among households contacts. Committee on Modeling Community Containment for Pandemic Influenza Board on Population Health and Public Health Practice, Institute of Medicine of the National Academies, "Modeling Community Containment for Pandemic Influenza, A Letter Report." (Washington, D.C.: 2006).

[90] Hatchett, Mecher, and Lipsitch, 5, and Bootsma and Ferguson, 7592.

[91] R.J. Blendon, L.M. Koonin, J.M. Benson, M.S. Cetron, W.E. Pollard, E.W. Mitchell, et. al, "Public response to community mitigation measures for pandemic influenza, *Emerging Infectious Diseases*, vol. 14 (2008): 778-786.

[92] Robert J. Blendon, Catherine M. DesRoches, Martin S. Cetron, John M. Benson, Theodore Meinhardt, and William Pollard, "Attitudes Toward the Use of Quarantine In a Public Health Emergency in Four Countries," *Health Affairs*, vol. 25 (2006): W22.

[93] Department of Health and Human Services, *U.S. Department of Health and Human Services Pandemic Influenza Communications Plan* (Washington, D.C.: November 2006).

[94] The following individuals have been identified as primary spokespeople for the medical response in a pandemic—HHS Secretary, HHS Deputy Secretary, Assistant Secretary for Health, Assistant Secretary for Preparedness and Response, Deputy Assistant Secretary for Preparedness and Response, HHS Science Advisor, Director of the National Vaccine Program Office, Director of CDC, Director of the National Institute of Allergy and Infectious Diseases at the National Institutes of Health, Assistant Secretary for Public Affairs, Deputy Assistant Secretary for Public Affairs, Director of the HHS Press Office, and Director of Media Affairs (regional media).

[95] A tabletop exercise is a facilitated analysis of a hypothetical emergency situation. The purpose of the exercise is to have participants examine problems based on current plans and to identify where those plans need to be refined.

[96] Messages are written to a sixth grade reading level and presented in 3 short sentences that convey 3 key messages in 27 words. The approach is based on surveys showing that lead or front page media and broadcast stories usually convey only three key messages, typically in less than 9 seconds for broadcast media or 27 words for print.

[97] HHS has developed planning checklists for state and local jurisdictions, medical offices and clinics, emergency medical service and non-emergent (medical) transport organizations, home health care services, individuals and families, businesses, school districts (K-12), childcare and preschool facilities, colleges and universities, faith-based and community organizations, long-term care and other residential facilities, the travel industry, and health insurers.

[98] In addition, we have cited concerns about multiple and potentially confusing or conflicting messages coming from many agencies at all levels of government during a pandemic. See GAO-08-36, 5.

[99] Harvard School of Public Health Project on the Public and Biological Security, "Pandemic Influenza and the Public: Survey Findings," presentation at the Institute of Medicine (Oct. 26, 2006).

[100] Department of Homeland Security, *National Response Framework* (Washington, D.C.: January 2008).

[101] Pub. L. No. 93-288 § 101, 88 Stat. 143 (1974) (as amended) (codified as amended at 42 U.S.C. § 5121).

[102] Homeland Security Council, *National Strategy for Pandemic Influenza* (Washington, D.C., Nov. 1, 2005).

[103] Homeland Security Council, *National Strategy for Pandemic Influenza Implementation Plan* (Washington, D.C.: May 3, 2006).

[104] Homeland Security Council, *National Strategy for Pandemic Influenza Implementation Plan One Year Summary* (Washington, D.C.: July 17, 2007).

[105] Department of Health and Human Services, *HHS Pandemic Influenza Plan* (Washington, D.C.: November 2005).

[106] Department of Health and Human Services, *Pandemic Influenza Implementation Plan* (Washington, D.C.: November 2006).

[107] White House, Homeland Security Presidential Directive-21: Public Health and Medical Preparedness (Washington, D.C.: Oct. 18, 2007).

[108] Department of Health and Human Services and Department of Homeland Security, *Guidance on Allocating and Targeting Pandemic Influenza Vaccine* (Washington, D.C.: July 23, 2008).

[109] See Departments of Labor, Health and Human Services, and Education, and Related Agencies Appropriations Act, 2006. Pub. L. No. 109-149, 119 Stat. 2833, 2857 (funds not limited to purposes related to pandemic or avian influenza); Department of Defense, Emergency Supplemental Appropriations to Address Hurricanes in the Gulf of Mexico, and Pandemic Influenza Act, 2006, Pub. L. No. 109-148, 119 Stat. 2680, 2783, 2786; Emergency Supplemental Appropriations Act for Defense, the Global War on Terror and Hurricane Recovery, 2006, Pub. L. No. 109-234, 120 Stat. 479 (includes $30 million to be transferred to the U.S. Agency for International Development). HHS also received appropriations specifically available for pandemic-inflenza-related purposes, among other purposes, totaling $50 million in fiscal year 2004, $182 million in fiscal year 2005, and $100 million in fiscal year 2007. 2004: Consolidated Appropriations Act, 2004, Pub. L. No. 108-199, 118 Stat. 3, 251; 2005: Consolidated Appropriations Act, 2005, Pub. L. No. 108-447, 118 Stat. 2809, 3138, Emergency Supplemental Appropriations Act, 2005. War on Terror, and Tsunami Relief, 2005, Pub. L. No. 109-13, 119 Stat. 231, 276, 280; 2007: Revised Continuing Appropriations Resolution, 2007, Pub. L. No. 110-5, 121 Stat. 8, 33. Many of these appropriations are available without fiscal year limitation.

[110] Also, approximately $179 million of the appropriated funds was dedicated to international collaboration, with the remainder going to other areas, such as state and local preparedness and risk communications.

[111] GAO, *Influenza Pandemic: Efforts Under Way to Address Constraints on Using Antivirals and Vaccines to Forestall a Pandemic*, GAO-08-92 (Washington, D.C.: Dec. 21, 2007), 26.

In: Influenza Pandemic - Preparedness and Response to …   ISBN: 978-1-60692-953-7
Editor: Emma S. Brouwer pp.159-200   © 2010 Nova Science Publishers, Inc.

Chapter 6

U.S. Policy Regarding Pandemic-Influenza Vaccines

Congressional Budget Office

Summary

Public health officials are concerned that a particular strain of influenza, known as H5N1, or "avian flu," which has caused widespread infection of poultry flocks in Asia, Europe, the Near East, and Africa, might become easily transmissible among humans, causing illness and death at rates unseen at least since the early 20th century. In the "Spanish flu" pandemic of 1918 and 1919, more than 500,000 people died in the United States and some 50 million perished worldwide. By contrast, in a typical year, seasonal influenza causes about 36,000 deaths in the United States. Public health officials worry that an influenza pandemic today could cause some 2 million deaths in the United States. It also could lead to substantial adverse economic consequences both here and abroad (CBO 2005, 2006a).

Against the prospect of such an event, the Department of Health and Human Services (HHS) has developed a plan to prepare for and combat an influenza pandemic and has budgeted about $7.9 billion since 2004 for influenza preparedness activities (HHS 2005b). Most of that money— about $5.6 billion—was provided through supplemental appropriation bills in 2006 in response to the HHS plan. About $3.2 billion of the supplemental funds, along with some additional funds that are part of HHS's annual appropriation, is being spent for vaccine-related activities, reflecting the strong consensus among public health officials that vaccination is the best tool for reducing the consequences—and the costs—of an influenza pandemic.[1]

HHS planners initially confronted two problems: inadequate capacity for vaccine production and delays in producing vaccine. The emergence of H5N1 as a human health risk found a U.S. production base that had been reduced to a single domestic manufacturer, using an egg- based process developed in the 1940s to produce the vaccine. The current process for delivery of seasonal- influenza vaccine takes about six months from the initial step of isolating the virus strain to the final delivery of the vaccine to the clinic or doctor's office.

Step one in HHS's plan was to promote an increase in capacity as rapidly as possible by encouraging the expansion and refurbishing of existing plants. The second, and current, step is to introduce cell-based manufacturing technology to the domestic production of influenza vaccine. (That method uses cells rather than chicken eggs as the medium in which to grow the active ingredient in the vaccine; it is a standard method for manufacturing most vaccines against childhood diseases, for example.)

Because production requires about six months, and an influenza pandemic could spread much faster than that, HHS's plan includes short- and longer-term approaches to the problem of making vaccines available quickly. In the short run, a small stockpile of vaccines could be used for a limited initial response. Longer-term plans call for the development of "next-generation vaccines," which will draw on advances in biotechnology to speed production. Because developing safe and effective vaccines could take years—perhaps a decade or more—HHS is encouraging pharmaceutical manufacturers to start development now.

In parallel with the efforts to scale up production of egg- and cell-based vaccines, HHS is funding the development of new adjuvants, substances that can be added to influenza vaccines to reduce the amount of active ingredient (also called antigen) needed per dose of vaccine. The use of adjuvants for egg-based and cell-based vaccines could allow domestic manufacturers to produce more doses in existing facilities, and so fewer new facilities would be needed to manufacture cell-based formulations. Moreover, smaller stockpiles could be used to protect larger numbers of people. But adjuvanted vaccines can induce more pronounced side effects than ordinary vaccines can, a definite downside because vaccines, unlike most other pharmaceuticals, are given to healthy people. To date, the Food and Drug Administration has not approved an adjuvanted vaccine for influenza. In contrast, adjuvanted influenza vaccines have been approved for use in Europe.

This paper from the Congressional Budget Office (CBO) focuses on the government's role, under HHS's plan, in the development of new vaccines and the capacity to manufacture them. It provides information on progress and on the potential cost of achieving HHS's vaccine- related goals, the continuing expenditures that are likely to be needed to maintain preparedness, and the experience of other countries in preparing for a possible pandemic. It also presents options for modifying HHS's 2005 plan. The work is based on a review of the academic literature, on industry data, and on interviews with government and industry experts who are working to improve the response of vaccine producers to a potential influenza pandemic.

Findings

The manufacturers of currently approved influenza vaccines made in the United States cannot produce vaccines of sufficient effectiveness, in sufficient quantities, or in the time required to meet public health needs in the event of an influenza pandemic. Several companies, some with funding from HHS, are developing adjuvants that could boost the effectiveness of influenza vaccines and thus reduce the amount of active ingredient needed per dose. In the short term, adjuvants offer the best hope for achieving HHS's goal of inoculating 300 million people within six months of the onset of an influenza pandemic; adjuvants could allow manufacturers to increase the number of doses produced in existing domestic manufacturing facilities, and their development would substantially affect the cost of most other aspects of HHS's plan. The extent to which manufacturers can develop safe and effective adjuvanted vaccines will have a major effect on the scope of preparations for a possible pandemic.

Additional Capacity and New Cell-Based Vaccines

By 2011, companies that receive funding from HHS plan to more than triple domestic capacity for production of egg-based influenza vaccines. To augment private investment, HHS has obligated $176 million to provide a year-round egg supply and to retrofit existing facilities. If, in addition to the increased capacity, manufacturers also can develop adjuvanted egg-based vaccines, it is possible that they could make enough to inoculate 225 million people or more. If not, the same facilities could be expected within six months to produce enough vaccine for only 38 million people.

HHS intends to support the modernization of influenza vaccine production by helping manufacturers shift from egg-based to cell-based technology, which HHS believes is more reliable. HHS has obligated $1.3 billion, an amount experience suggests is sufficient to support development of cell-based influenza vaccines.

New facilities would have to be built to produce the vaccines—although less capacity would be necessary for adjuvanted vaccines. CBO estimates that it would cost between $1.2 billion and $1.8 billion to build new production facilities for adjuvanted cell-based vaccines and between $7.6 billion and $11.4 billion for facilities for cell-based vaccines without adjuvants. Pharmaceutical manufacturers are not likely to create that much new capacity on their own because the capacity would exceed that necessary to meet demand for seasonal-influenza vaccine. Moreover, because building those facilities is a complex matter, it is not likely any would be finished in time to meet HHS's goal of 2011.

The additional capacity would be in excess of that needed in years when there is no pandemic. To keep the factories ready to operate, continuing federal support—in the form of purchases for the stockpile or direct payments— would probably be necessary.

Stockpiles

If safe and effective adjuvanted vaccines can be developed, the current stockpile could be stretched to vaccinate well more than HHS's initial goal of 20 million people. (Information from HHS indicates that it would cost about $350 million annually to replace expired vaccine and adjuvants.) Even if the development of adjuvants is not successful, the stockpile holds enough to vaccinate about 6 million people, and it would cost about $1.1 billion to purchase the remainder necessary to inoculate 20 million people. Once the stockpile is full, annual replenishment of expired vaccine should cost about $1.1 billion. Continued spending to maintain the stockpile could occupy excess manufacturing capacity and obviate much of the need for direct government payments to pharmaceutical manufacturers. However, because it was manufactured with a virus strain that differs from that likely to cause a pandemic, no one knows how effective the vaccine in the stockpile will be for protecting people in the event of a pandemic.

Next-Generation Vaccines

In the long-term, the public health community hopes that entirely new vaccines and production technologies will substantially reduce vaccine production times and create vaccines that offer broad protection against many—or all—strains of influenza virus. Developers expect to use recombinant DNA techniques to manufacture next-generation vaccines that might someday approach the lifetime effectiveness of currently available vaccines against many childhood diseases. HHS's plan has relatively few incentives for manufacturers to develop new products or production technologies because its funds go largely to support the expansion of existing production facilities for egg-based vaccines and for the development of new cell-based vaccines. Moreover, HHS's plans now call for supporting the creation of more production capacity than can be sustained by current demand. The excess supply could easily saturate the market, substantially driving down prices for influenza vaccine. Low prices could make the market look unattractive to companies developing next-generation vaccines. Consequently, government funding is likely to be needed to help bring next-generation vaccines to the marketplace.

Activities in Other Nations

Several European countries are entering into advance supply agreements with manufacturers to provide vaccines in the event of a pandemic; those governments agree to make advance payments to guarantee the supply of vaccine in the event of an influenza pandemic. It is unknown whether the companies can produce the vaccines promised under their agreements. Several European countries also are stockpiling vaccines, although the size of the stockpiles relative to national populations varies substantially. International organizations and other nations' governments also are funding the development of influenza vaccines, although not to the extent seen in the United States.

Options

In at least one important regard, the world's circumstances have changed since HHS published its plan in 2005: Several manufacturers have reported success using adjuvants in influenza vaccines, and some of them have been approved in Europe. Adjuvants have the potential to substantially reduce the amount of antigen needed per dose. That development raises questions about whether the current policy is the most cost-effective approach to meeting HHS's goals. CBO examined several other options, briefly outlined here.

Scale Back Support for Cell-Based Manufacturing Technology

One option that HHS might consider if adjuvanted vaccines prove successful is to reduce the capacity targeted for manufacturing cell-based influenza vaccine. A reduction could save the $600 million that HHS currently has budgeted for the construction of facilities for producing cell-based vaccines, and it would reduce the amount of spending needed to maintain the new facilities. The resulting reliance on a small number of manufacturers and facilities and on poultry flocks, however, could increase the risk of supply disruptions.

Add Resources to Develop Next-Generation Vaccines

Success with adjuvanted vaccines could have implications for the use of resources devoted to development of the next generation of vaccines and for the mechanisms the government uses to accomplish its objectives. Specifically, if adjuvanted vaccines reduced the near-term risk posed by pandemic influenza because they stretched available and planned production capacity, more resources might be made available to support the development of next- generation vaccines.

Alternative mechanisms for providing that support also could be considered for next-generation vaccines. HHS could use demand-side rather than supply-side incentives to accomplish its goals. For example, HHS could commit to stockpiling next-generation vaccines that proved successful rather than choosing which specific companies and technologies to support. Such an approach would help HHS reduce the likelihood of encountering pitfalls associated with active government intervention in decisionmaking about private investment and commercial production.

Early success in developing next-generation influenza vaccines is unlikely, however. Most of the formulations are in early stages of development, at the start of a long and risky path to approval.

Consider Advance Supply Agreements

HHS could consider entering into advance supply agreements like those used in Europe for procuring the quantities of vaccine necessary to immunize the U.S. population in the event of a pandemic. Such agreements could pro-vide a contractual obligation for manufacturers to supply vaccines to public health officials or physicians in the United States. Although the current U.S. approach of directly subsidizing vaccine development and additional production capacity could result in a more abundant supply of vaccine, it does not ensure that the United States would be able to buy enough vaccine to meet its need in a pandemic. Manufacturers could exhaust their supplies when fulfilling their European agreements before they have the chance to sell any to the United States. If the United States does pursue advance supply agreements, it might be necessary to structure them to recognize that other nations' governments could temporarily restrict or prohibit exports of pandemic-influenza vaccine until their own populations have been immunized.

The Size of the Vaccine Stockpile

The current goal of 20 million doses for the stockpile could be too large or too small: If, for example, the strain that causes the pandemic influenza does not respond to the stockpiled vaccine formulation, the stockpile could be wastefully large. But it could be too small if a pandemic were to spread through the population more quickly than new vaccines could be manufactured.

Successful development of adjuvanted vaccines could alter the balance of risks in determining the size of the stockpile and potentially reduce the cost of mitigating those risks. Some recent research indicates that adjuvanted vaccines could provide protection against more than one strain of virus, thereby improving the chances that the vaccines in the stockpile would be effective in a pandemic. Moreover, because adjuvants would reduce the amount of antigen required, HHS either could retain its current goal of maintaining a stockpile sufficient to inoculate 20 million people while reducing the amount of stockpiled antigen or it could plan to expand the population it would inoculate with prepandemic vaccine.

1. THE MARKET FOR SEASONAL-INFLUENZA VACCINE AND THE CHALLENGE OF PROVIDING VACCINE IN A PANDEMIC

The prospect of an influenza pandemic—a global outbreak of influenza that leads to serious illness or death in large numbers of people—is cause for concern among policymakers, public health experts, and the public at large. Pandemics are not new: There were three in the 20th century, the deadliest of which, the "Spanish flu" of 1918, caused global devastation, killing more than 500,000 people in the United States and about 50 million people worldwide. According to the World Health Organization (WHO), an influenza pandemic requires three conditions: First, a new virus emerges to which people have little natural immunity. Second, infection leads to significant rates of illness or death. And third, the virus is transmitted efficiently from one person to another (WHO 2006, p. 1).

Although a pandemic could be caused by any of several influenza strains, policymakers and public health experts are particularly worried about the persistence of the currently circulating H5N1 strain (the "avian flu" or "bird flu"), which has caused high mortality among poultry in Asia and has spread in poultry from Southeast Asia to Central Asia, Europe, and Africa.[2] The H5N1 virus meets two of the three conditions for a pandemic: First, people have little natural immunity to H5N1 because it has not widely circulated among the human population. And second, it has caused significant illness in the 385 people who have become infected, and 243 of those people have died. The mortality rate from the H5N1 virus is thus in excess of 60 percent of known cases (WHO 2007a).[3] So far, WHO's third condition has not been met: The H5N1 virus is not transmitted efficiently from one person to another. Close contact with infected poultry is thought to be required for human infection. However, the danger exists that the virus will evolve in a way that allows for efficient human-to-human transmission, perhaps leading to a pandemic. Depending on the virulence of the particular strain of influenza, a pandemic could have substantial consequences for human health and for economic activity around the world (CBO 2005, 2006a). Because infectious diseases are unpredictable, public health authorities cannot say for sure when a pandemic will arise, whether it will involve H5N1 or some other strain, or whether it will be mild or virulent.

Against the prospect of a pandemic like the 1918 Spanish flu, the Department of Health and Human Services (HHS) since 2004 has budgeted about $7.9 billion for activities to support a research and preparedness plan for an influenza pandemic (see Table 1-1). A large portion of that amount—nearly $5.6 billion—came in supplemental appropriations for 2006 to fund HHS's plan for coping with an influenza pandemic (HHS 2005b).[4] The department's national response plan includes support for research and development in new vaccines and new vaccine formulations, an increase in production capacity, and the establishment of vaccine stockpiles. The plan also encompasses the stockpiling of existing antiviral drugs as well as other medical supplies (including surgical masks, respirators, ventilators, and syringes) and the development of new antiviral drugs. In addition, HHS's recommendations address the coordination of state and local preparedness and response and methods for monitoring influenza viruses that have the potential to cause a pandemic.

Table 1-1. HHS's Funding for Influenza Preparedness, 2004 to 2008

(Budget authority, in millions of dollars)							
	2004	**2005**	**2006**	**2006ᵃ**	**2007**	**2008**	**Total, 2004–2008**
Office of the Secretary	43	101	4	5,152	0	76	5,377
Centers for Disease Control and Prevention	198	323	295	400	73	73	1,361
Food and Drug Administration	3	5	5	20	33	38	103
National Institutes of Health	113	164	207	18	271	271	1,044
Total	**357**	**592**	**511**	**5,590**	**377**	**458**	**7,885**

Source: Congressional Budget Office based on data collected from HHS.

Note: HHS = Department of Health and Human Services.

a. Additional funds were provided in the form of emergency supplemental appropriations.

HHS has budgeted $3.2 billion of its 2006 supplemental appropriations (plus some of its appropriated funds from other years) for vaccines (see Table 1-2). Relying mainly on the supplemental funding provided in 2006, HHS has obligated almost $2.6 billion to promote the development of vaccines, increase the investment in new production capacity, and procure vaccine stockpiles (see Table 1-3). According to agency officials, HHS has yet to obligate about $1.3 billion of the supplemental appropriations provided in 2006. About $900 million of that amount is budgeted for vaccine-related activities. Officials at HHS note that although those funds have not yet been obligated, there are plans for their use.

The President's budgetary proposals for 2009 include $820 million for HHS to pursue its pandemic-influenza activities. Of that amount, $467 million is to procure vaccines for the stockpile and to fund vaccine production capability, $40 million is to stockpile other medical supplies, and $313 million is to fund preparedness activities at the Centers for Disease Control and Prevention (CDC), the Food and Drug Administration (FDA), the National Institutes of Health (NIH), and the Office of the Secretary in HHS.

The vaccine component of HHS's plan is motivated by concerns about the capacity and capabilities of the current group of manufacturers of seasonal-influenza vaccine to respond to the threat of a pandemic. Because current vaccines and manufacturing capacity are inadequate to protect the U.S. population in the event of a pandemic, HHS is devoting much of its effort to developing new vaccines and expanding existing manufacturing capacity. Specifically, the first goal is to have in place by 2011 domestic production capacity sufficient to supply vaccine to the entire U.S. population within six months of the onset of a pandemic. The second goal is to stockpile enough doses of prepandemic vaccines to inoculate 20 million people. (Prepandemic vaccines are developed from strains that public health officials believe have the most potential to cause an influenza pandemic.) First priority for vaccination will be given to children and to people who are critical to maintaining security, health care, and essential services.

This Congressional Budget Office (CBO) paper examines several questions:

- What steps have been taken and what is the status of HHS's plan to improve manufacturers' response to an influenza pandemic?

Table 1-2. Supplemental Funding for HHS's Pandemic-Influenza Plan, 2006

	Budget Authority	
	Millions of dollars	Percentage
Vaccines	3,233	58
Antiviral Drugs	911	16
Medical Supplies	170	3
State and Local Preparedness[a]	770	14
Monitoring[b]	455	8
Other	51	1
Total	**5,590**	**100**

Source: Congressional Budget Office based on data from HHS (2006a).
Note: HHS = Department of Health and Human Services.
a. Includes funding for state subsidies for antiviral drugs.
b. Includes international and domestic activities.

- What changes have occurred in the vaccine industry, particularly as a result of expanded government involvement in the influenza vaccine market?
- What is the continuing role for the government in developing and producing influenza vaccines to meet the performance objectives specified under current policy, and how will that role affect federal spending?

The Market for Seasonal-Influenza Vaccine

The first line of defense against seasonal influenza, which results in the hospitalization of about 200,000 people and causes about 36,000 deaths each year in the United States, is annual vaccination.[5] About 100 million U.S. residents were inoculated in the 2006–2007 season. Vaccination is considered a principal strategy to combat pandemic influenza as well, but a pandemic will create huge surges in demand. The nation's response to an influenza pandemic will depend to a great extent on whether the manufacturers of seasonal-influenza vaccine can meet the challenge of providing a far larger number of doses of the correct vaccine quickly enough to inoculate the whole population.

As it is currently formulated, the seasonal-influenza vaccine contains 15 micrograms (a microgram is one one- millionth of a gram) of active ingredient, or antigen (the protein that elicits an immune response in the body) from each of three strains of influenza virus, for a total of 45 micrograms per dose. (By contrast, a pandemic vaccine would contain antigen from a single strain.) Since the 1 940s, manufacturers have made vaccines by injecting seed viruses into hens' eggs, growing them there, and then using the viruses grown in the fluids inside the eggs as the starter for the vaccine.

The FDA has licensed two main types of vaccine: One, called a subunit vaccine, uses purified proteins from killed viruses. The subunit vaccine is delivered by injection and accounts for 97 percent of the vaccine used in the United States. The other type uses a weakened live form of the influenza virus (often called live, attenuated virus). The vaccine made from the weakened live virus is administered in an intranasal spray, and just one company produces it for the U.S. market.

Table 1-3. HHS's Obligations for Pandemic- Influenza Vaccine Projects

	Obligations[a] (Millions of dollars)	Duration
Develop New Vaccines	1,435	2005 to 2012
Increase Capacity	176	2004 to 2012
Stockpile Vaccine	950	2004 to 2008
Total	**2,561**	

Source: Congressional Budget Office based on data from Robinson (2008).

Note: HHS = Department of Health and Human Services.

a. As of December 2007.

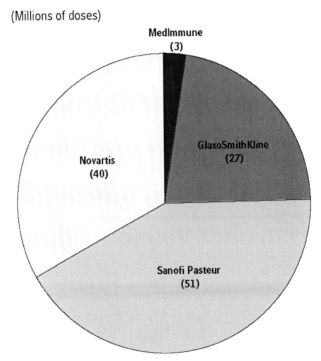

(Millions of doses)

MedImmune (3)

GlaxoSmithKline (27)

Novartis (40)

Sanofi Pasteur (51)

Source: Congressional Budget Office based on Health Industry Distributors Association (2007) and Novartis (2007).

Figure 1-1. Vaccine Production for the 2006–2007 Influenza Season in the United States

Because the genetic makeup of influenza viruses can change rapidly, the vaccine must be reformulated each year to confer immunity against the strains researchers believe will circulate that year. In February or March, the FDA announces the strains, which are chosen on the basis of surveillance data from CDC and WHO. Manufacturers then produce vaccine for delivery between November and March, the peak influenza season in the Northern Hemisphere. It takes about six months from the time the virus strains are isolated for the process to play out: manufacturing, purification, testing, filling, packaging, and delivery to clinics and physicians' offices.

The production of seasonal-influenza vaccine is characterized by high fixed costs—costs that do not change whether a manufacturer produces one dose of vaccine or millions. The most widely cited analysis puts the fixed cost of producing any vaccine at 60 percent of the total costs (exclusive of research and development costs), regardless of volume (Mercer Management Consulting 2002). Among the fixed expenses are depreciation, administration, quality assurance, and personnel.

Another 25 percent of the cost is fixed at the batch level regardless of batch size. Only 15 percent of the cost is truly variable, fluctuating directly with the number of doses produced.

The proportion of fixed costs suggests that the manufacturers with the largest market share will enjoy lower average costs—a condition that is conducive to market concentration among vaccine producers. As the number of producers declines, the potential for supply disruptions caused by contamination or other problems rises.

For the 2006–2007 season, there were only four manufacturers of influenza vaccine for the United States: GlaxoSmithKline (GSK), Sanofi Pasteur, Novartis, and MedImmune (see Figure 1-1). And only one of those, Sanofi Pasteur, actually produces the vaccine domestically. In all, those manufacturers produced about 120 million doses of vaccine for the 2006–2007 season, of which about 100 million were distributed (see Figure 1-2). (Because seasonal-influenza vaccine is reformulated each season, manufacturers must discard undistributed vaccine every year.)

The supply of seasonal-influenza vaccines has been disrupted several times in the recent past. In 2000–2001, manufacturers had difficulty growing one of the three influenza strains, and some facilities were shut down because of the FDA's concerns about compliance with good manufacturing practices (Danzon, Sousa Pereira, and Tejwani 2005; Government Accountability Office 2007). In the 2003–2004 season, Wyeth's decision to exit the market rather than incur the cost of upgrading its facility left just two manufacturers of injectable influenza vaccine. One of the two was unable to deliver any vaccine to the U.S. market for the 2004–2005 season because of contamination at its facility in the United Kingdom.

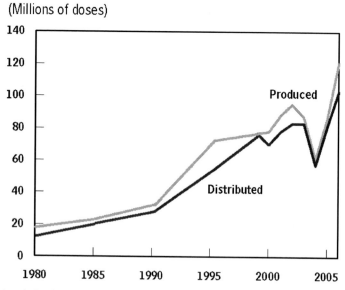

Source: Congressional Budget Office based on data from the Centers for Disease Control and Prevention.

Figure 1-2. Seasonal-Influenza Vaccine for the U.S. Market

Between 1999 and 2006, list prices (which are set by manufacturers and reported to CDC) for influenza vaccine jumped from about $2 to about $11 per dose. In general, individual clinicians, clinics, and hospitals pay list price or close to it; large groups, state consortia, and health plans often can negotiate for rebates and discounts (Institute of Medicine 2004, pp. 127–128). The number of doses distributed rose from 77 million in 1999 to 100 million in 2006 (see Figure 1-2).

WHO has estimated that, in 2007, manufacturers produced 565 million doses for the global market (WHO 2007d). That quantity would still fall well short of the number needed to inoculate the world's 6.6 billion people; by 2010, new production capacity could raise the global supply to 1 billion doses of seasonal-influenza vaccine.[6]

Supplying Vaccine in a Pandemic

If an influenza pandemic were to occur today, it would be impossible to meet HHS's goal of vaccinating the entire U.S. population of about 300 million people within the next six months. To begin with, current capacity for domestic production would be completely inadequate. (Only 50 million of the approximately 120 million doses produced for the domestic market during the 2006–2007 influenza season were manufactured in the United States.) In the event of a pandemic, moreover, it could be difficult to obtain supplies from overseas, especially if there are shortages in vaccine-producing countries or if those countries vaccinate their own populations before permitting exports to the United States (Osterholm and Branswell 2005).

It also is anticipated that the pandemic-influenza vaccine would have to be stronger than the seasonal version. Because of the lack of previous exposure to the H5N1 virus, humans would be expected to have no immunity at all. The only H5N1 vaccine currently approved for the U.S. market requires a course of two doses at 90 micrograms per dose (FDA 2007). (The seasonal vaccine is administered in a single dose of 45 micrograms of antigen— 15 micrograms against each of three strains. Most adults are exposed regularly to seasonal-influenza viruses and thus have some immunity, so the seasonal vaccine is in effect a booster shot. The course for children, who generally have less exposure and hence less immunity, typically is two doses.)

When all of those factors—uncertain availability of imports, higher content per dose, and more doses per course—are taken into consideration, current U.S. capacity to produce pandemic vaccine is only about 12.5 million courses (see Table 1-4). That estimate could be high; in the past, manufacturers have had difficulty growing pandemic-influenza strains. Moreover, given the six months it takes to produce and distribute current vaccines, experts fear that the pandemic-influenza vaccine would not be available until after the first wave of a pandemic had passed.

An influenza pandemic therefore would present a significant challenge for public health authorities and for manufacturers. About one-third of the U.S. population was vaccinated in the 2006–2007 season. If a pandemic were to occur, demand for vaccine would be much greater, even if vaccinating the entire U.S. population were not a policy goal. It would be a significant undertaking to increase output by so much, so quickly.

Overview of HHS's Plan

Because domestic vaccine manufacturers right now could not quickly provide enough vaccine to meet the threat of an influenza pandemic, HHS has focused on increasing domestic capacity for production. In the future, the agency plans to focus on reducing production time.

The emergence of H5N1 as a human health risk found a U.S. manufacturing base reduced to a single domestic manufacturer, producing the vaccine in an egg-based process developed in the 1940s. The first step in the HHS plan was to promote an increase in capacity as rapidly as possible by encouraging the expansion and refurbishing of existing plants. The second, and current, step is to introduce cell-based manufacturing technology to the domestic production of vaccine. Cell-based production uses animal cells to culture the virus, and it is a standard method for producing other vaccines, including several against childhood diseases.

It would be more expensive and time-consuming to initiate cell-based manufacturing than it would be to add capacity for egg-based production. But, HHS contends, adding cell-based capacity reduces the risk that is inherent in egg-based technology—that the laying hens could become infected with H5N1. HHS also argues that it allows for the possibility of producing the quantities of vaccine that would be needed in a pandemic.

HHS's plan includes short- and longer-term approaches to solving the problem of how to make the vaccine available quickly in the event of an influenza pandemic. In the short run, the procuring of a limited stockpile of vaccines would permit the government to expedite an initial response. But because stockpiled vaccines are made before a pandemic virus emerges, the formulations are not expected to perfectly match the pandemic virus, and they might not provide adequate protection. Moreover, the size of the current stockpile would permit inoculation of only a limited number of people.

Table 1-4. Domestic Production Capacity for Seasonal and Pandemic-Influenza Vaccine

	Adjustment Factors	Assumptions
Seasonal-Influenza Vaccine	50 Million Doses	
Adjustments for		
Strains per dose of pandemic vaccine	× 3	One strain instead of three
Antigen per dose of pandemic vaccine[a]	÷ 6	90 micrograms instead of 15 micrograms against a single strain[b]
Doses per course of pandemic vaccine	÷ 2	Two doses per course[c]
Pandemic Vaccine for U.S. Market	12.5 Million Courses	

Source: Congressional Budget Office.

a. Antigen is the active ingredient in a vaccine.

b. A microgram is one one-millionth of a gram.

c. For seasonal vaccines, a course generally consists of a single dose. Researchers believe the pandemic-influenza vaccine will require a course consisting of two doses.

HHS's long-term plans to promote the development of the next generation of vaccines—perhaps taking advantage of new methods in biotechnology—would address the problems of capacity shortage and of long production times. However, because developing safe and effective vaccines could take years, perhaps a decade or more, HHS's plan would encourage pharmaceutical manufacturers to start development now so that they are more likely to be able to produce vaccines quickly if a pandemic occurs in the future.

In parallel with those efforts, HHS is funding the development of adjuvants, substances that could boost the potency of the antigen in vaccines, thus reducing the amount of active ingredient needed per dose. Their successful development could affect many areas of HHS's plan. The use of adjuvants for egg-based and cell-based vaccines could allow for the production of more doses of vaccine from existing facilities, and fewer new manufacturing facilities would need to be built. Moreover, smaller stockpiles could be set aside to protect larger numbers of people.

Risks Associated with HHS's Plan

Any program that targets a problem as complex as an influenza pandemic entails risks and costs. The technology for cell production, for example, has been expensive to develop, and building the necessary facilities will require yet more resources. Yet, should technology develop successfully for the next generation of vaccines, the newly refurbished production facilities for egg-based products and the newly constructed facilities for cell-based vaccines would no longer be needed for producing influenza vaccine. The egg-based production facilities could become obsolete and perhaps be discarded while the facilities for cell-based production could be put to other uses.

A strategy of building up egg-based capacity while focusing on next-generation technology could avert some of the expense associated with modernizing the manufacturing technology. The trade-off would come with the possible exposure of the country to risk if the development of next-generation technology vaccines were delayed or never occurred at all.

Governments abroad have chosen different strategies in the face of the possibility of an influenza pandemic. Several member states of the European Union have entered into advance supply agreements with vaccine manufacturers. The governments agree to pay the manufacturers in advance, and the vaccine makers guarantee they will provide a specified number of doses of vaccine within a set period, such as six months. The governments' expectation is that the manufacturers (or the U.S. government) will develop the requisite vaccines and manufacturing technology. Other governments have given much less support for technology development than has the U.S. government. Given that seasonal-influenza vaccine is largely privately purchased in the United States, some analysts have asked whether substantial federal support for technology development is appropriate, especially compared with other governments' investments.

Although the threat of a pandemic on the scale of the Spanish flu of 1918 looms large in public health calculations, public health officials also recall the prospect in 1976 of an outbreak of what was known as the swine flu. In that instance, there was a widely perceived threat, and a federal vaccine program was initiated rapidly (Allen 2007, p. 261; Kolata 1999, pp. 121–185). The government determined it would inoculate 200 million U.S. residents within six months. In the end, some 40 million people received the vaccine, double the number ever vaccinated in a single year. However, the pandemic never appeared, and within months the vaccine became associated in public opinion—possibly incorrectly—with Guillain-Barré syndrome, a rare neurological disorder. The federal government ended up paying $100 million in compensation. Because of that history of premature response and backlash, and because vaccines are drugs that are given to healthy people, the public health community is cautious about introducing new vaccines into the market even in anticipation of a global health threat.

Additional Public Health Questions

The government's role in the vaccine market under HHS's plan also raises important questions for the medical and public health communities about whether the plan provides adequate protection against the threat of a pandemic. For example, HHS will need to ensure that it has mechanisms in place to identify the recipients and distribute the vaccines from the stockpile and from manufacturers as the vaccines are being produced. Policy- makers must decide who will pay for pandemic vaccines. Currently, most influenza vaccine is purchased by the private sector. Would the same conditions obtain during a pandemic? Those issues are beyond the scope of this paper, which focuses on the development of new vaccines and the capacity to manufacture them.

2. DEVELOPING NEW VACCINES

Unlike a good deal of federally funded biomedical research, the work supported by the Department of Health and Human Services to develop new vaccines and new types of vaccine production is product-oriented. The objective of that applied work is to produce vaccines that are more effective and produced faster, more reliably, and in larger volumes than in the past. Rather than seeking to advance knowledge in the general hope that a cure or treatment might eventually emerge, HHS's efforts are directed at taking vaccines through clinical trails to approval for use.

HHS is concentrating on three specific development areas: The first involves the constraints imposed by limited capacity for production, which could be overcome by the use of adjuvants, substances that can be added to a vaccine to boost its ability to produce an immune system response. If manufacturers can develop and use adjuvanted vaccines, they should be able to produce more doses of vaccine with current domestic capacity because each dose can contain a smaller amount of antigen, or active ingredient. The second area of research involves manufacturing influenza vaccines through cell-based technology, which now is in wide use for other kinds of vaccines. The third area focuses on long-term alternatives to current vaccines and their manufacturing processes. That work aims to develop next-generation vaccines, and it includes efforts to reduce the time necessary to produce large quantities of vaccine that would be needed in the event of an influenza pandemic.

Projects supported by HHS are in various stages of development. Some projects have not entered the clinical-trial phase; others in Phase III (the final stage of clinical trials) in the

United States have been approved in Europe. HHS hopes to accelerate the typical drug approval process by funding clinical trials and testing to arrive more quickly at the licensing phase. Typically, clinical trials can last five to seven years (see Box 2-1). HHS is encouraging the development of vaccines based on H5N1 (the "bird flu" virus) and other currently circulating virus strains with pandemic potential so that manufacturers gain experience producing pandemic-like vaccines. Then, if a pandemic occurs, HHS hopes that within six months of onset, manufacturers will be in a position to deliver vaccines based on the correct virus strain.

Although this paper considers them separately, in practice it is difficult to distinguish the development of a vaccine from the development of its production facility. The regulatory process requires at least some of the vaccine used in Phase III clinical trials to be manufactured at full- scale production volumes in facilities that meet industry standards for manufacturing. The Food and Drug Administration must approve both the vaccine and the manufacturing facility.

Adjuvanted Vaccines

The pandemic-influenza vaccine that is currently licensed in the United States at best offers poor to moderate protection against the H5N1 virus, even though a course contains 12 times the amount of antigen used to combat a single seasonal-influenza virus strain (Poland 2006). HHS therefore considers the H5N1 vaccine a good candidate for research in adjuvanted vaccines, which offer the promise of requiring smaller amounts of antigen per dose and provide some hope of protection against virus strains that are different from but related to the strain used to make the vaccine.

2-1. Vaccine Development: Typical Time and Cost

On average, it takes a little over a decade for a drug to move from preclinical development to the market-place, and it is an expensive undertaking. The cost for clinical trials alone—only a portion of the process—can exceed $100 million. The analysis presented here assumes that the schedules and costs of developing pharmaceutical drugs and vaccines are similar, although industry observers often focus on pharmaceutical drugs, which are chemically synthesized, rather than on biopharmaceuticals, which are derived from living sources. (Influenza vaccines, for example, come from viruses grown in hens' eggs). The Web site of the Food and Drug Administration (FDA) explains the development process for vaccines.[1]

Development Timeline for a Vaccine

Before a vaccine enters human testing, the developer conducts laboratory (in vitro) and laboratory animal (in vivo) testing to determine whether the product will be safe enough for researchers to proceed to clinical trials. The developer must obtain the FDA's approval to begin clinical trials through the submission of an investigational new drug, or IND, application.

Clinical trials typically have three phases. Phase I focuses on the vaccine's safety and generally involves fewer than 100 human subjects. The purpose of Phase II, which typically involves several hundred subjects, is to expand Phase I safety data and identify whether and at what dose the vaccine elicits a protective immune response. Phase III typically involves thousands of people and is used to document effectiveness and develop additional safety data (notably concerning the incidence and severity of side effects) required for licensing. Clinical trials generally last five to seven years. If all three phases of the clinical development are successful, the developer may submit a biologics license application, or BLA, to the FDA for review. If the FDA approves the application, the developer launches the new vaccine, a process that includes training its sales force and increasing production capabilities to meet the anticipated demand.

Costs of Clinical Trials

Researchers at the Federal Trade Commission have analyzed the cost of clinical trials (Adams and Brantner, 2008). They report that drug trials can cost from $12 million annually at the 25th percentile to $26 million annually at the 75th percentile. That is, in 25 percent of the cases, the manufacturers spent $12 million or less; in 25 percent of the cases, they spent $26 million or more; and in 50 percent of the cases, they spent between $12 million and $26 million per year for a drug in clinical trials. The researchersalso reported average spending per drug of $38 million per year (see the table to the right).

The researchers calculated that the total cost to take a drug through clinical trials ranges from $78 million at the 25th percentile to $166 million at the 75th percentile. They also reported that average spending (of $239 million) exceeded spending at the 75th percentile, which suggests that average spending is heavily influenced by a relatively small share of drugs that are very expensive to develop. (The Congressional Budget Office converted the published estimates, which were expressed in 1999 dollars, to 2007 values using the consumer price index for all urban consumers for medical expenditures. That index was used instead of the gross domestic product deflator or the producer price index because medical costs, including the costs of clinical trials, have risen much faster than the rate of inflation.)

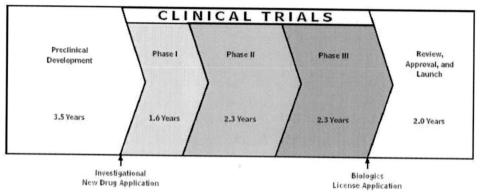

Source: Congressional Budget Office based on Adams and Brantner (2006, 2008); DiMasi and Grabowski (2007); DiMasi, Hansen, and Grabowski (2003); and Struck (1996).

The Cost of Clinical Trials for an Investigational New Drug, by Percentile

(Millions of dollars)	Percentile			Average
	25	50	75	
Annual Spending	12	21	26	38
Total Spending	78	127	166	239

Source: Congressional Budget Office based on data reported by Adams and Brantner (2008).

The cost of developing influenza vaccines is more likely to fall in the range between the 25th and 75th percentiles than it is to be comparable to average spending for drug development. Other types of clinical trials (those for some cancer drugs, for example) require expensive hospital stays for study participants or involve drugs that are expensive to manufacture. Clinical trials for influenza vaccines, by contrast, are relatively simple: In Phases I and II, subjects are given the flu shot; after a few weeks, laboratory tests determine the blood concentrations of antibodies to the virus, and subjects are assessed for side effects. In Phase III, subjects are given the injection and assessed later to determine whether they have become sick with influenza or have developed any health complications.

Clinical trials account for something between onefifth and one-third of the total costs of developing a drug. Other expenses include research and preclinical development; opportunity costs incurred by forgoing the return a developer might receive from a different investment; and the costs of drugs that do not proceed through the development and approval process. See CBO (2006b) for a review of pharmaceutical research and development costs.

[1] See "Vaccine Product Approval Process," www.fda.gov/Cber/vaccine/vacappr.htm.

Successful development of adjuvanted vaccines could affect many aspects of HHS's plan. If they are used with the older egg-based vaccines or with those produced by cell-based techniques, the success of adjuvanted vaccine could mean that a smaller stockpile could protect a larger number of people and that existing manufacturing capacity might be stretched to provide enough vaccine for a larger share of the population.

The adjuvanted vaccines currently licensed for use in the United States—against diphtheria, tetanus, hepatitis A, and hepatitis B—are made with aluminum (Vogel and Hem 2004, p. 70). But aluminum adjuvants do not reduce the amount of antigen needed by enough to substantially increase the amount of vaccine that would be available during a pandemic. Some other influenza vaccines formulated with proprietary adjuvants—mainly emulsions containing special oils in water—have shown the ability to allow significant reductions in the amount of antigen required, however, and they might be sufficient to confront the challenge of an influenza pandemic. Even though some of those influenza vaccines formulated with proprietary adjuvants have been approved in Europe, the FDA's approval is likely to require the manufacturers to supply additional data on the safety of adjuvanted vaccines. The FDA has not approved a human vaccine containing a new type of adjuvant in many years. Other types of adjuvants have thus far produced too many side effects to meet the FDA's standards, and, in at least one case in Europe, an approved adjuvanted influenza vaccine had to be withdrawn because of its association with Bell's palsy (Kenney and Edelman 2004, pp. 215–216).[7] The FDA's requirements for additional data are likely to increase the costs of development and delay approval.

HHS has awarded contracts, for a total of $133 million, to three companies (GlaxoSmithKline, Novartis Vaccines and Diagnostics, and Iomai Corporation) to support the development of H5N 1 influenza vaccines with adjuvants (see Table 2-1). The contracts support work through Phase III clinical trials in the United States aimed at obtaining U.S. licensure for the products. Each company must provide its proprietary adjuvant for government-sponsored, independent evaluation with influenza vaccines from other manufacturers.

Novartis is working on a proprietary adjuvanted H5N1 influenza vaccine that has demonstrated an acceptable immune response when administered in a course of two doses of 7.5 micrograms of antigen each, about one-twelfth the dose of the currently licensed H5N 1 vaccine. In May 2007, the European Commission approved the vaccine for use in the event that a pandemic is officially declared by the World Health Organization or the European Union (European Medicines Agency 2007b). The manufacturer will produce a formulation that contains the influenza strain causing the pandemic. Novartis also sells a seasonal-influenza vaccine that contains the same adjuvant that is in its H5N1 vaccine. That formulation is licensed for use in most of Europe in people over the age of 64. Since its approval, about 30 million doses have been distributed (Novartis 2007, p. 39).

GSK also formulated a prepandemic H5N1 influenza vaccine with its proprietary adjuvant. (The vaccine, developed from a virus strain that has the potential to cause a pandemic, is called prepandemic because it would be produced before a pandemic begins. It is intended for use before or in the early stages of a pandemic.) The adjuvanted vaccine was documented to elicit an acceptable immune response when administered in two doses of 3.8 micrograms of antigen each, a 24-fold decrease in the amount of antigen required relative to the currently licensed pandemic vaccine (GSK 2007). In May 2008, the European Commission approved the vaccine (European Medicines Agency 2008). By the end of 2008, the company plans to submit the vaccine to the FDA for U.S. approval (Whalen 2008a).

GSK also has a pandemic-influenza vaccine formulated with an aluminum adjuvant.[8] That adjuvanted vaccine, which was approved by the European Commission in March 2007, elicited an acceptable immune response when administered in two doses of 15 micrograms of antigen each, which is one-sixth the dosage of the currently licensed H5N1 vaccine (European Medicines Agency 2007a).

Iomai is developing a skin patch that contains an adjuvant for use in tandem with an injected vaccine formulation; the product is still in the early stages of clinical trials. According to the company, in a recently completed Phase I/II clinical trial, the combination vaccination elicited an acceptable immune response when administered in a single dose of 45 micrograms of antigen, a fourfold decrease in the amount of antigen required relative to the currently licensed pandemic vaccine (Iomai 2008b).[9] Iomai announced in April 2008 that it is working with HHS on a budget for a new Phase II trial (Iomai 2008a).

Sanofi Pasteur currently is funding its own early clinical trials for a vaccine formulated with its proprietary adjuvant. The company stated that, in Phase I clinical trials, the compound elicited an acceptable immune response when administered in two doses of 1.9 micrograms of antigen each (Lewcock 2007c).

Table 2-1. Egg-Based Pandemic-Influenza Vaccines, with and without Adjuvants

	HHS Obligations (Millions of dollars)	Adjuvant	Dose (Micrograms)[a]	Approval Status[b]
Sanofi Pasteur	0	None	90.0	Approved in U.S.
Iomai	14	Proprietary	45.0	Phase II
GlaxoSmithKline	0	Aluminum	15.0	Approved in EU
Novartis	55	Proprietary	7.5	Approved in EU
GlaxoSmithKline	63	Proprietary	3.8	Approved in EU
Sanofi Pasteur	0	Proprietary	1.9	Phase I
Total	**133**			

Source: Congressional Budget Office based on European Medicines Agency (2007a, b; 2008), HHS (2007a), Iomai (2008a, b), NIH (2008c), and Sanofi Pasteur (2007a, c).

Note: HHS = Department of Health and Human Services; EU = European Union.

a. All vaccines other than that produced by Iomai (which is administered as a combination of a patch and a single injection) are administered in two injected doses. A microgram is one one-millionth of a gram.

b. See Box 2-1 for a discussion of the various steps in the approval process.

HHS has budgeted more funding for the development of adjuvanted vaccines even though only about $5 million of the $133 million obligated to date has been spent. Specific amounts have not been announced, but an agency press release stated that Iomai may receive an additional $114 million in funding upon successful completion of Phase I trials (HHS 2007).

Manufacturers could decide to develop two distinct vaccines: a seasonal vaccine without adjuvants and a pandemic-influenza vaccine with adjuvants. The benefit– risk calculus, and therefore the regulatory landscape, is likely to change in the event of a pandemic. Because of the lower risk associated with seasonal influenza, those vaccines are held to high standards: They must be absolutely safe; extremely well-tolerated; and elicit few, if any, side effects. By contrast, because the risk of illness and death from whatever virus causes a pandemic is much higher, a higher risk of side effects from a vaccine could be acceptable. Adjuvanted vaccines might also be used in the United States, as in Europe, for patient groups that do not respond well to the conventional vaccines against seasonal influenza (for example, elderly people).

Cell-Based Vaccines

HHS's funding for the development of cell-based influenza vaccines is motivated by the potential drawbacks of egg-based production, particularly the need for large supplies of eggs (and the hens to produce them) and specialized manufacturing facilities. According to HHS, the domestic supply would be inadequate in the event of a pandemic, and the specialized manufacturing facilities are not easily duplicated. The egg supply also could be threatened by influenza viruses, including H5N1, that infect poultry flocks.

Cell-based vaccines use antigens from viruses grown in purified strains (or lines) of cells, for example, from the kidneys of dogs. Cell-based production technology is widely used to manufacture vaccines against polio, chicken pox, measles, mumps, and rubella. Policymakers at HHS believe that cell-based production could offer a more reliable and flexible method of producing influenza vaccines that can be scaled up to meet pandemic needs. Unlike eggs, which are perishable and must be ordered months in advance, cell lines can be kept frozen indefinitely, a benefit should it prove necessary to scale up a major manufacturing capability on short notice (HHS 2006c, p.7).

Some industry analysts believe that HHS's planning emphasis should not be on cell-based production because it does not substantially reduce production times (Matthews 2006). Rather, they believe HHS should focus on bringing next-generation vaccines to market. In addition, some of the cell lines that have the potential to produce large volumes of influenza vaccine also could cause tumors (Homeland Security Council 2006, footnote 16, p. 105).

To date, HHS has obligated $1.3 billion to promote the development of new influenza vaccines based on cell culture (see Table 2-2). The agency is contracting with several manufacturers in the hope of diversifying and expanding the supply of influenza vaccine for the United States. In the past, dependence on a few suppliers has contributed to shortages of seasonal vaccine when one or another has experienced disruptions in supply. In May 2006, HHS added to the $97 million contract signed earlier with Sanofi Pasteur when it awarded five contracts worth $1 billion in all. To reinforce the commitment, in November 2007 HHS extended its contract with DynPort Vaccine and Baxter International for another $201 million.

The manufacturers are at various points along the path toward approval for cell-based vaccines (see Table 2-2). Some have products that are still in preclinical development; others have cell-based vaccines moving through Phase III clinical trials. Novartis expects to submit an application for a U.S. license in 2008 for a seasonal- influenza vaccine, already approved in the European Union, and to make it available in Europe for the 2008– 2009 influenza season (Lewcock 2007a). DynPort Vaccine is managing a Phase III clinical trial for a cell-based seasonal-influenza vaccine and a Phase I clinical trial for a cell-based pandemic-influenza vaccine, both developed and manufactured by Baxter (Computer Sciences Corporation 2007).

Rather than using an adjuvant to cut the amount of antigen needed per dose of vaccine, Baxter's pandemic- influenza vaccine uses the whole virus. Whole-virus vaccines have been shown to be more effective than subunit vaccines that consist of just the purified proteins from the virus. However, because whole-virus vaccines also have been more prone to cause adverse reactions, all injectable seasonal-influenza vaccines licensed in the United States are subunit vaccines.

Baxter is developing another whole-virus, cell-based, pandemic-influenza vaccine that, according to the company, can be produced in three months instead of the typical six months (Ehrlich and others 2008; Wright 2008). Baxter's production process for that vaccine is faster largely because it uses a "wild-type" virus (one that circulates in nature). Other companies first modify the H5N1 virus so it can be grown in eggs without killing the embryo; that modification and the associated safety testing take about two months. The disadvantages of using the wild-type virus include increased risks of infection among production workers and of the virus's escaping the production facility. Thus, facilities for manufacturing wild-type vaccines must meet stricter safety standards than are required for seasonal-influenza-vaccine manufacturing. HHS's contracts support the development of cell-based pandemic vaccines using modified H5N 1, but not wild-type, viruses (see Table 2-2).

Table 2-2. HHS's Contract Awards and Development Status for Cell-Based Influenza Vaccines

	Obligations (Millions of dollars)	Vaccine	
		Seasonal	Pandemic
DynPort Vaccine and Baxter[a]	242	Phase III	Phase I
GlaxoSmithKline	275	Preclinical Development	Preclinical Development
MedImmune	169	Phase I	Preclinical Development
Novartis Vaccines and Diagnostics	221	Phase III	Preclinical Development
Sanofi Pasteur	97	Phase II	Phase I
Solvay Pharmaceuticals	299	Phase I	Phase I
Total	**1,302**		

Source: Congressional Budget Office based on Computer Sciences Corporation (2007), HHS (2005a, 2006b), NIH (2008b), Novartis (2007, p. 35), Program for Appropriate Technology in Health (2007, p. 13), Sanofi Pasteur (2007b), and WHO (2007c).

Notes: HHS = Department of Health and Human Services.

See Box 2-1 for a discussion of the various steps in the development and approval process.

a. DynPort Vaccine is the prime contractor; it manages the clinical trials. Baxter is developing the candidate vaccines; it will manufacture the vaccines and own all clinical data and licenses.

In general, the vaccines for which HHS is providing support are somewhere between Phase I and Phase II clinical trials (see Table 2-2). Phase II and Phase III studies take a little over two years each (see Box 2-1 on page 10); submitting the product for the FDA's review and launching it in the marketplace can add another year or two.[10] So it is likely to be another six years before most of the companies that were awarded contracts from HHS can complete development of their cell-based influenza vaccines and bring them to market.

Results of a study by researchers at the Federal Trade Commission suggest that manufacturers' expenditures for a single drug in clinical trials typically range between $12 million and $26 million per year, although clinical trials for some drugs can cost much more (see Box 2-1). Those estimates do not include the cost of failures or return on private investment. On that basis, for each successful vaccine, the additional costs incurred in the remaining four years for Phase II and Phase III clinical trials would add between $48 million and $104 million to what is already spent, with a median value of $84 million. On the basis of that calculation, the estimated remaining cost to develop 12 vaccines—one seasonal and one pandemic version of a cell-based vaccine for each of the six companies—is likely to range between $600 million and $1.2 billion.

The $1.3 billion obligated to date could be sufficient to ensure the development of cell-based vaccines. As of January 2008, the contracting companies had requested that HHS reimburse them for $160 million (roughly 12 percent of the total contracts). The contracts' balance of $1.1 billion would cover the remaining costs of clinical trials, as long as those costs do not approach or exceed the high end of the estimated range.

Next-Generation Vaccines

The six months that it takes to produce egg-based or most cell-based vaccines could be too long to respond to an influenza pandemic: Past outbreaks have reached the United States within two to five months of emerging in Asia, and some experts believe that the increase in international travel could facilitate an even faster transmission from abroad. After the egg-based and cell-based techniques, the next generation of vaccine manufacturing, based on the use of recombinant-DNA technology, offers the prospect of increased efficacy, shorter production times, and perhaps broader protection against some or all influenza strains for years or even a lifetime (see Box 2-2), although the vaccines could be 10 years or more away from the market. HHS has yet to fund their development for use against influenza, in part because it has chosen to build on the decades of experience in using cell culture to produce other vaccines.

However, HHS plans to award contracts worth $155 million for the development of next-generation vaccines (Robinson 2007). Even without contracts from HHS, several companies have been working on next-generation vaccines, sometimes with help from agencies within HHS, including the National Institutes of Health (NIH) and the Centers for Disease Control and Prevention (CDC). One article in a medical journal in 2007 enumerated 29 next-generation influenza vaccines in development, concluding that the "pipeline for new influenza vaccines is robust" (Belshe 2007, pp. 746, 748). With one exception, however, next-generation vaccines have not advanced past early-stage clinical trials.

The funding of the development of cell-based vaccines and the expansion of egg-based capacity (discussed in Chapter 3) could solidify the hold of those technologies on the market for seasonal-influenza vaccine. Once plants open, it will be difficult for new entrants to compete, unless their costs are markedly below those of existing producers. Increases in capacity could saturate the market and drive down the price of seasonal vaccine, making the market less attractive to newcomers. New technology alone will not be sufficient to increase market share. The newer live influenza virus vaccine, for example, has not captured a significant portion of the market, even though it offers greater cross-protection against different virus strains. It also is administered as a nasal spray, rather than by injection, which can be a benefit to people who find shots unpleasant or painful.

2-2. WHAT CONSTITUTES THE NEXT GENERATION OF INFLUENZA VACCINES?

Vaccine manufacturers hope to make extensive use of recombinant DNA techniques to produce large amounts of vaccine more quickly than is possible with egg-based or cell-based production. Universal vaccines that protect against a range of strains—or perhaps all strains—could protect the population in advance of an influenza pandemic.

Recombinant Vaccines

Recombinant vaccines are made by splicing antigen-producing genes into the DNA of another organism. The modified organisms then reproduce to provide bulk quantities of antigen (the active ingredient in the vaccine). Recombinant techniques are already in use to make vaccines against hepatitis B and human papillomavirus (CDC 2006, FDA 2006). The hepatitis B vaccine is made by splicing the genes that produce the antigen into plasmids—viruslike DNA molecules—inserting the modified plasmids into yeast cells, and then growing the recombinant yeast cells to produce more antigen. One manufacturer has a recombinant seasonal-influenza vaccine in Phase III clinical trials (NIH 2008a). However, most recombinant influenza vaccines have not yet advanced past early-stage clinical trials.

Universal Vaccines

Even though many vaccines last years or a lifetime, people now must be vaccinated every year to maintain immunity against seasonal influenza. Current influenza vaccines target hemagglutinin, a protein on the surface of the virus, and the vaccines "train" the immune system to react to that protein. Because the hemagglutinin protein changes rapidly as influenza viruses mutate, however, the pattern the immune system tries to recognize is not the same from year to year. Scientists are investigating vaccines that target other proteins that do not change so rapidly and that are present in all strains of influenza. At least one company has reported promising results in Phase I clinical trials (Gray 2008).

To be sure, next-generation vaccines could replace egg- or cell-based formulations if they proved substantially better than current formulations. In some years, the seasonal vaccine does not confer good protection against seasonal influenza because the strains in the vaccine are different from the strains that happen to be circulating that year. The mismatch is the result of the long production timeline, which requires manufacturers and public health officials to choose the strains far in advance of the season. Some next-generation vaccines in development hold the promise of much-shortened production timelines, allowing for the decision about which strains to include in a given year's vaccine to be made much closer to the flu season so as to reduce the probability of strain mismatches.

Even more desirable would be a vaccine that protects against all influenza strains. The hope is that someday it will be possible to be vaccinated just once for a lifetime of immunity against all strains of influenza.

If, in the end, the private sector does not find that next- generation vaccines are an attractive investment, then the federal government probably would need to supply well more than $155 million to bring the new formulations to market. The discussion of development costs in Box 2-1 illustrates the point: Getting one next-generation vaccine through clinical trials could cost well over $100 million, exclusive of the costs of capital or of the costs associated with the failure of a given vaccine to advance to the regulatory finish line of FDA approval. Because the principal characteristics of next-generation vaccines are still largely unknown, it is likely that there will be many failures, which will in turn drive up the costs of bringing those products to market. Moreover, because most next-generation vaccines are still in the earlier stages of development, additional research will be necessary before clinical trials can begin.

International Efforts at Funding the Development of Vaccines

The European Commission funds research on the development of influenza vaccines under its Sixth Framework Programme, which supports a multinational consortium of vaccine specialists who are trying to develop an H5N1 vaccine (Cordis 2007; European Commission 2007). The program announced a grant of $5.5 million.[11] The schedule for the four-year effort calls for clinical trials to begin within two years. The effort is part of a longer program that has spent $102 million on all aspects of influenza research, not just vaccines, since 2001. Of that amount, $55 million has gone to research on vaccines, including some veterinary vaccines. Although CBO has not been able to ascertain the specific funding by individual countries' ministries of health, a BBC News (2006) report stated that Germany is spending $313 million on vaccine development.

3. INVESTING IN NEW CAPACITY FOR PRODUCTION

Current manufacturing capacity for the only licensed pandemic-influenza vaccine in the United States is about 25 million doses, or enough vaccine to protect about 12.5 million people (see Table 1-4 on page 6). The goal the Department of Health and Human Services set for vaccine production in an influenza pandemic is 24 times the amount available in the United States— manufacturers would have to produce enough vaccine for each of the nation's 300 million people. (In an influenza pandemic, a course of immunization would consist of two doses for each person). Policymakers at HHS do not believe the goal can be achieved solely by expanding capacity for egg-based production. However, because it is the dominant technology, the agency has awarded contracts to domestic manufacturers of egg-based influenza vaccines to substantially expand capacity (see Table 3-1).

Another goal is to shift the production of influenza vaccine from egg-based to cell-based technology. Manufacturers of cell-based vaccines developed under the advanced-development contracts will be eligible for additional funding from HHS to build new facilities. Cell- based technology does not work substantially faster than egg-based methods, however, and shortened production time is another goal of HHS's plan. In the ideal case, HHS calls for the new egg- or cell-based capacity that is being funded today to be retired when next-generation vaccines are ready to come to the market or, in the case of capacity for cell-based production, put to some other use. It is expected that the new vaccines will be produced more quickly than are current formulations and that they will provide broader protection against many or even all strains of influenza viruses.

The process of putting manufacturing capacity into place is more difficult for vaccines than it is for most other drugs. During the final phases of clinical development, the manufacturer must seek approval of the proposed manufacturing facility from the Food and Drug Administration. The vaccine maker also must expand the capacity of its production processes from that used for quantities required in clinical trials to that appropriate for commercial production. The FDA's approval process includes facility inspections and it requires the company to demonstrate that its product elicits immune responses that are consistent from batch to batch. That requirement for dual certification limits manufacturers' flexibility in altering either the process or the facility to boost production. HHS hopes to provide manufacturers with incentives to begin now to assemble new facilities in advance of an influenza pandemic. Then, if a pandemic occurs, the new vaccines can be produced within six months of the onset.

Egg-Based Manufacturing Capacity

HHS has taken several actions to increase domestic capacity for egg-based manufacturing of influenza vaccine. In 2004, the agency signed a $43 million contract with Sanofi Pasteur to ensure a year-round supply of eggs for that company's domestic manufacturing facility, to stockpile other vaccine-manufacturing supplies, and to supply pandemic-influenza vaccine for clinical trials. A year-round supply of eggs makes it possible for Sanofi Pasteur to produce pandemic vaccine even if a pandemic occurs outside of the company's annual production cycle. Because that contract expires in 2008, HHS has requested $42 million for 2009 to maintain a year-round egg supply for the next five years.

In 2007, HHS signed contracts totaling $133 million with two companies (about $77 million to Sanofi Pasteur and $55 million to MedImmune) to retrofit their domestic vaccine-manufacturing facilities. The facility upgrades will allow Sanofi Pasteur to produce prepandemic vaccine for the stockpile year-round. Currently, Sanofi Pasteur produces prepandemic vaccine for the stockpile only during the three months of the year that it is not producing seasonal vaccine. MedImmune does not produce pre- pandemic vaccine for the stockpile. Its live, attenuated vaccine (made with a weakened form of the virus) against H5N1 has not been successful in early clinical trials (WHO 2008). Furthermore, there is fear that stockpiling prepandemic vaccine made with a live, attenuated virus could increase the chances of a pandemic's occurring by providing the opportunity for a virus with pandemic potential to mix with a seasonal strain, creating a deadly transmissible virus (McKenna 2007a).

Sanofi Pasteur is working to triple its production capacity by 2011. The company is set to pay $25 million of the $102 million cost of retrofitting an existing facility, and it has added a second facility, at a cost of $150 million, to its complex in Swiftwater, Pennsylvania (*Vaccine Weekly* 2007). When both facilities are approved by the FDA— which is expected by 2011— the company's annual production capacity for seasonal-influenza vaccine will approximately triple, from 50 million to 150 million doses of 45 micrograms each. That expected capacity could allow the manufacturer to produce 75 million doses of its licensed pandemic-influenza vaccine, or enough vaccine for about 38 million people (at 90 micrograms per dose for a two-dose course). If the company's experimental adjuvanted vaccine proves safe and effective, then its capacity would increase because the amount of antigen (the active ingredient in a vaccine) it had to produce would drop. For example, its expected capacity would be 450 million doses of an adjuvanted pandemic vaccine (at 15 micrograms of antigen per dose), enough to inoculate 225 million people, but even larger capacity increases are also possible. However, additional manufacturing facilities would still have to be built to produce the adjuvants.

By 2011, MedImmune is expected to have emergency capacity to produce 50 million doses of pandemic vaccine.[12] MedImmune's manufacturing facility in the United Kingdom produces bulk seasonal-influenza vaccine for the U.S. market, but it prepares the seasonal seed strain at its facility in California. MedImmune will use its award to retrofit its California facility to produce bulk quantities of pandemic-influenza vaccine in case of an emergency. The company will contribute $14 million to the project.

The contract also included options in later years that would keep the new capacity in reserve and ready to produce in the event of a pandemic by manufacturing at least one commercial-scale lot of vaccine each year to maintain licensure. The size of a lot depends on the facility, but typically it would be hundreds of thousands of doses. The cost of production in the contract is about $15 million per year for a capacity of 50 million doses of pandemic-influenza vaccine.

Cell-Based Manufacturing Capacity

Each of the six companies that won advanced development contracts for cell-based vaccines was required to commit to establishing a U.S.-based cell-manufacturing facility with a production capacity of at least 150 million doses of pandemic-influenza vaccine within the first six months after the onset of a pandemic, although the awards do not cover the cost of building new manufacturing facilities.

HHS does not expect that each of the six contracts will lead to additional capacity that can produce 150 million doses of pandemic-influenza vaccine. Instead, it forecasts the possibility of a total of 475 million doses from the additional domestic capacity, and it plans to award additional contracts totaling $600 million to the most successful companies. That funding will defray the costs of building new facilities for cell-based manufacturing.

Because the expanded capacity would not be needed to meet the demand for seasonal vaccine, some government funding would probably be required to induce producers to build more factories. The contracts for retrofitting the egg-based production facilities involve cost sharing between the government and the two companies, each of which would provide at least 25 percent of the total cost. HHS has said that the contracts for cell-based vaccine facilities will require manufacturers to provide a higher percentage.

Initial Costs

Production facilities for cell-based influenza vaccine are newly under construction, so estimates of the cost to build and obtain the FDA's approval should be considered preliminary. According to the company, the Novartis plant in North Carolina will cost more than $600 million and will have a production capacity of 50 million doses of seasonal vaccine (Lewcock 2007b; Whalen 2006). That estimate includes the cost of bringing the plant online and the cost of seeking the FDA's approval for the facility, which can take two years. Other industry sources have estimated a cost of about $320 million—bringing the plant online and obtaining the FDA's approval would add to that total—to build a plant with an annual capacity of 50 million doses of cell-based seasonal vaccine. On the basis of discussions with industry experts, CBO anticipates that bringing the plant online and submitting to the FDA's approval process would add 25 percent to the capital cost of that plant, making the total cost about $400 million.

Table 3-1. HHS's Funding for Capacity to Produce Influenza Vaccine

	Obligations (Millions of dollars)	Duration
Provide Year-Round Egg Supply	43	2004–2008
Retrofit Existing Egg-Based Manufacturing Facilities	133	2007–2012
Build New Cell-Based Manufacturing Facilities	TBD	TBD
Total	176	

Source: Congressional Budget Office based on Robinson (2008).

Notes: HHS = Department of Health and Human Services,

TBD = to be determined. HHS has not yet awarded contracts to build new facilities for manufacturing cell-based vaccines. HHS has stated that it will award $600 million for that purpose.

Most vaccine producers are developing adjuvants, substances that can be added to vaccine formulations to reduce the amount of antigen needed per dose. (The first calculations that follow assume that the use of adjuvants will cut the amount of antigen needed from 90 micrograms to 15 micrograms per dose for the pandemic- influenza vaccine.[13]) That amount, which equals the amount of antigen for each strain of seasonal-influenza vaccine, is easily being bested in published clinical trials (see Table 2-1 on page 12). To the extent that producers achieved a larger antigen savings than assumed, the costs described here would overstate the cost of the program.

A plant with a capacity of 50 million seasonal-influenza doses (45 micrograms per dose) could produce 150 million pandemic-influenza doses at 15 micrograms per dose. It would take about three plants with that capacity to produce 475 million doses. If the cost of construction, bringing the plant online, and obtaining the FDA's approval averaged $400 million per plant, the total cost of the expanded capacity would be $1.2 billion. If each plant cost $600 million, the total would be $1.8 billion.

HHS's goal of diversifying the sources of the U.S. influenza vaccine supply would be met if, in addition to the existing domestic plants that produce egg-based vaccines, three plants were built for cell-based manufacturing. The nation's reliance on a small number of manufacturers has resulted in several recent disruptions in supply. If adjuvants fulfill the promise of sharply cutting the amount of antigen needed for pandemic-influenza vaccines, policy- makers might face a choice between reducing the cost of the program and ensuring a diversity of supply.

If no adjuvanted vaccine proves safe and effective, then the initial costs of construction would rise substantially. It would take 19 plants, rather than 3, to produce 475 million doses (at 90 micrograms of antigen per dose). The initial costs of construction would rise proportionately, to between $7.6 billion and $11.4 billion.

In either case, it is unlikely that enough capacity could be available in time to meet the target date of 2011. Only Novartis has begun construction of a domestic facility for making cell-based vaccine. The company anticipates its plant will be in operation by 2012 and will have an annual production capacity of 50 million doses of seasonal vaccine (Pink Sheet 2007). MedImmune has announced its intention to convert an existing plant in Frederick, Maryland, that currently manufactures monoclonal antibodies into a manufacturing facility for seasonal-influenza vaccine that would serve domestic and international markets with an expected capacity of 50 million to 60 million doses of cell-based seasonal vaccine. The influenza vaccine operations are unlikely to begin before 2012–2013. GlaxoSmithKline has purchased a vaccine-manufacturing facility in Pennsylvania that it plans to modernize to develop and produce cell-based seasonal- and pandemic-influenza vaccines (Megget 2007). Sanofi Pasteur, Baxter, and Solvay have not announced plans to manufacture cell-based vaccine in the United States.

Continuing Costs

If U.S. demand for seasonal-influenza vaccine grows by 4 percent per year (continuing the trend observed from 1999 to 2006; see Figure 1-2 on page 4), demand will reach nearly 130 million doses of vaccine by 2011. By itself, Sanofi Pasteur's projected capacity for egg-based vaccine, at 150 million seasonal doses by 2011, would exceed projected U.S. demand. So if all the new capacity for manufacturing egg-based and cell-based vaccines were built as called for by HHS, there would be excess capacity to serve the domestic demand for seasonal vaccine.

Cell-based technology might have technical advantages over egg-based production, but its economic advantages are less clear; the resulting vaccines could be more expensive for the near term (Lash and Wang 2006). Plants that manufacture cell-based vaccines will have alternative uses; plants that make egg-based formulations do not. Consequently, unless they have some federal incentives to remain, the excess capacity in the seasonal-influenza vaccine market could drive manufacturers of cell-based vaccine from the market first. If the costs for cell-based production facilities to remain in reserve are similar to those for producers of egg-based vaccines—$15 million annually per 50 million doses—then the capacity to produce 475 million cell-based doses of pandemic-influenza vaccine would cost about $140 million per year to remain operational at 15 micrograms per dose. If no company developed adjuvanted vaccines, the continuing costs would be about $850 million at 90 micrograms per dose.

Purchases of vaccine for the stockpile could go a long way toward supporting the reserve capacity. It could cost between $350 million and $1.1 billion annually to purchase replacement vaccine for the stockpile as the contents expired (as described in Chapter 4). The new manufacturing capacity also could be supported through exports of seasonal vaccine and through increased domestic demand for seasonal vaccine.

Some experts have suggested that the additional cell-based production facilities could be used to manufacture other products during years when there is not an influenza pandemic. Then, if a pandemic did occur, a plant could switch to manufacturing vaccine against the pandemic-influenza strain. The caveat about dual-use facilities involves safety. Manufacturing facilities would have to be cleaned to prevent cross-contamination and then subjected to a new FDA approval process, which could easily take months. If HHS's objective of a maximum delay of six months from the identification of a pandemic to the inoculation of the public is to be met, the recertification process could prove impractical. It also might not be cost-effective to build dual-use facilities that required specialized equipment and processes for the manufacture of different products.

International Efforts to Build Capacity

An alternative way to encourage private-sector construction of capacity is for governments to sign advance supply agreements with producers. The Department of Health in the United Kingdom has agreements with several suppliers to deliver 150 million doses of vaccine as soon as possible in the event a pandemic is identified (Donaldson 2006). The French government has an agreement with Sanofi Pasteur to deliver 28 million doses of vaccine in the event of a pandemic, and Italy has signed agreements for 36 million doses of vaccine (BBC News 2006; Sanofi Pasteur 2006). Several other countries also have signed such agreements. Although the terms have not been revealed, the Canadian government has signed an agreement with GSK, which has a plant producing influenza vaccine in Quebec. There is no public information about whether the companies have the capacity to produce the vaccines promised in the advance supply agreements.

The European and U.S. strategies for developing and maintaining capacity entail costs and risks. Under the European approach, the manufacturers might not have the capacity to fulfill the advance supply agreements in the event of a pandemic. And despite the U.S. subsidies for vaccine development and capacity building, in the event of a pandemic, the United States would not have a committed supply and would have to spend additional money to buy vaccine. Moreover, the manufacturers could exhaust their supplies in the act of meeting their obligations under the European advance supply agreements and have nothing left to distribute in the United States.

The World Health Organization has made several small grants to help build vaccine-manufacturing capacity in very poor countries (P. Taylor 2007). The funding is limited ($2 million to Thailand, for example) and is not likely to be adequate to support new production facilities. Total funding for such construction in all countries is $18 million, $11 million of which is provided by HHS.

Private companies also are increasing their investments in other countries in response to the growing demand for seasonal-influenza vaccines. Microbix, a Canadian company, has just signed a contract to build a $200 million manufacturing facility in China (N. Taylor 2008a). The project will be jointly financed by the company and the government of China, which has indicated an interest in increasing its seasonal vaccination rate from the current 2 percent to 20 percent of its population. Sanofi also recently completed building a manufacturing plant in China (Whalen 2008b), and press reports indicate that the other major companies hope to garner a share of that market. More generally, Sanofi is expanding its worldwide capacity and has launched a multiyear, multi-billion-dollar construction effort to create vaccine-manufacturing capacity against a variety of diseases, including influenza (N. Taylor 2008b).

4. STOCKPILING VACCINE

One goal of the Department of Health and Human Services' plan for an influenza pandemic is to stockpile—as soon as possible and within the constraints of industrial capacity—enough vaccine to immunize 20 million people against the strains that present a pandemic threat (HHS 2005b, p. 24). It is far-fetched to think that a prepandemic vaccine—so called because it is produced before the onset of a pandemic—would be a perfect match for the virus causing the pandemic, but policymakers and public health officials hope that it would offer at least some protection to people who are essential to maintaining security; to health care providers; to those who provide essential products and services; and to infants, young children, and pregnant women before a vaccine specific to the pandemic can be produced.[14]

Since 2004, HHS has obligated more than $950 million to procure roughly 26 million doses of prepandemic-influenza vaccine (90 micrograms of antigen per dose) for the stockpile (see Table 4-1). The stockpile is intended to meet changing threats to public health; as new influenza strains are identified as having the potential to cause a pandemic, they will be added to the stockpile. So far, HHS has stockpiled vaccines against two variants of the H5N1 virus, the "bird flu." The first variant, called clade 1, consists of the virus that is circulating in Cambodia, Thailand, and Vietnam. The second, clade 2, consists of the virus circulating in China and Indonesia (WHO [no date]). (A clade is a group of viruses descended from a single ancestor.) Although HHS currently is treating the stockpile as one entity, the cost of stockpiling vaccine would rise if it was determined that each strain required a separate stockpile with enough vaccine to immunize 20 million people.

At two doses per course (the recommendation for pandemic-influenza vaccine), the stockpile would hold enough to inoculate about 13 million people. Because there already are standards for how long seasonal- influenza vaccines can be stored, HHS has begun studies to determine how long the stockpiled prepandemic vaccines can be counted on to be safe and effective. Currently, HHS assumes a two-year shelf life, which is consistent with industry data for the shelf life of seasonal- influenza vaccine. About 15 million of the 26 million doses in the stockpile have already expired or are now reaching expiration, so the approximately 11 million doses left in the stockpile would be enough to inoculate only about 5.6 million people.

Production of vaccine for the stockpile currently is limited to the three months of the year when the manufacturers are not making seasonal-influenza vaccine. However, HHS has signed a contract with Sanofi Pasteur to retrofit its domestic vaccine-manufacturing facility so it can produce prepandemic-influenza vaccine year-round for the stockpile.

Cost to Complete and Maintain the Stockpile

Several factors drive the cost of completing and maintaining the stockpile: the ability of adjuvants to reduce the amount of antigen needed in a dose of vaccine, the shelf life of stockpiled antigen and adjuvants, and the number of virus strains against which stockpiles must be established.

Stockpiling Adjuvanted Vaccines

Most of the vaccine in the stockpile is being stored in bulk at company sites. From there, it must be put into its final formulation and packaged for shipping to doctors' offices and clinics. Part of HHS's plan for a response to an influenza pandemic includes the use of any available adjuvants; the agency wants to be able to consider adjuvanted vaccines as it determines optimal dosage.

Table 4-1. U.S. Stockpile of H5N1 Vaccine, by Year of Purchase

(Millions of doses)					
	2004	2005	2006	2007	Total
Clade 1	0.5	7.1	0.9	0	8.4
Clade 2	0	0	6.4	11.2	17.6
Total	**0.5**	**7.1**	**7.4**	**11.2**	**26.0**

Source: Congressional Budget Office based on Robinson (2008).
Note: H5N1 is the virus that causes the "bird flu." A clade is a group of viruses descended from a single ancestor. One dose contains 90 micrograms of antigen. (A microgram is one one-millionth of a gram; antigen is the vaccine's acitve ingredient). Influenza vaccine typically expires after two years; 15 million doses have expired or will expire soon.

If the use of adjuvants substantially reduced the need for antigen, the current stockpile could surpass HHS's goal of providing enough for 20 million people. If adjuvants made it possible for a dose to consist of 15 micrograms of active ingredient—which would match the amount for each strain of seasonal-influenza vaccine—rather than the 90 micrograms called for with the pandemic-influenza formulation, then the 11 million doses remaining in the stockpile could be stretched to 66 million, or enough to inoculate about 33 million people. In that event, the stockpile would not need to be made larger, although adjuvant would have to be produced and purchased.

Like the vaccines they augment, adjuvants have a limited shelf life—HHS assumes that adjuvants will expire after three years. On the basis of information from the agency, CBO estimates that it would cost $350 million per year to replace expiring antigen and adjuvants with enough new material to maintain a stockpile for 20 million people through 2020, assuming 15 micrograms of antigen per dose. However, the costs would be less if HHS determined that the stockpiled antigen had a longer shelf life: If it lasted three years instead of two, the cost of annual maintenance would drop to about $300 million.

Because adjuvants are not stand-alone drugs, approval by the Food and Drug Administration for adjuvanted versions of the vaccines already in the stockpile would be contingent on completion of additional clinical trials (some are in the planning stages). If the stockpiled vaccines and the adjuvants were made by different companies, however, additional hurdles could arise concerning intellectual property rights (McKenna 2007b). However, if an influenza pandemic were to occur, the FDA could permit the use of unlicensed adjuvanted vaccines even if they had not completed the full cycle of clinical trials. Unlicensed vaccines could be administered under an emergency use authorization or under FDA's Investigational New Drug provisions (Lister 2007, p. 30).

Stockpiling Vaccines without Adjuvants

If there is no success in using adjuvants to substantially cut the amount of antigen required, then about 29 million doses of vaccine will be needed to complete the stockpile. Information from HHS indicates that the cost would be about $1.1 billion. However, if HHS found that the stockpiled antigen had a shelf life longer than two years, that cost would be reduced. For example, if antigen could be kept in the stockpile for three years, the cost of completing the stockpile would fall to about $790 million. After completion, it would cost about $1.1 billion annually to replace expired antigen and to maintain a stockpile for 20 million people through 2020.

Additional Considerations

The vaccine in the stockpile is a combination of vaccines made from different strains of the H5N 1 virus. Vaccine made from one strain might not provide protection against viruses from different strains. If HHS maintained a stockpile of vaccine for 20 million people for each circulating strain then the cost of the stockpiles would rise. For example, it would cost about $2.2 billion annually for HHS to maintain a complete stockpile for two circulating strains without adjuvants and about $700 million annually with adjuvants.

The results of recent studies show that adjuvants can increase the ability of influenza vaccines to protect against viruses from different but related virus strains that are not contained in the vaccine (WHO 2008). Thus, if adjuvants can be used with the stockpile, the number of virus strains against which stockpiles must be built can be reduced (WHO 2007b).

The annual cost of maintaining the stockpile would be greater than the cost of funding reserve capacity. Instead of paying $160 million to $870 million per year in subsidies to keep the additional capacity for egg-based or cell-based production ready, most of that excess capacity could be used to produce vaccine for the stockpile, at an additional annual cost of $350 million to $1.1 billion.[15] However, not all of the reserve capacity would be suitable for making vaccine for the stockpile (see Chapter 3).

International Efforts to Stockpile Vaccine

The World Health Organization has proposed a global stockpiling plan that would focus on developing nations, mostly those without domestic manufacturing capacity or sufficient resources, to purchase vaccines from abroad (Lewcock 2007d). Several manufacturers (Baxter, GlaxoSmithKline, and Sanofi Pasteur) have pledged to donate or sell at a discount millions of doses of pre- pandemic vaccine over the next several years. As with the domestic stockpile, the success with adjuvants will determine the number of people who can be immunized. In addition, like policymakers in the United States, WHO will have to decide what to do about stored, but expired, vaccines.

Individual countries are procuring stockpiles, although many more are planning to rely on advance supply agreements (Mounier-Jack, Jas, and Coker 2007, p. 925). The United Kingdom's Department of Health (2008) has announced that it is stockpiling 3 million doses; France and Italy have announced plans for stockpiling 2 million doses each (Mackenzie 2005). In all, those supplies would contain enough vaccine to inoculate about 2 percent of the populations of those countries. By contrast, Ireland has announced its intention of creating a stockpile of 8.5 million doses, and Austria has signed a contract for 16 million doses; enough in each case to inoculate the entire population of the country (Raymond 2006). The amount in the stockpiles, relative to the size of the population, varies greatly from one nation to another, and different countries could be purchasing vaccine with different amounts of antigen per dose.

5. OPTIONS FOR MODIFYING HHS'S PLAN

The vaccine component of the plan developed by the Department of Health and Human Services in 2005 would provide some amount of immediate insurance against an influenza pandemic, more protection when vaccines produced with cell culture technology are approved and facilities are built, and at some point in the indefinite future a much-reduced risk if next-generation vaccines are successful. This analysis by the Congressional Budget Office indicates that additional spending will be necessary for the indefinite future and that it is unlikely that the objective of providing enough vaccine to immunize 300 million people will be met by 2011. The environment in which the original plans were made has changed in at least one important regard: Policymakers have more information today than they did in 2005 when the plan was formulated. In particular, the likelihood has increased that adjuvants could be used to reduce the amount of antigen needed to provide immunity. That information raises several questions about whether the course of current policy is the most cost-effective and whether it should be altered:

- Does progress in developing adjuvanted vaccines suggest that the current plan supports too much expansion of production capacity?
- In light of the prospects for adjuvanted vaccines, would providing more support for early and advanced development for next-generation vaccines ultimately provide more protection against an influenza pandemic?
- Should the United States consider adopting a strategy similar to that of several governments in the European Union? (Instead of giving direct government support to new production facilities, some European governments have entered into advance supply agreements to purchase vaccine in the event of an influenza pandemic.)
- Does the prospect of successfully developing an adjuvanted vaccine change the optimal size of the stockpile of prepandemic vaccines?

Adjuvanted Vaccines and Adequate Capacity

One option HHS might consider if adjuvanted vaccines fulfill their promise is to reduce targets for domestic cell- based manufacturing capacity. Such a reduction could initially save $600 million that HHS has budgeted for the construction of the facilities, and it could reduce the spending that will be necessary to keep manufacturers in a state of readiness.[16]

European regulatory authorities have approved adjuvanted vaccines against seasonal and pandemic influenzas. Drug companies are reporting encouraging results for other adjuvanted influenza vaccines in clinical trials in Europe and the United States. The arithmetic of pandemic vaccination changes dramatically, as discussed in Chapter 2, if adjuvanted vaccines are developed and approved. An extrapolation of the results from clinical trials leads to the preliminary conclusion that, by 2011, domestic egg-based manufacturing could produce enough antigen within six months of the onset of a pandemic to immunize 225 million people with adjuvanted vaccines at 15 micrograms per dose. Data from the most successful clinical trials for adjuvanted vaccines show that the projected U.S. capacity would make it possible to produce enough antigen within six months of the onset of a pandemic to immunize the U.S.

population several times over. However, if adjuvanted vaccines were not used, the projected capacity could produce enough antigen only to inoculate about 38 million people (see Table 2-1 on page 12).

In light of that wide range of estimates of the possible domestic volume of production for egg-based vaccines, it might be prudent for the federal government to slow its support for additional capacity and focus more effort on developing adjuvants. If adjuvant development is successful, the capacity for egg- or cell-based production that is currently available or under construction would be enough to meet HHS's goal of vaccinating every U.S. resident within six months of the onset of a pandemic. If development is not successful, however, the current plan for $600 million in subsidies would be just a fraction of the $7.6 billion to $11.4 billion needed to build enough cell-based production capacity to meet HHS's goal.

Current and announced capacity already exceeds what could be supported by demand for seasonal vaccine. Creating additional (possibly unneeded) capacity could compound the risk that the industry would expand too much and then would need to contract, with the result that some companies would exit the market, as has occurred in the past.

Such a change in policy would come with risks, however. The decision not to support the building of new plants for cell-based production would leave the domestic supply still concentrated in a few facilities that are producing egg-based vaccine. Contamination of just one facility or of associated poultry flocks during an influenza pandemic could grievously hamper the federal response and leave the U.S. population at risk. Although manufacturers adhere to strict practices to ensure that their flocks are protected from disease, the risk remains. Adjuvants would lessen that risk, however, because their use would mean there is less capacity and fewer flocks to protect.

Creating additional capacity to produce cell-based vaccines would improve the government's ability to immunize people who cannot be vaccinated with adjuvanted vaccines. If even a fraction of people required the unadjuvanted vaccine, the supply of antigen could be quickly exhausted. Policymakers could conclude that the side effects from adjuvants, which to date have been minor, are outweighed by the need to immunize a majority of the population. But such a decision would be likely to reduce compliance.

HHS could be optimistic in its goals for manufacturing capacity for cell-based vaccine, in any event. The manufacturers have had incentives to develop adjuvanted prepandemic vaccines in order to win premium-priced contracts from governments around the world for vaccine stockpiling. Absent a market in which to sell the additional seasonal cell-based vaccine, large federal subsidies are likely to be needed to support construction of such facilities, an eventuality that might require additional appropriations.

Next-Generation Vaccines

Next-generation vaccines are needed to reduce the production time required to manufacture the current set of vaccines. Development of adjuvanted vaccines also could have implications for the resources devoted to next- generation vaccines and for the mechanisms the government chooses to accomplish its objectives. Specifically, if adjuvanted vaccines reduce the near-term risk posed by an influenza pandemic by stretching the available and the planned capacity, then resources might be available to support more development of next-generation vaccines. Moreover, there might be enough time to work through markets to use guaranteed purchases or other mechanisms to promote the development of next-generation vaccines, where manufacturers with successful products would be ensured sales into the stockpile.

However, policymakers cannot count on easy and rapid success with next-generation vaccines. Those formulations are, in many cases, based on truly novel concepts and are largely in the early stages of development. It is likely that there will be many failures, which will prolong the process and increase the costs of bringing those products to market.

Advance Supply Agreements

European governments have chosen to enter into advance supply agreements with companies to provide vaccine in the event of a pandemic. The U.S. approach differs: Policymakers here have chosen to provide direct support to manufacturers for the development of vaccines and the construction of new production facilities. The U.S. government could consider entering into advance supply agreements, which are seen in Europe as economically attractive because each side can concentrate on what it does best: Governments track public health needs, and businesses develop vaccines and manufacturing facilities.

Also, with the advance supply agreements, the governments actually purchase some specified amount of vaccine for their populations. The U.S. government, in contrast, would not have a committed supply of vaccine and would need to spend additional funds to acquire vaccine for an influenza pandemic. Companies may have to fulfill the European advance supply agreements first before selling vaccine to the United States, possibly exhausting their supplies. It might be necessary for the United States to structure agreements to recognize that other nations' governments could temporarily restrict or prohibit exports of pandemic-influenza vaccine until their own populations have been immunized. Even if the United States enters into advance supply agreements, there remains the risk that manufacturers will not have the capacity to fulfill those agreements.

Some analysts question the ability of advance supply agreements to stimulate the development of technology, especially given the lengthy process of ushering vaccines through approval. The European governments, they argue, are beneficiaries of U.S. efforts in technology development. Other analysts point to Sanofi Pasteur's independent development of an as-yet-unapproved adjuvant as one example of technology development that occurs in response to government demand (in this case for the national stockpiles) but without direct subsidies.

The Size of the Stockpile

The potential success of adjuvanted vaccines could provide a rationale for HHS to reconsider the size of the stockpile. The current policy calls for building and maintaining a stockpile of prepandemic vaccines large enough to immunize 20 million people. In the event of a pandemic, that supply would be distributed first to health care workers and first responders; to providers of public safety and critical infrastructure; and to infants, young children, and pregnant women.

Determining the optimal size of the stockpile poses a challenge for a variety of reasons that are related to the public health risks that the stockpile is designed to reduce. The current goal of 20 million doses for the stockpile could be too large or too small: If, for example, the strain that causes the pandemic influenza does not respond to the stockpiled vaccine formulation, the stockpile could be wastefully large. But it could be too small if a pandemic were to spread through the population more quickly than new vaccines could be manufactured. The size of the stockpile, moreover, is linked to other elements of the HHS plan that are related to antiviral drugs, medical supplies, and state and local preparedness measures.[17]

Successful development of adjuvanted vaccines could alter the balance of risks in determining the size of the stockpile and potentially reduce the cost of mitigating those risks. Some recent research indicates that adjuvanted vaccines could provide protection against more than one strain of potential pandemic virus, thereby improving the chances that the vaccines in the stockpile would be effective in a pandemic. Moreover, because adjuvants would reduce the amount of antigen required to immunize any target population, HHS either could retain its current goal of maintaining a stockpile sufficient to inoculate 20 million people while reducing the amount of stockpiled antigen or expand the number of people that could receive the prepandemic vaccine. Doing the latter would reduce the risk that a pandemic would move through the population more quickly than new vaccines could be manufactured, and it might provide enough protection in the population to reduce the severity of the pandemic.

REFERENCES

Abrantes-Metz, R. M., Adams, C. P. & Metz, A. D. (2006). "Pharmaceutical Development Phases: A Duration Analysis." *Journal of Pharmaceutical Finance, Economics, and Policy, vol. 14*, no. 4, 19-41.

Adams, Christopher P. & Van V. Brantner. (2006). "Estimating the Cost of New Drug Development: Is It Really $802 Million?" *Health Affairs,* vol. 25, no. 2, pp. 420–428.

———. 2008. "Spending on New Drug Development." Working paper, Social Science Research Network. March 14. http://papers.ssrn.com/sol3/papers.cfm ?abstractjd= 869765.

Allen, Arthur. (2007). *Vaccine: The Controversial Story of Medicine's Greatest Lifesaver.* New York: W.W. Norton.

BBC News. (2006). "Bird Flu: Country Preparations." February 21. http://newsvote.bbc.co.uk/mpapps/ pagetools/print/news.bbc.co.uk/2/hi/health/ 43800 14.stm.

Belshe, R. B. (2007). "Translational Research on Vaccines: Influenza as an Example." *Clinical Pharmacology and Therapeutics, vol. 82*, no. 6, pp. 745–749.

Berndt, Ernst, R. & others. (2005). "Industry Funding of the FDA: Effects of PDUFA on Approval Times and Withdrawal Rates." *Nature Reviews, Drug Discovery, vol. 4* (July), 545-554.

CBO (Congressional Budget Office). (2005). "A Potential Influenza Pandemic: Possible Macroeconomic Effects and Policy Issues." Letter to the Honorable William H. Frist. December 8, 2005; revised July 27, 2006.

———. (2006a). "A Potential Influenza Pandemic: An Update on Possible Macroeconomic Effects and Policy Issues." Letter to the Honorable William H. Frist and the Honorable Judd Gregg. May 22; revised July 27.

———. (2006b). *Research and Development in the Pharmaceutical Industry*. October. CDC (Centers for Disease Control and Prevention). 2005. "Avian Influenza (Flu)." www.cdc.gov/flu/ avian/gen-info/flu-viruses.htm.

———. (2006). "Hepatitis B Vaccine: Fact Sheet." www.cdc.gov/NCidod/diseases/hepatitis/b/ factvax.htm.

———. (2008). "Questions and Answers: Seasonal Influenza." www.cdc.gov/flu/about/qa/disease.htm.

Computer Sciences Corporation. (2007). "U.S. Department of Health and Human Services Completes Funding of 2006 Contract Award to CS C's DVC and Baxter." Press release. November 27. www.csc.com/ investorrelations/news/ 11 589.shtml.

Cordis. (2007). "New EU Project to Develop a Novel Pandemic Influenza Vaccine." *Cordis: News*. September 27. http://cordis.europa.eu/ fetch?CALLER=EN_NEWS&ACTION =D&SESSION=&RCN=2842 1.

Couch, Robert, B. (2004). "Nasal Vaccination, *Escherichia coli* Enterotoxin, and Bell's Palsy." *New England Journal of Medicine, vol. 350*, no. 9, 860-861.

Danzon, Patricia M., Nuno Sousa Pereira, & Sapna S. Tejwani. (2005). "Vaccine Supply: A Cross- National Perspective." *Health Affairs,* vol. 24, no. 3, pp. 712–715.

Department of Health (U.K.). (2008). "Bird Flu and Pandemic Influenza: What Are the Risks?" www.dh.gov.uk/en/ Aboutus/MinistersandDepartmentLeaders/ ChiefMedicalOfficer/Features/DH_4 102997.

DiMasi, Joseph A. & Henry G. Grabowski. (2007). "The Cost of Biopharmaceutical R&D: Is Biotech Different?" *Managerial and Decision Economics, vol. 28*, no. 4–5, pp. 469–479.

DiMasi, Joseph A., Ronald, W. Hansen, & Henry, G. Grabowski. (2003). "The Price of Innovation: New Estimates of Drug Development Costs." *Journal of Health Economics, vol. 22,* no. 2, pp. 15 1–185.

Donaldson, Liam. (2006). "*Global Health Strategies for Global Health Threats*." Department of Health (U.K.), Wood Memorial Lecture for the Royal Naval Dental Services, Fort Blockhouse, Gosport, Hants. June 30.

Ehrlich, Hartmut J. & others. (2008). "A Clinical Trial of a Whole-Virus H5N 1 Vaccine Derived from Cell Culture." *New England Journal of Medicine, vol. 358*, no. 24, pp. 2573–2584.

European Commission. (2007). *Influenza Research: EU Funded Projects 2001–2007.* EUR22822. Brussels: European Commission, Directorate-General for Research. http://ec.europa.eu/research/health/ poverty-diseases/doc/influenza-research_en.pdf.

European Medicines Agency. (2007a). "European Public Assessment Report (EPAR): Daronrix, EPAR Summary for the Public." March. www.emea.europa.eu/ humandocs/PDFs/EPAR/daronrix/H-706-en 1 .pdf.

———. (2007b). "European Public Assessment Report (EPAR): Focetria, EPAR Summary for the Public." May. www.emea.europa.eu/humandocs/PDFs/EPAR/ focetria/H-7 10-en 1 .pdf.

————. (2008). "European Public Assessment Report (EPAR): Prepandrix, EPAR Summary for the Public." March. www.emea.europa.eu/humandocs/PDFs/ EPAR/prepandrix/H-822-en1 .pdf.

FDA (Food and Drug Administration). (2006). *"FDA Licenses New Vaccine for Prevention of Cervical Cancer and Other Diseases in Females Caused by Human Papillomavirus."* Press release. June 8. www.fda.gov/bbs/topics/NEWS/2006/ NEW0 1385 .html.

————. (2007). "FDA Approves First U.S. Vaccine for Humans Against the Avian Influenza Virus H5N1 ." Press release. April 17; updated April 19. www.fda.gov/bbs/topics/NEWS/2007/ NEW0 161 1.html.

Fedson, David S. (2003). "Pandemic Influenza and the Global Vaccine Supply." *Clinical Infectious Diseases, vol. 36,* no. 12, 1552-1561.

Ferguson, Neil M. & others. (2006). "Strategies for Mitigating an Influenza Pandemic." *Nature (London), vol. 422,* no. 7101, p. 448.

Fukuda, Keiji, & others. (2004). "Inactivated Influenza Vaccines." In *Vaccines,* 4th ed. Stanley A. Plotkin and Walter A. Orenstein, eds., with assistance of Paul A. Offit. Philadelphia: Saunders, 339-369.

Government Accountability Office. (2007). *Influenza Vaccine: Issues Related to Production, Distribution, and Public Health Messages.* Report to the Committee on Oversight and Government Reform, House of Representatives. GAO-08-27.

Gray, Alistair. (2008). "Trial Results Give Acambis Boost in Race for Pandemic Flu Vaccine." *Financial Times.* January 4. www.ft.com/cms/s/0/c72ba9ea-ba67-d1dcabcb-0000779fd2ac.html?nclick_check= 1.

GSK (GlaxoSmithKline). (2007). "GlaxoSmithKline Files its New Pre-Pandemic Influenza Vaccine in Europe." Press release. January 29. www.gsk.com/media/ pressreleases/2007/2007_0 1_29_GSK96 1 .htm.

Health Industry Distributors Association. (2007). *2006– 2007 Influenza Vaccine Production & Distribution: Market Brief.* Alexandria, Va.

HHS (Department of Health and Human Services). (2005a). *"HHS Awards $97 Million Contract to Develop Cell Culture-Based Influenza Vaccine: Effort Designed to Diversify and Accelerate Vaccine Production to Enhance Pandemic Preparedness."* Press release. April 1. www.hhs.gov/news/press/ 2005pres/2005040 1 .html.

————. (2005b). *HHS Pandemic Influenza Plan. www.hhs.gov/pandemicflu/plan/pdf/* HHSPandemicInfluenzaPlan.pdf.

————. (2006a). "Adapting Manufacturing Facilities for Production of Pandemic Influenza Vaccines." Request for proposal. DHHS-ORDC-VB-06-07. July 24.

————. (2006b). "HHS Awards Contracts Totaling More Than $1 Billion to Develop Cell-Based Influenza Vaccine." Press release. May 4. www.hhs.gov/news/ press/2006pres/20060504.html.

————. (2006c). *HHS Pandemic Planning Update II: A Report from Secretary Michael O. Leavitt.* June 29.

————. (2007). "HHS Funds Advanced Development of H5N1 Influenza Vaccines: Three New Contracts Will Focus on Antigen-Sparing Vaccines." Press release. January 17. www.hhs.gov/news/press/2007pres/01/ 20070 1 17b.html.

Homeland Security Council. (2006). *National Strategy for Pandemic Influenza.* May. www.whitehouse.gov/ homeland/nspi_implementation.pdf.

Institute of Medicine. (2004). *Financing Vaccines in the 21st Century.* Report of the Board on Health Care, Committee on the Evaluation of Vaccine Purchase Financing in the United States. Washington, D.C.: National Academy Press.

Iomai. (2008a). "*Iomai Receives HHS Approval to Begin Phase 2 Trial of H5N1 Influenza Adjuvant Patch.*" Press release. April 15. http://investors.iomai.com/ phoenix.zhtml?c= 178326&p=irol-newsArticle &ID=1 129568&highlight.

———. (2008b). "*Study Finds Single Dose of Iomai Patch with Pandemic Flu Vaccine Achieves Protective Levels.*" Press release. March 20. http://investors.iomai .com/phoenix.zhtml?c=178326&p=irol-newsArticle &ID= 1120501 &highlight.

Kenney, Richard & Robert Edelman. (2004). "Adjuvants for the Future." In *New Generation Vaccines,* 3rd ed. Myron Levine and others, eds. New York: Marcel Dekker.

Kolata, Gina. (1999). *Flu: The Story of the Great Influenza Pandemic of 1918 and the Search for the Virus That Caused It.* New York: Farrar, Straus, and Giroux.

Lash, Lyle, III, and Henry Wang. 2006. "Economic Comparison of Egg and Cell Culture for Influenza Vaccine Manufacturing." Presentation. American Chemical Society annual meeting, Division of Biochemical Technology. San Francisco. September 14.

Lewcock, Anna. (2007a). "Cell-Based Flu Jab Gets EU Go Ahead." *In-Pharma Technologist. com.* June 13. www.in-pharmatechnologist.com/news/ng.asp ?n=77338&m= 1 IPE6 1 3&c=fvaksanwurcxpyl.

———. (2007b). "First US Cell-Based Flu Vaccine Plant Underway." *In-Pharma Technologist. com.* August 28. www.in-pharmatechnologist.com/news/ ng.asp?n=79288_novartis-vaccine-cell-based.

———. (2007c). "Low Dose Bird Flu Shot Promises Pandemic Protection." *Outsourcing-Pharma. com.* September 18. www.outsourcing-pharma.com/news/ ng.asp?n=79839&m= 1 OSP9 1 8&c=fvaksanwurcxpyl.

———. (2007d). "Manufacturers Back WHO Avian Flu Stockpiling Plans." *In-PharmaTechnologist.com.* June 14. www.in-pharmatechnologist.com/news/ ng.asp?n=7738 1 &m= 1 IPE6 14&c=fvaksanwurcxpyl.

Lister, Sarah. (2007). *Pandemic Influenza: Domestic Preparedness Efforts.* CRS Report for Congress RL33145. Congressional Research Service. February 20.

Mackenzie, Deborah. (2005). "Stockpile Bird Flu Vaccine Now." *New Scientist Online.* February 17. www.newscientist.com/channel/health/bird-flu/ dn7012.

Matthews, James. (2006). "*Egg-Based Influenza Vaccine Production—30 Years of Commercial Experience and Our Future Expectations for Cell Culture.*" Presentation. National Academy of Engineering and Institute of Medicine conference, Vaccine Production Engineering Approaches to a Pandemic. Washington, D.C. April 10–11.

McKenna, Maryn. (2007a). "The Pandemic Vaccine Puzzle." *CIDRAP News.* University of Minnesota, Center for Infectious Disease Research and Policy. October– November. www.cidrap.umn.edu/cidrap/content/ influenza/panflu/news/nov1 507panvax.html.

———. (2007b). "The Pandemic Vaccine Puzzle; Part 4: The Promise and Problems of Adjuvants." *CIDRAP News.* University of Minnesota, Center for Infectious Disease Research and Policy. October 30. www.cidrap.umn.edu/cidrap/content/influenza/ panflu/news/oct3007panvax4.html.

Megget, Katrina. (2007). "GSK Increases H5N1 Vaccine Presence in US." *In-PharmaTechnologist.com.* August 7. www.in-pharmatechnologist.com/news/ng.asp?id =78815.

Mercer Management Consulting. (2002). *Lessons Learned: New Procurement Strategies for Vaccines. Final Report to the GA VI Board.* Geneva, Switzerland: GAVI Alliance Secretariat. June 28.

Mounier-Jack, Sandra, Ria Jas & Richard Coker. (2007). "Progress and Shortcomings in European National Strategic Plans for Pandemic Influenza." *Bulletin of the World Health Organization, vol. 85,* no. 12, pp. 923–929.

Mutsch, Margot & others. (2004). "Use of the Inactivated Intranasal Influenza Vaccine and the Risk of Bell's Palsy in Switzerland." *New England Journal of Medicine, vol. 350,* no. 9, pp. 896–903.

NIH (National Institutes of Health). (2008a). "Immunogenicity, Safety, Reactogenicity, Efficacy, Effectiveness and Lot Consistency of FluBlok." *Clinical Trials.gov.* http://ClinicalTrials.gov/show/NCT00539981.

———. (2008b). "Safety and Tolerability of a Cell- Derived Influenza Vaccine in Healthy Adults Aged 18 Years and 49 Years." *ClinicalTrials.gov.* http://clinicaltrials.gov/show/nct00599443.

———. (2008c). "Study of Different Formulations of an Intramuscular A/H5N1 Inactivated, Split Virion Influenza Adjuvanted Vaccine." *ClinicalTrials.gov.* http://clinicaltrials.gov/show/NCT00664417.

Novartis. (2007). *Annual Report.* Basel, Switzerland.

Osterholm, Michael, and Helen Branswell. (2005). "Emerging Pandemic: Costs and Consequences of an Avian Influenza Outbreak." Presentation. Woodrow Wilson International Center for Scholars. September 19. www.wilsoncenter.org/index.cfm?event_id = 142787&fuseaction =events.event_summary.

Pink Sheet. (2007). "Novartis Vaccines Unit Looks to Make Its Presence With New Technologies." *Prescription Pharmaceuticals and Biotechnology, vol. 69,* no. 48 (November 26), p. 27.

Poland, Gregory A. (2006). "Vaccines Against Avian Influenza—A Race Against Time." *New England Journal of Medicine, vol. 354,* no. 13, pp. 141 1–1413.

Program for Appropriate Technology in Health. (2007). *Influenza Vaccine Strategies for Broad Global Access: Key Findings and Project Methodology.* October. www.path.org/files/VAC_infl_publ_rpt_10-07.pdf.

Raymond, Emilie. (2006). "Baxter Signs Austrian Flu Vaccine Contract." *DrugResearcher. com.* November 23. www.drugresearcher.com/news/ng.asp?n=72275 -baxter-austria-influenza.

Robinson, Robin. (2007). "*U.S. Pandemic Preparedness Medical Countermeasures: Forecasts for Development, Stockpiling, and Infrastructure Building.*" Presentation. HHS Public Health Emergency Medical Countermeasures Enterprise Stakeholders Workshop. Washington, D.C. August 2. www.medicalcountermeasures.gov/video_content/ day3.html.

———. (2008). "*U.S. Government Progress on Next Generation Medical Countermeasures for Pandemic Influenza.*" Presentation. Phacilitate Vaccine Forum, Focus Session 1. Washington, D.C. January 28.

Sanofi Pasteur. (2006). "*Sanofi Pasteur Supplies Prototype Vaccine for Italian Government Pandemic Initiatives.*" Press release. February 28. www.sanofipasteur.com/ sanofi-

pasteur/front/index.jsp?siteCode=AVPI
_US&codeRubrique=80&codePage=PressRelease _15_12_2005_3.

———. (2007a). "*FDA Licenses First U.S. Vaccine for Humans Against Avian Influenza.*" Press release. April 17. http://en.sanofi-aventis.com/Images/20070417_h5n 1_fda_en_tcm24-1 7270.pdf.

———. (2007b). "*Sanofi Pasteur Initiates Phase II Trial of Cell Culture-Based Seasonal Influenza Vaccine.*" Press release. November 7. http://1 98.73.159.214/ sanofi-pasteur/ImageServlet?imageCode=206 13 &siteCode=SP_HQ.

———. (2007c). "*Sanofi Pasteur's Investigational H5N1 Influenza Vaccine Achieves High Immune Response at Low Dosage.*" Press release. September 18. www.sanofipasteur.com/sanofi-pasteur/front/index.jsp?codeRubrique=131 &lang=EN&siteCode =SP_HQ.

Struck, Mark-M. (1996). "Vaccine R&D Success Rates and Development Times." *Nature Biotechnology, vol. 14,* pp. 591–593.

Taylor, Nick. (2008a). "*Microbix Chinese Vaccine Plant Boosts Global Capacity by 20%.*" In-PharmaTechnologist. com. June 25. www.in-pharmatechnologist.com// news/ng.asp?n=86 1 26&c=0D7Cw4Nu 12 o0Ujt0QSIq3g%3D%3D.

———. (2008b). "*Sanofi Launches $6.25bn Vaccine Battle Plan.*" In-Pharma Technologist. com. June 26. www.in-pharmatechnologist.com/news/ng.asp?id=86 1 56-sanofi-aventis-vaccine-plant.

Taylor, Phil. (2007). "WHO to Help Fund Bird Flu Vaccine Plants in Developing World." *In -Pharma Technologist .com.* April 26. www.in-pharmatechnologist.com/ news/ng.asp?n=76070-who-bird-flu-vaccine.

Vaccine Weekly. (2007). "Flu Vaccines; Sanofi Pasteur Announces Completion of Construction of New U.S. Influenza Vaccine Manufacturing Facility." August 8, p. 16.

Vogel, Frederick & Stanley Hem. (2004). "Immunologic Adjuvants." In *Vaccines,* 4th ed. Stanley A. Plotkin and Walter A. Orenstein, eds., with assistance of Paul A. Offit. Philadelphia: Saunders, pp. 69–79.

Whalen, Jeanne. (2006). "Novartis Plans North Carolina Flu-Vaccine Facility." *Wall Street Journal.* July 19, p. D13.

———. (2008a). "European Regulators Back Bird-Flu Vaccine." *Wall Street Journal.* February 22, p. B4.

———. (2008b). "Sanofi Sees Global Vaccine Sales Doubling." *Wall Street Journal.* June 26, p. B5.

WHO (World Health Organization). 2006. *Global Pandemic Influenza Action Plan to Increase Vaccine Supply.* www.who.int/vaccines-documents/DocsPDF06/ 863.pdf.

———. (2007a). "Epidemic and Pandemic Alert and Response, Cumulative Number of Confirmed Human Cases of Avian Influenza A/(H5N1) Reported to WHO." June 19. www.who.int/csr/disease/ avian_influenza/en/.

———. (2007b). "Global Stockpile of H5N1 Vaccine 'Feasible.'" Press release. April 26. www.who.int/ mediacentre/news/releases/2007/pr2 1 /en/index.html.

———. (2007c). "Initiative for Vaccine Research (IVR): Tables on the Clinical Trials of Pandemic Influenza Prototype Vaccines, Complete Data Set." July 19. www.who.int/vaccine_research/diseases/influenza/ flu_trials_tables/en/index3.html.

———. (2007d). "Projected Supply of Pandemic Influenza Vaccine Sharply Increases." Press release. October 23. www.who.int/mediacentre/news/releases/2007/ pr60/en/index.html.

————. (2008). *4th WHO Meeting on Evaluation of Pandemic Influenza Prototype Vaccines in Clinical Trials.* Geneva, Switzerland. February 14–15. www.who.int/vaccine_research/diseases/influenza/ meetingi40208/en/print.html.

————. No date. "Avian Influenza: Responding to the Pandemic Threat. Frequently Asked Questions." www.searo.who.int/LinkFiles/Avian_Flu_FAQs_II.pdf.

Wright, Peter F. (2008). "Vaccine Preparedness—Are We Ready for the Next Influenza Pandemic?" *New England Journal of Medicine, vol. 358*, no. 24, pp. 2540–2543.

End Notes

[1] The remainder of the spending in HHS's plan is for developing and stockpiling antiviral drugs that might prevent the spread of a pandemic or diminish the severity of illness in people who become infected; creating stockpiles of other medical supplies, such as surgical masks, respirators, ventilators, and syringes; coordinating state and local preparedness; and monitoring the spread of disease.

[2] Influenza viruses that affect humans, birds, and other animals are named for two surface proteins, hemagglutinin and neuraminidase. The surface of H5N1, accordingly, has one type 5 (of the possible 16) hemagglutinin protein and one type 1 (of 9) neuraminidase protein (CDC 2005).

[3] The mortality rate, however, might in fact be substantially lower. Public health authorities do not know how many people with milder cases did not seek medical care or how many received care that was not reported.

[4] A supplemental appropriation is an act of Congress appropriating funds in addition to those already contained in the usual annual appropriation legislation.

[5] According to CDC, "Influenza is a respiratory illness. Symptoms of flu include fever, headache, extreme tiredness, dry cough, sore throat, runny or stuffy nose, and muscle aches. Children can have additional gastrointestinal symptoms, such as nausea, vomiting, and diarrhea, but these symptoms are uncommon in adults. Although the term 'stomach flu' is sometimes used to describe vomiting, nausea, or diarrhea, these illnesses are caused by certain other viruses, bacteria, or possibly parasites, and are rarely related to influenza" (CDC 2008).

[6] Recommendations for meeting potential global demand for pandemic vaccine are discussed by David Fedson (2003).

[7] The adjuvant in question belonged to a different family of adjuvants than those discussed for use in a pandemic-influenza vaccine (Couch 2004; Mutsch and others 2004).

[8] That vaccine is a whole-virus vaccine; seasonal-influenza vaccines licensed in the U.S. are subunit vaccines. Vaccines formulated from whole viruses can be more effective at lower doses, but they also generally cause more side effects (Fukuda and others 2004, pp. 346–347).

[9] Phase I/II clinical trials combine the objectives of Phases I and II to examine both the safety of the vaccine and its ability to elicit a protective immune response.

[10] Several research groups have examined drug development times, including Adams and Brantner (2006, 2008); DiMasi and Grabowski (2007); DiMasi, Hansen, and Grabowski (2003); and Struck (1996). However, some of that work tracked the development of drugs from as early as 1983, before the enactment in 1992 of the Prescription Drug User Fee Act (PDUFA), which has since been reauthorized several times, most recently in 2007. Many analysts, including Berndt and colleagues (2005) and Abrantes-Metz, Adams, and Metz (2006), concur that PDUFA and its reauthorizations have sped development.

[11] Values shown are converted from euros at an exchange rate of 1.57 dollars to the euro, the average for May, June, and July 2008.

[12] MedImmune is not developing an adjuvant. That company's vaccine uses a live, attenuated virus (a weakened form of the virus), which reduces the amount of antigen needed per dose.

[13] HHS uses that assumption in its contracts for expanding egg-based capacity (HHS 2006a). However, in other planning, HHS has assumed that different amounts of antigen would be required for pandemic-influenza vaccine (Robinson 2008).

[14] For a listing of the priority groups, see "Draft Guidance on Allocating and Targeting Pandemic Influenza Vaccine," www.pandemicflu.gov/vaccine/prioritization.html.

[15] Of the total, $15 million per year would go to subsidize capacity for producing egg-based vaccine; the balance of roughly $140 billion to $850 billion annually would support expanded capacity for production of cell-based vaccine (see Chapter 3).

[16] Although HHS has budgeted $600 million to offer capital subsidies to manufacturers to build cell-based production facilities, no contracts have been signed as of this writing.

[17] For a discussion of the likely interactions of various public health policies during a pandemic, see Ferguson and colleagues (2006).

CHAPTER SOURCES

The following chapters have been previously published:

Chapter 1 – This is an edited, excerpted and augmented edition of a United States Congressional Research Service publication, Report Order Code RL33579, dated August 1, 2008.

Chapter 2 – This is an edited, excerpted and augmented edition of a United States Congressional Research Service publication, Report Order Code RL33145, dated February 20, 2007.

Chapter 3 – This is an edited, excerpted and augmented edition of a United States Congressional Research Service publication, Report Order Code RL34190, dated September 24, 2007.

Chapter 4 – This is an edited, excerpted and augmented edition of a United States Congressional Research Service publication, Report Order Code RL34724, dated October 20, 2008.

Chapter 5 – This is an edited, excerpted and augmented edition of a United States Government Accountability Office (GAO), Report to Congressional Committees. Publication GAO-08-671, dated September 2008.

Chapter 6 – This is an edited, excerpted and augmented edition of a United States Congressional Budget Office publication, Pub. No. 2928, dated September 2008.

INDEX

D

E

F

G

H

I

T

U

V

W

Y